Bill Jackson

Endothelial Mechanisms of Vasomotor Control

H. Drexler, A. M. Zeiher,
E. Bassenge, H. Just (eds.)

Endothelial Mechanisms of Vasomotor Control

With special Reference to the Coronary Circulation

Steinkopff Verlag Darmstadt
Springer-Verlag New York

The editors:
Dr. H. Drexler, Dr. A. Zeiher, Prof. Dr. H. Just
Klinikum der Albert-Ludwigs-Universität
Abteilung Innere Medizin
Hugstetter Straße 55
7800 Freiburg
Prof. Dr. E. Bassenge
Institut für angewandte Physiologie
Hermann-Herder-Straße 7
7800 Freiburg

Die Deutsche Bibliothek – CIP-Einheitsaufnahme
Endothelial mechanisms of vasomotor control: with special reference to the coronary circulation/
H. Drexler ... (ed.). – Darmstadt: Steinkopff; New York: Springer, 1991
(Supplement to Basic research in cardiology; Vol. 86, Suppl. 2)
ISBN 3-7985-0866-6 (Steinkopff) Gb.
ISBN 0-387-91392-0 (Springer) Gb.
NE: Drexler, Helmut [Hrsg.]; Basic research in cardiology/Supplement

Basic Res. Cardiol. ISSN 0300-8428
Indexed in Current Contents.

Medical editor: Sabine Müller – English editor: James C. Willis – Production: Heinz J. Schäfer

Printed in Germany

Typesetting and Printing: Brühlsche Universitätsdruckerei Gießen
Printed on acid-free paper

Preface

In recent years, we have witnessed a rapid expansion of our knowledge regarding the role of the endothelium in the control of vascular tone (and organ perfusion) in health and disease. Physiology, pharmacology, and molecular biology have uncovered a wealth of information on structure and function of this heretofore largely neglected "organ". Clinical medicine is now called upon to define the clinical significance of these observations that imply the mechanisms of blood coagulation, e.g., the interaction of thrombocytes with the endothelium, vasomotor control, and specifically, the regulation of smooth muscle tone with consequences for vascular resistance and conductance and organ blood flow. Finally, metabolism of lipids with the everlasting problem of atherosclerosis is an important aspect.

In a second step, implications regarding the improvement of current therapeutic concepts, as well as the development of new modalities of pharmacotherapy will have to be discussed.

The topic addressed by the 1990 Gargellen Conference: Endothelial Mechanisms of Vasomotor Control, clearly is of interest for both basic scientists and clinicians.

It has been the aim of the organizers, the Society for Cooperation in Medical Science (SCMS) with this and the previous symposia to foster and support both basic science *and* clinical research.

Research in medicine today shows two major directions of development: on the one hand, increasing involvement of the basic sciences and their methodology. On the other hand, statistical validation of concepts and therapeutic strategies in large scale population- and multicenter-studies.

These conceptually divergent developments call for cooperation with clinical medicine. Progress will have to be tested at the bedside. Clinical observation and understanding will always form the basis of new avenues for development and needs for therapy.

The 1990 Gargellen Conference was unanimously considered a valuable "state-of-the-art" assessment of a rapidly developing field. The work presented uncovered new implications of the endothelium's function and metabolism, and has given insights into the mechanisms of vascular growth and angiogenesis.

It was, therefore, deemed necessary to publish the proceedings, inspite of and in clear recognition of the large volume of current medical literature.

We were grateful to the editor of Basic Research in Cardiology, in particular to G. Elzinga for his enthusiastic support of this supplement to the journal.

We likewise wish to thank B. Lewerich and S. Müller of the publishers Dr. Dietrich, Steinkopff Verlag, Darmstadt, for their assistance.

It should not go unnoticed that scientists from both the pharmaceutical industry and from universities have authored the original contributions of this monograph. The chairmen of the symposium have led us from basic science to clinical medicine. We owe particular thanks to the organizers of the symposium, PD Dr. Helmut Drexler and PD Dr. Andreas Zeiher of the Medizinische Universitätsklinik, Innere Medizin III in Freiburg.

Our particular thanks go to the corporate sponsors of the conference and of the proceedings volume: Bayer AG, Leverkusen (Dr. Bertschig), Cassella-Riedel AG, Höchst (Dr. Leonhardt), Gödecke AG, Freiburg (Drs. Kapp and Bahrmann), and MSD Sharp & Dohme, München (Dr. Bestehorn). Their generous and personal support has made this progressive step possible for the entire scientific community.

Eberhard Bassenge, MD
Professor of Medicine
Institute for Applied Physiology
Freiburg

Hanjörg Just, MD
Professor of Medicine
Med. Univ.-Klinik
Freiburg
Society for
Cooperation in Medical
Science (SCMS)

Contents

Endothelial function in pathological conditions

Endothelial function in the clinical setting

Basic Physiology of EDRF

Introduction

H. Just

The function of the endothelial monolayer, which continuously envelops the circulating blood, has since Brücke (1857) and Lister (1909) been associated with the maintenance of the liquidity of the blood. Only in 1976, when Moncada et al. discovered prostacyclin (17), and 1980, when Furchgott and Zawadzki (7) described the essential role of the intact endothelium for the vasodilatory action of acetylcholine, was the significance of this organ for vasomotor control recognized.

The interaction of the function of the endothelium with neurohumoral influence has been particularly well studied in the coronary vascular system. The endothelial modulation of coronary tone has been recently reviewed by Bassenge and Busse (1).

In order to maintain the fluidity of the blood and the patency of the blood vessels, the endothelial cells synthetize many active substances; e.g., fibronectin, heparansulfate, interleukin-I, tissue plasminogen activator, several growth factors influencing angiogenesis, prostacyclin, platelet activating factor, endothelium-derived relaxing factor, EDRF, known to be nitric oxide, and various vasoconstrictor substances, such as endothelin.

The production of these substances, acting on the luminal, and/or the abluminal side, interacts with platelets or leukocytes in the streaming blood; on the abluminal side it interacts with the vascular smooth muscle cells or mastcells. Intracellular messengers like cyclic adenosine monophospate, cyclic guanosine monophosphate, and/or calcium modulate the action of the endothelial cell products.

For example, shear stress forces of the streaming blood will initiate the production of EDRF within the cell, and as consequence the smooth muscle cells will relax instantaneously, thereby adapting vessel size to the demand for blood flow (1). A further example: The production of prostacyclin will be stimulated by thrombin, contact with activated leukocytes, prostaglandin peroxides emerging from plateles, or, likewise, stretching of the arterial wall, to name a few.

These remarkable functions are brought about by the endothelial cell lining of the entire vasculature – and possibly the heart. The total cell mass of the endothelium has been estimated to amount to approximately 2.5 kg. This is about one-half of the blood volume or approximately equal to the blood cell mass. It exceeds by about five times the weight of the heart, and equals the weight of the liver, the organ considered to have the highest intensity of metabolic activity in the body.

Structure

The endothelial cell monolayer is continuous in arteries and veins; the cells are polygonal. In vessel segments with laminar flow they attain a longitudinal orientation and stretch in length. The mechanism of this reversible and seemingly repeated action possibly changes the configuration and shape of the cells, as well as the underlying intracellular structural elements, but remains to be elucidated.

Contact to the cellular components of the blood on the luminal side is highly variable in relation to flow modalities, be it laminar or turbulent. In laminar flow conditions endothelial function can be expected to be more pronounced towards the abluminal side, i.e., vascular smooth muscle. Indeed, flow-dependent vasodilation seems to be most prominent in conductance vessels with laminar flow, where and when coagulation processes are of lesser importance. Nothing is known about a possible relationship between endothelial function and poststenotic dilation.

Flow-dependent vasomotion can be expected to occur anywhere in the vascular system. Morphologic differences in the endothelial cell lining in different vascular segments have so far not been demonstrated. Flow-dependent vasomotion seems to be most significant, however, in vascular resistance vessels with an internal diameter down to 70 μm (8).

Towards the abluminal side the basement membrane separates the endothelium from the thick smooth muscle layers of the media. Active substances, especially small molecules like EDRF (=NO), endothelin (a small peptide) will easily pass the multiply perforated basement membrane. It is, however, uncertain how the deeper layers of the media can be reached and how signal transmission is achieved.

Function under normal conditions

With respect to endothelium-dependent vasodilator effects, Schretzenmayer (1933) was the first to observe flow-dependent vasodilation (19); he studied the femoral artery in dogs. We know today that several mechanisms influence arterial width and tone; at the level of the resistance vessels sympatho-adrenergic alpha-constrictor and beta-2-dilator effects dominate. In addition, myogenic autoregulation mediated through metabolic products of the working organ adapts flow regionally to the need.

Coordination of intra-organ blood flow is difficult to eludicate; one, upstream-oriented coordinating mechanism, reaching into the feed arteries was described by Segal and Duling (20). Large artery size seems to be determined mainly by the vascular renin-angiotensin-system (6, 9) and the function of the endothelium.

As long as blood flows a basal production of EDRF seems to determine basal vascular tone (18). At rest, organ blood flow is dependent of intra-parenchymal resistance vessels. With functional hyperemia the pressure gradient between resistance and conductance vessels decreases. Conductance vessel size is almost instantaneously adapted to the increased flow; with cessation of flow increase the effect will be reversed, and basal tone will determine vessel size and tone again. The amplitude of caliber change under normal conditions is not well known for every segment; it can be estimated to vary between and as much as 20%.

The duration of time over which maximal flow-dependent dilation can be maintained is not known. However, longer duration of dilation seems to lead to structural changes, i.e., a larger vessel. The role of growth factors, derived from the endothelium or elsewhere in the vascular wall under these conditions, is currently under investigation.

The mechanisms for tissue perfusion are regionally confined and are subject to conditioning and deconditioning. For example, tennis players will increase their peak reactive hyperemic blood flow in the playing arm, as opposed to the non-playing one. With chronic increase in flow, release of EDRF is increased (16). Therefore, it has been speculated that the increase in blood-flow response with training may be due to enhanced release of EDRF. The role of endothelial constrictor mechanisms (endothelin) in this respect is still unclear. Conversely, chronic decreases in flow, e.g., during immobilization, heart failure or high-grade stenosis, will likewise reduce blood-vessel size, an effect which appears to be endothelium-dependent (13). Augmentation or reduction of flow-dependent vasodilation is reversible, as long as the endothelium remains intact. Under pathologic conditions other factors influencing vascular tone, compliance and size will interfere.

Dysfunction of the dilator mechanism

Dysfunction of the endothelium has been reported for several pathological conditions, directly involving or even destroying the endothelium, and is associated with impaired flow-dependent dilation (4) and paradoxical vasoconstriction to acetylcholine in vivo (14). Here, complete reversibility may be impossible (morphologic destruction, even after endothelial re-growth) or questionable (metabolic diseases, hypercholesterolemia, atherosclerosis).

Endothelial dysfunction of this type my be regionally localized (damage, atherosclerosis) or generalized (hypertension, hypercholesterolemia). Regional involvement may seriously impair parenchymal nutrition. Preliminary data suggest that adaptation of myocardial microperfusion depends on endothelial function of the coronary circulation in humans (22). Myocardial ischemia under exercise may, in part be evoked or aggregated by endothelial dysfunction. The role of the endothelium in the syndrome X and in atypical chest pain syndromes needs to be elucidated. The coronary vasomotion of conductance vessels in response to sympathetic stimulation depends on the functional status of the endothelium (21). It is controversial whether systemic endothelial dysfunction with a generalized failure of the arterial system to dilate in response to increased flow may be involved in the development of hypertension, or be a secondary phenomenon (15).

In congestive heart failure, reduced blood flow under exercise or even at rest characterizes the disease and limits organ function and exercise capacity (23). Improved cardiac pumping does, however, not readily reverse, for example, skeletal muscle function. Reduced dilatory capacity of the vascular system, as one part of this phenomenon, relates to several factors: activated renin-angiotensin-system, alpha-adrenergic tone, reduced endothelial function (5, 11), and increased sodium content of the vascular wall (stiffness factor) (23).

There is indirect evidence that exaggerated nitric oxide (NO) synthesis e.g., derived from both the vascular wall and blood cells (e.g., monocytes and neutrophils) may play a role in the decreased systemic vascular resistance in septic shock (3, 10, 12). Indeed, inhibition of NO-formation by synthesis from L-arginine has been shown to restore the vascular responsiveness in the experimental setting (12).

At present, disturbances of endothelial function of primary or secondary nature are of largely unanticipated clinical significance, but may offer new avenues for therapeutic strategies. The following contributions to this supplement to Basic Research in Cardiology attempt to describe today's knowledge in this important and rapidly evolving field.

References

1. Bassenge E, Busse R (1988) Endothelial modulation of coronary tone. Prog Cardiovasc Dis 30:349–380
2. Bassenge E, Münzel T (1988) Consideration of conduit and resistance vessels in regulation of blood flow. Am J Cardiol 62:40E–44E
3. Beasley D (1990) Interleukin 1 and endotoxin activate soluble guanylate cyclase in vascular smooth muscle. Am J Physiol 259:R38–R44

4. Drexler H, Zeiher AM, Wollschläger H, Bonzel T, Just H (1989) Flow-dependent coronary dilation in man. Circulation 80:466–474
5. Drexler H, Hayoz D, Münzel T, Zeiher AM, Hornig B, Just H, Brunner HR, Zelis R (1991) Characterization of endothelial function in patients with chronic heart failure. J Am Coll Cardiol (in press)
6. Dzau VJ, Safar ME (1988) Large conduit arteries in hypertension. Circulation 77:947–954
7. Furchgott RF, Zawadski JV (1980) The obligatory role of endothelial cells in the relaxation of arterial smooth muscle by acetylcholine. Nature 288:373–376
8. Griffith TM, Edwards DH, Davies RLI, Harrison TJ, Evans KT (1987) EDRF coordinates the behaviour in vascular resistance vessels. Nature 329:442–445
9. Holtz J, Busse R, Sommer O, Bassenge E (1987) Dilation of epicardial arteries in conscious dogs induced by angiotensin-converting enzyme inhibition with enalaprilat. J Cardiovasc Pharmacol 9:348–355
10. Julou-Schaffer, G, Gray GA, Fleming I, Schott C, Parratt JR, Stoclett J-C (1990) Loss of vascular responsiveness induced by endotoxin involves l-arginine pathway. Am J Physiol 259:H1038–H1043
11. Kaiser L, Spickard RC, Olivier NB (1989) Heart failure depresses endothelium-dependent response in canine femoral artery. Am J Physiol 256:946–991
12. Kilbourn RG, Gross SS, Jubran A, Adams J, Griffith OW, Levi R, Lodato RF (1990) NG-methyl-L-arginine inhibits tumor necrosis factor-induced hypotension: implications for the involvement of nitric oxide. Proc Natl Acad Sci 87:3629–3632
13. Langille L, O'Donnel F (1986) Reductions in arterial diameter produced by chronic decreases in blood flow are endothelium-dependent. Science 231:405–407
14. Ludmer PL, Selwyn AP, Shook TL, Wayne RR, Madge GH, Alexander RW, Ganz P (1986) Paradoxical vasoconstriction induced by acetylcholine in atherosclerotic coronary arteries. N Engl J Med. 315:1046–1051
15. Lüscher TF (1990) The endothelium. Target and promotor of hypertension? Hypertension 15:482–485
16. Miller VM, Vanhoutte PM (1988) Enhanced release of endothelium-derived factor(s) by chronic increases in blood flow. Am J Physiol 255:H446–H451
17. Moncada S, Gryglewski R, Bunting S, Vane JR (1976) An enzyme isolated from arteries transforms prostaglandin endoperoxides to an unstable substance that inhibits platelet aggregation. Nature 263:663–665
18. Rees DD, Palmer RMJ, Moncada (1989) Role of endothelium-derived nitric oxide in the regulation of blood pressure. Proc Natl Acad Sci 86:3375–3378
19. Schretzenmayr A (1933) Über kreislaufregulatorische Vorgänge an den großen Arterien bei der Muskelarbeit. Pflüger's Arch Ges Physiol 232:743–748
20. Segal SS, Duling BR (1986) Communication between feed arteries and microvessels in hamster striated muscle: Segmented vascular responses are functionally coordinated. Circ Res 59:283–290
21. Zeiher AM, Drexler H, Wollschläger H, Saurbier B, Just H (1989) Coronary vasomotion in response to sympathetic stimulation in humans: Importance of the functional integrity of the endothelium. J Am Coll Cardiol 14:1181–1190
22. Zeiher AM, Drexler H, Wollschläger H, Just H (1990) Endothelial dysfunction alters the linkage of myocardial oxygen demand to microvascular tone in humans (abstr). Circulation 82:III–247
23. Zelis R, Flaim SF (1982) Alterations in vasomotor tone in congestive heart failure. Prog Cardiovasc Dis 24:437–459

Author's address:
Prof. Dr. H. Just
Medizinische Universitätsklinik
Abt. Innere Medizin III
Hugstetter Str. 55
W-7800 Freiburg, FRG

Cellular mechanisms controlling EDRF/NO formation in endothelial cells

R. Busse, A. Lückhoff, and A. Mülsch

Department of Applied Physiology, University of Freiburg, FRG

Summary: We investigated the molecular mechanisms whereby Ca^{2+} enters the endothelial cytosol and regulates endothelial nitric oxide synthesis L-arginine-dependent nitric oxide synthesis by isolated endothelial cytosol as quantified by activation of a purified soluble guanylate cyclase was concentration-dependently enhanced by free Ca^{2+} (EC_{50} 0.3 μM). The Ca^{2+}-dependent activation was inhibited by the calmodulin antagonists mastoparan, melittin, and calcineurin (IC_{50} 450, 350, and 60 nM, respectively) in a calmodulin-reversible manner. After removal of endogenous calmodulin the Ca^{2+}-dependency of endothelial NO synthase was lost, but could be reconstituted with exogenous calmodulin. The results indicate that Ca^{2+}-calmodulin directly activates the endothelial nitric oxide synthase, thereby transducing agonist-induced increases in intracellular free Ca^{2+} concentration to nitric oxide formation from L-arginine, K^+-induced depolarization of the endothelial cells markedly inhibited the sustained, but not initial phase of the intracellular Ca^{2+} response to bradykinin, indicating that K^+-induced depolarization depresses the transmembrane Ca^{2+} influx. On the contrary, the K^+ channel activator Hoe 234 which elicits hyperpolarization of the endothelial cell membrane, augmented the sustained phase of the agonist-induced intracellular Ca^{2+} signal, but not the resting intracellular Ca^{2+} level. The effects of K^+ and Hoe 234 on the agonist-induced Ca^{2+}-response were reflected by corresponding changes in agonist-induced EDRF/NO release. From these data, we suggest that the endothelial membrane potential may play an important role for the extent of agonist-induced Ca^{2+} influx and, thereby, the endothelial EDRF/NO synthesis.

Key words: Endothelial nitric oxide synthesis; intracellular free Ca^{2+}; calmodulin; membrane potential; hyperpolarization; K^+ channel activator; Hoe 234

Introduction

In the last 10 years it has become increasingly clear that the vascular endothelium plays a crucial role in the adjustment of vascular tone, as well as in the control of platelet activation. A predominant part of these endothelial functions is mediated by the endothelium-derived relaxing factor (EDRF) (4, 11), a labile compound that acts by a direct stimulation of the soluble guanylate cyclase in the target cells (10). There is compelling evidence that EDRF is identical with (32) or at least closely related (29) to nitric oxide (NO). Formation of NO/EDRF has been recently demonstrated in several other mammalian cell types, including activated macrophages (14, 17), neutrophils (37), neuronal cells (18), kidney epithelial cells (36), and carcinoma cells (2). It has been shown in immunostimulated macrophages that endogenous L-arginine is metabolized in a NADPH-dependent manner by a cytosolic enzyme system that yields citrulline and NO (24). Although, in principle, the so-called "oxidative L-arginine pathway" itself seems to be identical in macrophages and endothelial cells, the cellular regulation of NO synthesis is quite different. NO release does not occur immediately after immunostimulation of macrophages, but requires a lag phase of several hours during which NO synthase is expressed (25). Furthermore, induction and activity of NO synthase in macrophages are independent of the intracellular calcium level (15). In contrast, an elevation in the intracellular free calcium concentration ($[Ca^{2+}]_i$) has been shown to be a prerequisite for the formation of NO in endothelial cells, no matter whether it was induced by receptor-dependent stimuli like acetylcholine, ATP, and bradykinin, or by receptor-independent substances like calcium ionophores or thimerosal (21). Furthermore, sustained increases in $[Ca^{2+}]_i$ required the presence of extracellular Ca^{2+} and transmembrane Ca^{2+} influx that, however, could not be inhibited by blockers of voltage-gated Ca^{2+} channels like nifedipine or verapamil (7, 19, 26).

In this review, we summarize our recent experimental work on the molecular mechanisms whereby the cytosolic Ca^{2+} concentration regulates endothelial NO production. Furthermore, we present some recent concepts on the control of Ca^{2+} entry into endothelial cells.

Materials and Methods

Measurements of cytosolic free Ca^{2+} concentration ($[Ca^{2+}]_i$)

Endothelial cells from bovine aorta were kept in culture for 1 to 3 subcultures as previously described (20).

$[Ca^{2+}]_i$-measurements were performed in cultured cells grown on quartz coverslips by means of the fluorescent probe indo-1. The cells were loaded with indo-1 by incubation (60–75 min, 38° C) with 0.8 µmol/l indo-1/AM and 0.025% (w/v) Pluronic F-127, a non-ionic detergent. Thereafter, the coverslips were washed and transferred into cuvettes filled with HEPES buffer. Fluorescence was recorded in a temperature-controlled (37° C) spectrofluorometer (Schoeffel RRS 1000). The excitation wavelength was set to 350 nm, emission was simultaneously measured at 400 nm and 450 nm (450 nm is the isosbestic wavelength). The signals were digitized and stored in a computer. The intracellular free calcium concentration ($[Ca^{2+}]_i$) was calculated on a second-to-second basis from the ratio of both fluorescence intensities (R) (12).

Preparation of endothelial cytosol

Endothelial cells were isolated from fresh porcine aortae by digestion with dispase, as described recently (28). Suspended endothelial cells were washed twice (1000 × g, 5 min, 4° C) in 1 ml of 15 mM HEPES buffer pH 7.5 by sonication (3 times 10 s, 100 W). The cytosol was prepared by centrifugation (1 h 100000 × g supernatant). For removal of endogenous calmodulin, the cytosol was loaded on a Mono Q column (Pharmacia, Freiburg, FRG) and NO synthase was eluted with a salt gradient (0 to 0.5 M NaCl). Aliquots were stored at −30° C. Protein was determined by the Biorad assay (Biorad, Munich, FRG).

Detection of cytosolic NO formation by activation of soluble guanylate cyclase (GC)

Cytosol (0.05–0.5 mg of cytosolic protein per ml) was incubated (30 min) at 37° C (final volume 50 µl) in a buffer containing GC (1 µg protein per ml) purified to apparent homogeneity from bovine lung and L-arginine 1 mM, NADPH 0.1 mM, [α-^{32}P]GTP

0.1 mM (0.2 μCi), cGMP 0.1 mM, glutathione 2 mM, HEPES 15 mM pH 7.5, $MgCl_2$ 4 mM, 3-isobutyl-1-methylxanthine 1 mM, creatine phosphate 3.5 mM, creatine phosphokinase 4.8 units, bovine γ-globulin 0.1 mg/ml and EGTA 0.1 mM. The reaction was stopped by addition of 0.5 ml zinc acetate (120 mM) and 0.5 ml sodium carbonate (120 mM). [^{32}P]cGMP was isolated by chromatography on acid alumina and GC activity (nmol cyclic GMP formed per min per mg purified GC) was calculated as described (27)).

Results and Discussion

Ca^{2+}-calmodulin-dependent activation of NO synthase

The basal activity of purified soluble guanylate cyclase ($23.0 \pm 1.5\,nmol \cdot mg^{-1} \cdot min^{-1}$) was stimulated by endothelial cytosol (0.1 mg protein/ml) in nominally Ca^{2+}-free buffer (about 20 nM free Ca^{2+}) up to 2.4 fold (n = 20) (Fig. 1). Guanylate cyclase activity was further increased to 5.6 fold of basal activity (n = 20) by 2 μM free Ca^{2+}, indicating a direct Ca^{2+}-dependency of endothelial nitric oxide synthase. Addition of the peptide calmodulin inhibitor melittin as well as the Ca^{2+}-calmodulin-dependent phosphatase calcineurin potently inhibited Ca^{2+}-dependent NO formation (Fig. 1 a). This inhibition was reversed by addition of porcine brain calmodulin (Fig. 1 a). Calcineurin was the most potent inhibitor with an IC_{50} of 60 nM as compared to melittin (IC_{50} 350 nM) and mastoparan (IC_{50} 450 nM). In contrast, the pharmacological calmodulin inhibitors such as calmidazolium, fendiline, and trifluoperazine had virtually no inhibitory effect up to 10 μM (see Fig. 1 b). Removal of endogenous calmodulin from the cytosol by anion exchange chromatography completely abolished cytosolic NO formation. However, NO synthase activity could be reconstituted in the presence, but not in the absence of Ca^{2+} by addition of calmodulin (Fig. 2). These results suggest that the Ca^{2+}-dependent activation of NO synthesis in endothelial cells is mediated by calmodulin that transfers Ca^{2+}-sensitivity to endothelial NO synthase.

Voltage-driven Ca^{2+} influx

As mentioned in the introduction, calcium entry blockers do not inhibit Ca^{2+} influx into endothelial cells. Therefore, it is concluded that voltage-gated Ca^{2+} channels activated by membrane depolarization do not play a major role in endothelial Ca^{2+} homeostasis. In contrast, studies in several laboratories have recently revealed that depolarization markedly inhibits Ca^{2+} influx (1, 6, 23, 33–35). A representative example is shown in Fig. 3. In a control experiment (Fig. 3 a), stimulation of endothelial cells with bradykinin evoked an immediate rise in $[Ca^{2+}]_i$ that was sustained over several minutes. It is known that endothelial cells possess membrane receptors for bradykinin of the B_2-type that are coupled to phospholipase C. Hence, the initial peak in $[Ca^{2+}]_i$ may be attributed to mobilization of Ca^{2+} from intracellular stores, mediated by the hydrolysis-product of phospholipase C activity inositol 1,4,5 trisphosphate. However, the sustained phase of the increase in $[Ca^{2+}]_i$ depends on extracellular Ca^{2+} and was abolished in Ca^{2+}-free medium (Fig. 3 b). Likewise, in a medium containing a normal Ca^{2+} concentration (1 mM) but 90 mM K^+ (substituted for Na^+), the initial bradykinin-induced increase in $[Ca^{2+}]_i$ was preserved but the sustained response was much shorter than under control conditions (Fig. 3 c). This indicates that K^+-induced depolarization depresses transmembrane Ca^{2+} influx.

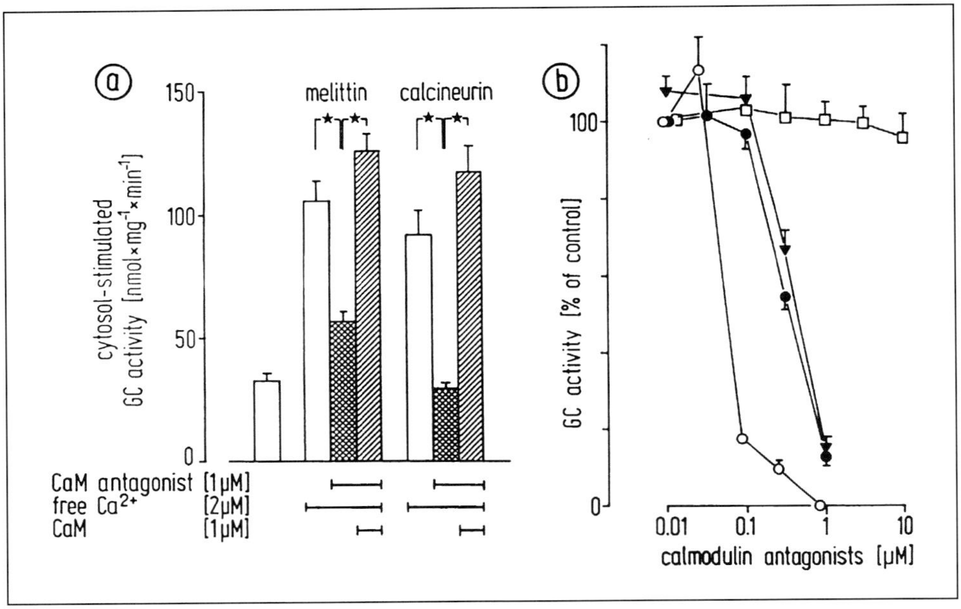

Fig. 1 a. Free Ca^{2+} (2 µM) increases the guanylate cyclase (GC) stimulation by endothelial cytosol (0.1 mg protein/ml) in the presence of L-arginine (0.3 mM) and NADPH (0.1 mM) (open columns). Calmodulin (CaM) antagonists (melittin, calcineurin, both 1 µM) significantly inhibit Ca^{2+}-cytosol-stimulated GC activity ($p<0.05$; $n=20$; cross-hatched columns). Porcine brain calmodulin (1 µM) significantly reverses this inhibition (hatched columns). **b** Effects of calmodulin inhibitors (calcineurin (○), mellitin (▽), mastoparan (○) and calmidazolium (□) on nitric oxide formation by endothelial cytosol. Effects were quantified by inhibition of guanylate cyclase (GC) activity (% of control in the absence of inhibitors). Endothelial cytosol was incubated with purified GC at different concentrations of calmodulin inhibitors in the presence of L-arginine (0.3 mM) and NADPH (0.1 mM) for 30 min at 37° C. Results from at least three independent experiments performed in triplicate

After we had demonstrated that endothelial Ca^{2+} fluxes are inhibited by depolarization, we tested the hypothesis that they may be enhanced by hyperpolarization. Indeed, we found that activators of K^+ channels like cromakalim and pinacidil which induce hyperpolarization in cultured endothelial cells (23) also augmented agonist-induced Ca^{2+} influx (22). So far the most potent substance tested is the novel compound Hoe 234. Preincubation with this K^+ channel opener enhanced and prolonged the increases in $[Ca^{2+}]_i$ under stimulation with bradykinin (Fig. 4). The effects of Hoe 234 were completely inhibited in a K^+-rich medium, indicating that Hoe 234 augmented $[Ca^{2+}]_i$ as a consequence of its activation of K^+ channels that leads to membrane hyperpolarization.

However, Hoe 234 did not markedly affect $[Ca^{2+}]_i$ in resting endothelial cells. Hence, it appears unlikely that hyperpolarization alone is sufficient to elicit Ca^{2+} influx that would be large enough for increases in $[Ca^{2+}]_i$. Obviously, an enhanced transmembrane Ca^{2+} turnover must already exist, induced by a separate stimulus like bradykinin, probably involving the opening of specific (yet unidentified) membrane channels. However, in the presence of bradykinin, it appears that Ca^{2+} influx is mainly determined

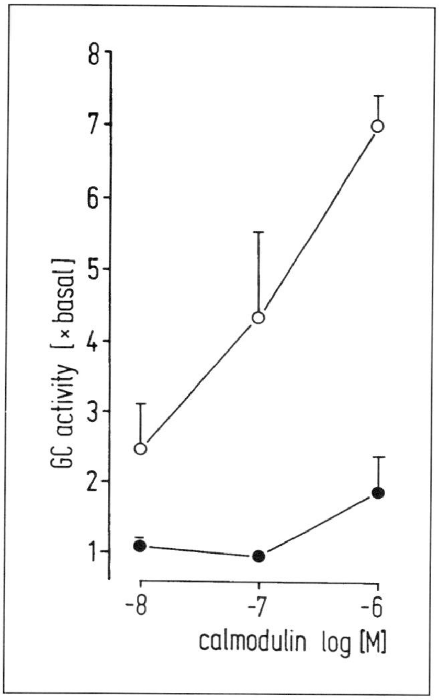

Fig. 2. Ca^{2+}-calmodulin-dependence of NO formation by partially purified NO synthase. The cytosol fraction eluted with 0.1–0.2 M NaCl from the Mono Q column was incubated with purified guanylate cyclase (GC) in the presence of L-arginine (0.3 mM), NADPH (0.1 mM) 20 nM (o) or 2 μM (o) free Ca^{2+}, and with increasing concentrations of calmodulin for 30 min at 37° C. Data are means ±SEM of three independent experiments

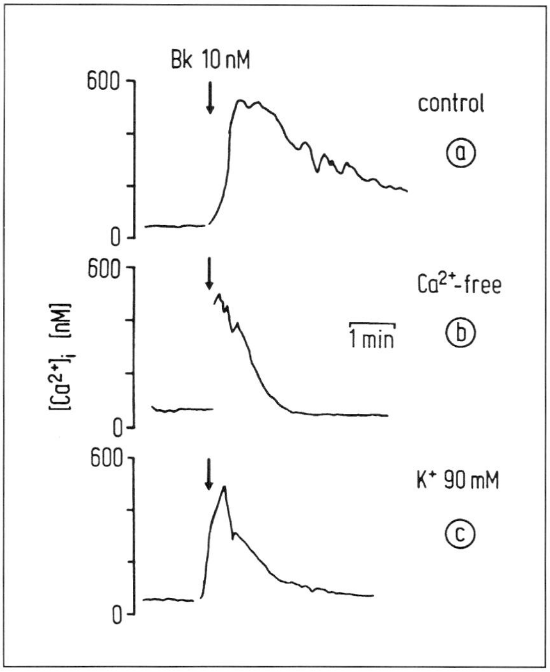

Fig. 3 a–c. Effects of removal of extracellular Ca^{2+} and of K^+-depolarization on bradykinin-induced increases in the intracellular free calcium concentration ($[Ca^{2+}]_i$) in endothelial cells. **a** Control. Bradykinin (Bk, final concentration 10 nM) was added (arrow) to cultured endothelial cells from porcine aorta loaded with the fluorescent indicator indo-1. **b** Stimulation with bradykinin was performed in a Ca^{2+}-free medium. **c** Stimulation with bradykinin was performed in a medium containing 90 mM K^+ (substituted for Na^+). Original tracings from three experiments performed with cells from the same batch

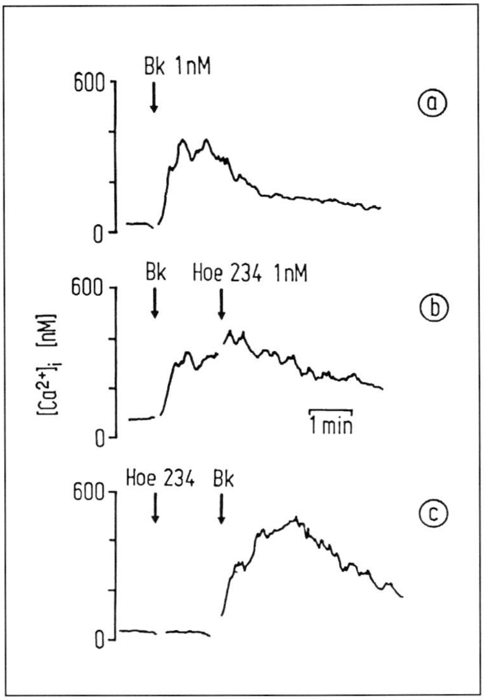

Fig. 4 a–c. Effects of the K^+ channel activator Hoe 234 on bradykinin-induced increases in $[Ca^{2+}]_i$ in endothelial cells. **a** Control. Stimulation was performed with bradykinin (Bk, final concentration 1 nM). **b** and **c** Hoe 234 (final concentration 1 nM) was added to the cell shortly after (**b**) or before (**c**) stimulation with bradykinin. Original tracings from three experiments performed with cells from the same batch

by the electrochemical driving force, i.e., the membrane potential and the transmembrane Ca^{2+} concentration gradient. The relative contribution of both factors may be estimated from the Goldman-Hodgkin-Katz current equation (16). According to this equation, Ca^{2+} influx would be enhanced by 45% when the membrane potential is shifted from -40 to -60 mV, whereas Ca^{2+} influx would be reduced to 30% by a depolarization to 0 mV.

Thus, the experiments presented in Fig. 3 are consistent with the view that bradykinin opens Ca^{2+} channels that are not gated by the potential. It should be noted, however, that definite experimental proof of those putative chanels has not yet been provided in electrophysiological studies.

Effects of membrane depolarization and hyperpolarization on EDRF release

From the findings that cytosolic NO synthesis in endothelial cells depends on $[Ca^{2+}]_i$ and that transmembrane Ca^{2+} influx is driven by the membrane potential, one should expect that modifications of the membrane potential may have dramatic effects on EDRF release. In order to test this hypothesis, we compared EDRF release in resting and bradykinin-stimulated endothelial cells under control conditions with that during depolarization, induced by raising the extracellular K^+ concentration to 70 mM, and during hyperpolarization, induced by the K^+ channel activator Hoe 234 (10 nM). The results are represented in Fig. 5. Bradykinin-induced EDRF release was almost com-

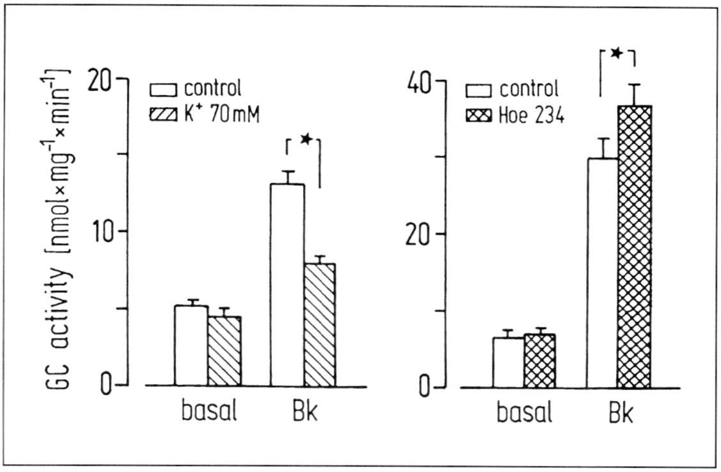

Fig. 5. Effects of depolarization with K^+ and of hyperpolarization with the K^+ channel activator Hoe 234 on EDRF release from endothelial cells. Endothelial cells cultured from porcine aorta were grown in 24-well plates. EDRF release (ordinate) is quantified as activity of purified soluble guanylate cyclase in the presence of samples from the medium covering the cells, obtained before (basal) and 90 s after application of bradykinin (Bk, final concentration 30 nM). Left: Comparison of EDRF release in a medium containing 4 mK K^+ (control) or 70 mM K^+. Right: Effects of preincubation with Hoe 234 (10 nM, 5 min). *Significantly different ($p<0.05$, paired *t*-test) from control

pletely abolished by depolarization, whereas it was significantly increased by the hyperpolarizing compound Hoe 234.

Hyperpolarization as physiological response to stimuli of EDRF release

Changes in the membrane potential of endothelial cells are not only elicited by changes in the extracellular K^+ concentration or by pharmacological activators of K^+ channels. To the contrary, hyperpolarization is an important factor by which endothelial Ca^{2+} fluxes are regulated under physiological conditions. A transient hyperpolarization has been shown (5, 8, 9, 23, 31) to be part of the endothelial response to various EDRF-releasing agonists (Fig. 6). This hyperpolarization is attributed to the opening of K^+ channels activated by $[Ca^{2+}]_i$, as demonstrated in patch-clamp studies in the cell-attached configuration (33). Furthermore, the endothelial response to shear stress, considered to be one of the most important physiological stimuli for EDRF release (4), is associated with increases in $[Ca^{2+}]_i$ and Ca^{2+}-dependent formation of EDRF/NO. Initial events after receptor occupation are mobilization of Ca^{2+} from internal stores as well as an increase in the transmembrane Ca^{2+} permeability, most likely by opening cation channels via yet unknown mechanisms which permit influx of Ca^{2+}. Thereafter, K^+ channels are activated by the initial rise in $[Ca^{2+}]_i$ and hyperpolarization ensues. Hyperpolarization, in turn, augments the driving force for Ca^{2+} influx, thus contributing to sustained increases in $[Ca^{2+}]_i$ which are the signal for the increases in NO synthesis.

This signal transduction mechanism in endothelial cells is clearly opposite to that in excitable cells like vascular smooth muscle cells. Here, Ca^{2+} influx occurs preferentially

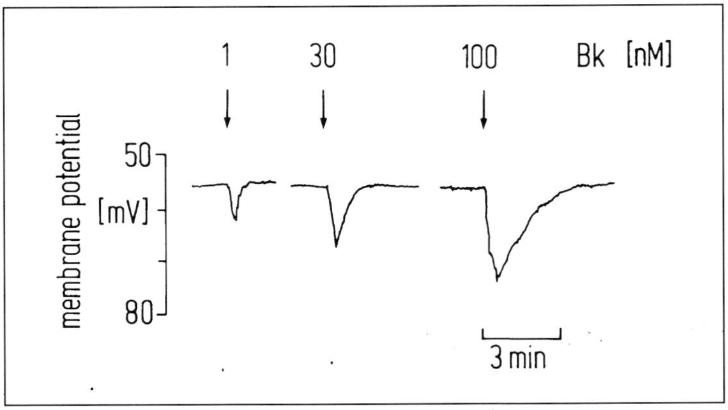

Fig. 6. Dose-dependent effects of bradykinin on the membrane potential of endothelial cells. Bradykinin (Bk, concentration 1-100 nM) was added to patch-clamped endothelial cells (whole-cell configuration, current clamped) cultured from porcine aorta

during depolarization because of the presence of voltage-gated Ca^{2+} channels. Hyperpolarization, in spite of augmenting the electrochemical gradient for Ca^{2+}, would diminish Ca^{2+} entry because the Ca^{2+} channels were closed under this condition. In fact, hyperpolarization is the principle by which K^+ channel activators induce relaxation of smooth muscle cells (13). Our studies have revealed that this class of drugs may have additional vasodilating effects by enhancing agonist-induced, $[Ca^{2+}]_i$-dependent formation of NO.

Therefore, in spite of the difference in the regulation of Ca^{2+} fluxes between endothelial and smooth muscle cells, the membrane potential exerts a functionally synergistic control function on both cell species of the vessel wall. Depolarization induces contraction, by direct activation of the contractile apparatus in smooth muscle cells, as well as by diminishing release of NO. On the other hand, hyperpolarization reduces the contractile responses of smooth muscle cells and is furthermoore a prerequisite for the formation of the powerful vasodilator NO in endothelial cells.

Conclusions

Synthesis of NO in endothelial cells is regulated by Ca^{2+} and by calmodulin at the level of a NO synthase system that has been partially purified from the cytosol. Sustained increases in the intracellular free calcium concentration in intact endothelial cells require the influx of extracellular Ca^{2+} that can be induced by several stimuli, such as bradykinin. This influx is regulated by the membrane potential in a way opposite to that in vascular smooth muscle cells: it is attenuated under depolarizing conditions, but enhanced under hyperpolarizing conditions. Therefore, the agonist-induced hyperpolarization, attributed to the opening of Ca^{2+}-dependent K^+ channels, may play an important role for EDRF release because hyperpolarization augments the driving force for Ca^{2+} influx and thereby contributes to longlasting increases in $[Ca^{2+}]_i$.

Acknowledgement. This work was supported by a grant from the Bundesministerium für Forschung und Technologie ("Biomaterialien und Hämokompatibilität")

References

1. Adams DJ, Barakeh J, Laskey R, van Bremen C (1989) Ion channels and regulation of intracellular calcium in vascular endothelial cells. FASEB J 3:2389–2400
2. Amber IJ, Hibbs JB, Taintor RR, Vavrin Z (1988) Cytokines induce an L-arginine-dependent effector system in nonmacrophage cells. J Leukocyte Biol 44:58–65
3. Ando J, Komatsuda T, Kamiya A (1988) Cytoplasmic calcium response to fluid shear stress in cultured vascular endothelial cells. In Vitro Cell Develop Biol 24:871–877
4. Bassenge E, Busse R (1988) Endothelial modulation of coronary tone. Prog Cardiovasc Dis 30:349–380
5. Busse R, Fichtner H, Lückhoff A, Kohlhardt M (1988) Hyperpolarization and increased free calcium in acetylcholine-stimulated endothelial cells. Am J Physiol 255:H965–H969
6. Cannell MB, Sage SO (1989) Bradykinin-evoked changes in cytosolic calcium and membrane currents in cultured bovine pulmonary artery endothelial cells. J Physiol (London) 419:555–568
7. Colden-Stanfield M, Schilling WP, Ritchie AK, Eskin SG, Navarro LT, Kunze DL (1987) Bradykinin-induced increases in cytosolic calcium and ionic currents in cultured bovine aortic endothelial cells. Circ Res 61:632–640
8. Danthuluri NR, Cybusky MI, Brock TA (1988) ACh-induced calcium transients in primary cultures of rabbit aortic endothelial cells. Am J Physiol 255:H1549–H1553
9. Daut J, Dischner A, Mehrke G (1989) Bradykinin induces a transient hyperpolarization of cultured guinea-pig coronary endothelial cells. J Physiol (London) 410:48P
10. Förstermann U, Mülsch A, Böhme E, Busse R (1986) Stimulation of soluble guanylate cyclase by an acetylcholine-induced endothelium-derived factor from rabbit and canine arteries. Circ Res 58:531–538
11. Furchgott RF (1983) Role of endothelium in responses of vascular smooth muscle. Circ Res 53:557–573
12. Grynkiewicz G, Poenie M, Tsien RY (1985) A new generation of Ca^{2+} indicators with greatly improved fluorescence properties. J Biol Chem 260:3440–3450
13. Hamilton TC, Weston AH (1989) Cromakalim, nicorandil and pinacidil: novel drugs which open potassium channels in smooth muscle. Gen Pharmacol 20:1–9
14. Hauschildt S, Bassenge E, Bessler W, Busse R, Mülsch A (1990) L-arginine-dependent nitric oxide formation and nitrite release in bone marrow-derived macrophages stimulated with bacterial lipopeptide and lipopolysaccharide. Immunol 70:332–337
15. Hauschildt S, Lückhoff A, Mülsch A, Kohler J, Bessler W, Busse R (1990) Induction and activity of NO synthetase in bone marrow-derived macrophage are independent of calcium. Biochem J 270:351–356
16. Hodgkin AL (1951) The ionic basis of electrical activity in nerve and muscle. Biol Rev 26:339–409
17. Iyengar R, Stuehr DJ, Marlette MA (1987) Macrophage synthesis of nitrite, nitrate, and N-nitrosamines: precursors and role of the respiratory burst. Proc Natl Acad Sci USA 84:6369–6373
18. Knowles RG, Palacios M, Palmer RMJ, Moncada S (1989) Formation of nitric oxide from L-arginine in the central nervous system – transduction mechanism for stimulation of the soluble guanylate cyclase. Proc Natl Acad Sci USA 86:5159–5162
19. Lückhoff A, Busse R (1986) Increased free calcium in endothelial cells under stimulation with adenine nucleotides. J Cell Physiol 126:414–420
20. Lückhoff A, Busse R, Winter I, Bassenge E (1987) Characterization of vascular relaxant factor released from cultured endothelial cells. Hypertension 9:295–303
21. Lückhoff A, Pohl U, Mülsch A, Busse R (1988) Differential role of extra- and intracellular calcium in the release of EDRF and prostacyclin from cultured endothelial cells. Br J Pharmacol 95:189–196
22. Lückhoff A, Busse R (1990) Activators of potassium channels enhance calcium influx into endothelial cells as a consequence of potassium currents. Naunyn-Schmiedebergs Arch Pharmacol 342:94–99

23. Lückhoff A, Busse R (1990) Calcium influx into endothelial cells and formation of EDRF is controlled by the membrane potential. Pflügers Arch 416:305–311
24. Marletta MA, Yoon PS, Iyengar R, Leaf CD, Wishnok JS (1988) Macrophage oxidation of L-arginine to nitrite and nitrate: nitric oxide is an intermediate. Biochemistry 27:8706–8711
25. Marletta MA (1989) Nitric oxide: biosynthesis and biological significance. Trends Bioch Sci 14:488–492
26. Morgan-Boyd R, Stewart JM, Vavrek RJ, Hassid A (1987) Effects of bradykinin and angiotensin II on intracellular Ca^{2+} dynamcis in endothelial cells. Am J Physiol 253:C588–C598
27. Mülsch A, Böhme E, Busse R (1987) Stimulation of soluble guanylate cyclase by endothelium-derived relaxing factor from cultured endothelial cells. Eur J Pharmacol 135:247–250
28. Mülsch A, Bassenge E, Busse R (1989) Nitric oxide synthesis in endothelial cytosol: evidence for a calcium-dependent and a calcium-independent mechanism. Naunyn-Schmiedebergs Arch Pharmacol 340:767–770
29. Myers RR, Minor RL, Guerra R, Bates JN, Harrison DG (1990) Vasorelaxant properties of the endothelium-derived relaxing factor more closely resemble S-nitrosocysteine than nitric oxide. Nature 365:161–163
30. Olesen SP, Clapham DE, Davies PF (1988) Haemodynamic shear stress activates a K^+ current in vascular endothelial cells. Nature 331:168–170
31. Olesen SP, Davies PF, Clapham DE (1988) Muscarinic-activated K^+ current in bovine aortic endothelial cells. Circ Res 62:1059–1064
32. Palmer RMJ, Ferrige AG, Moncada S (1987) Nitric oxide release accounts for the biological activity of endothelium-derived relaxing factor. Nature 327:524–526
33. Sauvé R, Parent L, Simoneau C, Roy G (1988) External ATP triggers a biphasic activation process of a calcium-dependent K^+ channel in cultured bovine aortic endothelial cells. Pflügers Arch 412:469–481
34. Schilling WP (1989) Effect of membrane potential on cytosolic calcium of bovine aortic endothelial cells. Am J Physiol 257:H778–H784
35. Schilling WP, Rajan L, Strobl-Jager E (1989) Characterization of the bradykinin-stimulated calcium influx pathway of cultured vascular endothelial cells. Saturability, selectivity, and kinetics. J Biol Chem 264:12838–12848
36. Schröder H, Schrör K (1989) Cyclic GMP stimulation by vasopressin in LLC-PK1 kidney epithelial cells is L-arginine-dependent. Naunyn-Schmiedebergs Arch Pharmacol 340:475–477
37. Wright CD, Mülsch A, Busse R, Osswald H (1989) Generation of nitric oxide by human neutrophils. Biochem Biophys Res Commun 160:813–819

Author's address:

Prof. Dr. R. Busse
Department of Applied Physiology
University of Freiburg
Hermann-Herder-Str. 7
W-7800 Freiburg, FRG

EDRF: nitrosylated compound or authentic nitric oxide

J. N. Bates, D. G. Harrison, P. R. Myers, and R. L. Minor

Departments of Anesthesia and Medicine and the Cardiovascular Institute
University of Iowa College of Medicine, Iowa City, USA

Summary: Endothelium-derived factor (EDRF) from bovine aortic endothelial cells was compared to solutions of authentic nitric oxide (NO) and to solutions of the nitrosothiol S-nitroso-L-cysteine. EDRF was produced from endothelial cells by basal release or by stimulation with the calcium ionophore A23187. Biological activity was measured as relaxation of porcine coronary arteries preconstricted with prostaglandin $F_{2\alpha}$, and chemical analysis was made of the nitrosyl content by measurement of NO released after chemical reduction with 1% sodium iodide in glacial acetic acid. EDRF, NO, and nitrosocysteine had identical half-lives, were all inactivated by hemoglobin and methylene blue, and were all augmented in their biological activity by superoxide dismutase. When solutions were analyzed for their biological activity as a function of the NO content (after NaI/acetic acid reduction), nitrosocysteine showed more vasodilation per amount of contained NO than did authentic NO.Solutions containing EDRF (basal release or by stimulation with A23187) subjected to the same analysis appeared similar to nitrosocysteine, and were distinct from solutions of NO. These experiments show that nitrosyl compounds other than NO can have properties very similar or identical to EDRF, and that in this system EDRF appears more similar to nitrosocysteine than to NO.

Key words: Endothelium-derived relaxing factor; nitric oxide NO; S-nitroso-L-cysteine; nitrosothiols; endothelial cells

Introduction

Endothelium-derived relaxing factor has the properties of a potent nitrovasodilator. It increases the activity of guanylate cyclase, it is inhibited by hemoglobin and methylene blue, arginine guanidino nitrogen-derived nitrite is produced as a stable metabolite from endothelial cells in parallel with EDRF, and inhibition of the nitrite production by competitive arginine analogs blocks EDRF release. The common feature of nitrovasodilators is their ability to enter into reactions that produce NO. NO can directly activate guanylate cyclase, and inhibition of the conversion to NO seems to block the vasodilatory effect of most or all nitrovasodilators. This led to the widely accepted theory that all nitrovasodilators act by the production of the common intermediate NO (16). The high potency of solutions of NO as a vasodilator, its great instability in the presence of oxygen, superoxide, and oxyhemoglobin, and its oxidation to nitrite are properties NO shares with EDRF which led to the hypothesis that EDRF and NO are identical (5, 11). The great potency of EDRF, which translates into its very low physiological concentrations, along with its great instability in biological preparations, has hindered success in collecting, isolating, and identifying EDRF as it is released from endothelial cells. Attempts at identification of EDRF have of necessity been really identifications of nitrite (or other nitrosyl), or demonstrations of reactions which are not entirely specific to NO (5, 9–11). Trace amounts of NO can be flushed from solutions of EDRF (9–11) without the use of reducing agents, but the amounts are insufficient to account for the bioactivity of EDRF. This small amount of NO could represent residual native EDRF (if EDRF is NO) or a decomposition product of another nitrosyl compound (if EDRF is another nitrovasodilator).

Several investigators have found that certain biological or biochemical assays of EDRF respond differently to EDRF than to authentic NO (1, 3, 7, 13, 14, 18). Myers et. al. (9) studied the similarity of EDRF and NO using bioassays of suspended preconstricted isolated porcine coronary arteries in parallel with NO measurement by a chemiluminescence technique after chemical reduction by acetic acid/iodide reflux. In this system nitric oxide (i.e., nitrite) production by endothelial cells was lower than that found in an equipotent (by bioassay) solution of authentic NO. This suggested that NO might be released from the endothelial cells in a form other than free NO, i.e., as a nitrosyl compound RNO that will release NO in the smooth muscle or will directly activate guanylate cyclase. To investigate this hypothesis, we have constructed model compounds that contain NO within their structure, release the NO readily, are potent vasodilators, and have other properties similar to EDRF. This report concentrates on one specific model compound, S-nitroso-L-cysteine (which has many properties similar to EDRF) and compares EDRF with NO and S-nitrosocysteine.

Methods

Measurement of nitric oxide

A chemiluminescence technique was used to specifically and quantitatively measure NO. Effluant from cultured endothelial cells, or standard solutions of known composition entered a 1% sodium iodide in glacial acetic acid reflux bath which was continually degassed by a stream of nitrogen directed to a nitric oxide analyzer. HI in the reflux bath quantitatively reduces nitrite and a variety of nitrosyl compounds to NO which is removed by the nitrogen. NO in the gas stream was measured by the chemiluminescent reaction of ozone and NO in an oxide of nitrogen analyzer (Dasibi, Glendale, California; model 2108). In experiments directly measuring NO in solution the sodium iodide and acetic acid were omitted from the reflux chamber.

Cultured cells

Cultured bovine aortic endothelial cells (BAEC) were grown on microcarrier beads using standard tissue culture techniques. Properties of the cell line have been previously published (4, 6). In each experiment, 100–500 million cells were transferred to a small glass chamber that was perfused with Kreb's buffer (37° C; 5% CO_2 and 95% O_2) at 44 cc/min. All studies were performed in the presence of 1 μM indomethacin. The effluant from the endothelial cells was directed to either a preconstricted bioassay ring or into the reflux flask attached to the NO analyzer.

Bioassay measurements

Porcine hearts were obtained fresh from a local slaughterhouse and immediately immersed in cold, oxygenated Kreb's saline. 2–4-mm segments of the left circumflex artery were isolated and the endothelium removed by gently rubbing the segment with forceps. The segments were then mounted on an apparatus coupled to a strain guage, and suspended in air. The segments were superfused with Kreb's buffer and stretched to their optimal length as determined by their response to 100 mM KCl. They were then preconstricted to 3–4 grams with 0.1–1.0 μM $PGF_{2\alpha}$, and their response was measured when superfused with the studied solution.

Preparation of nitric oxide solutions

Nitric oxide standards were prepared by injecting 25 μl of authentic nitric oxide gas into 25 cc of distilled water which had been deoxygenated by purging for greater than 30 min with helium. This produced a standard solution of 45 μM nitric oxide. The solution was prepared in a gas-tight syringe which was then mounted on a syringe pump for injection into the bioassay or reflux system.

Preparation of S-nitroso-L-cysteine

Two millimoles of nitric oxide (45 cc) were mixed with a slight excess of oxygen to allow complete oxidation to NO_2.This was condensed as N_2O_4 on the wall of the reaction vessel by immersion in dry ice/methanol. Only samples showing no visible blue coloration indicative of N_2O_3 were used. One millimole of L-cysteine was dissolved in a final volume of 1 ml of methanol to give 1 M cysteine in methanol. This solution was added to the reaction vessel containing N_2O_4 and allowed to warm to room temperature briefly. S-nitrosocysteine was produced by the reaction: $N_2O_4 + RSH \rightarrow RSNO + HNO_3$. The solution was diluted to 0.1 M nitrosocysteine in methanol, stored at $-20°$ C, and protected from oxygen and light; solutions were shown to be stable for several weeks under these conditions. Solutions of approximately 50 μM S-nitrosocysteine were prepared by dilution in deoxygenated distilled water and were discarded after several hours. Other nitrosothiols were prepared by the same method.

Chemicals and solutions

All drugs were prepared fresh daily except indomethacin which was maintained as a 1-mM stock. Kreb's buffer (118.3 mM NaCl, 4.7 mM KCl, 2.5 mM $CaCl_2$, 1.2 mM $MgSO_4$, 1.2 mM KH_2PO_4, 25 mM $NaHCO_3$) was aerated with 95% O_2 5% CO_2. Bradykinin, A23187, indomethacin, and all thiols were obtained from Sigma Chemical Co., St. Louis, Missouri. $PGF_{2\alpha}$ was purchased from Upjohn Co., Chicago, Illinois. Nitric oxide was from Matheson Scientific, Joliet, Illinois. Sodium iodide was from Aldrich Chemical Co., Milwaukee, Wisconsin.

Data analysis

Data are presented as the mean $\pm$ SEM. The concentration of NO was measured by chemiluminescence assay and compared to standard solutions of NO. Bioassay relaxations were expressed as a percent of the preconstricted tension. The amount of NO necessary to account for equivalent relaxation of the bioassay ring was compared with the amount of nitric oxide produced by cultured endothelial cells using paired *t*-tests with an appropriate Bonferroni correction for multiple comparisons.

Results

S-nitrosocysteine purity

S-nitrosocysteine, prepared as described, was assayed by ion-pair high-pressure liquid chromatography. The column was a C-18 reverse phase silica column with a mobile phase of 20% methanol, 80% (50 mM phosphoric acid, 1 mM octane sulphonic acid, pH 2.2). Ultraviolet detection at 210 nm was used to follow the sample. Analysis of the stock solutions showed virtually complete conversion of cysteine to S-nitrosocysteine (Fig. 1).

Solutions of S-nitrosocysteine in deoxygenated water at 10^{-7}M produced no measurable NO when flushed with nitrogen. In some experiments a small amount ($<5\%$) of the nitrosocysteine had decomposed prior to analysis and traces of NO appeared in the initial nitrogen flush. Continued flushing failed to detect any continuous NO release. Acidification with 1 M HCl did not result in NO release as would be expected if inorganic nitrite were present, but addition of 1% NaI/glacial acetic acid resulted in stoichiometric NO release.

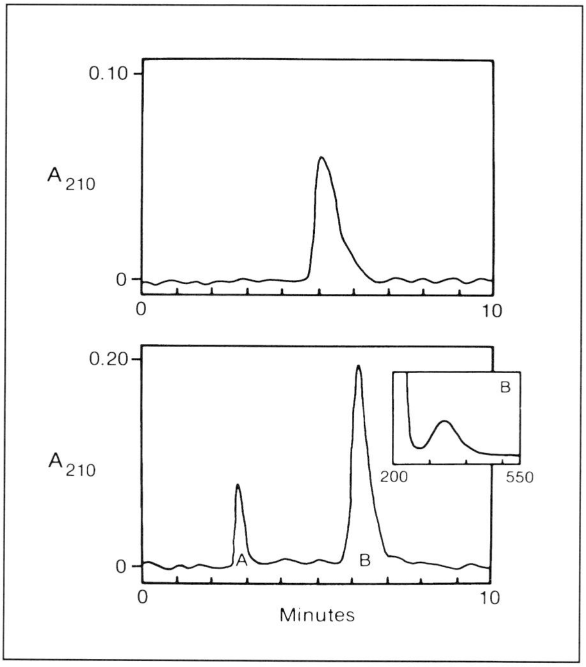

Fig. 1. HPLC analysis of S-nitrosocysteine. S-nitrosocysteine was prepared as described by the reaction of cysteine and NO_2 in methanol. Top: HPLC of cysteine by ion-pair chromatography on C-18 reversed phase silica column using a mobile phase of 20% methanol, 80% (50 mM phosphoric acid, 1 mM octane sulphonic acid, pH 2.2). Ultraviolet detection was at 210 nm. Bottom: HPLC of reaction mixture after addition of NO_2. Peak A migrates with nitric acid, peak B is S-nitrosocysteine. Inset: spectrophotometric analysis of peak B showing absorbance peak at 340 nm characteristic of nitrosothiols

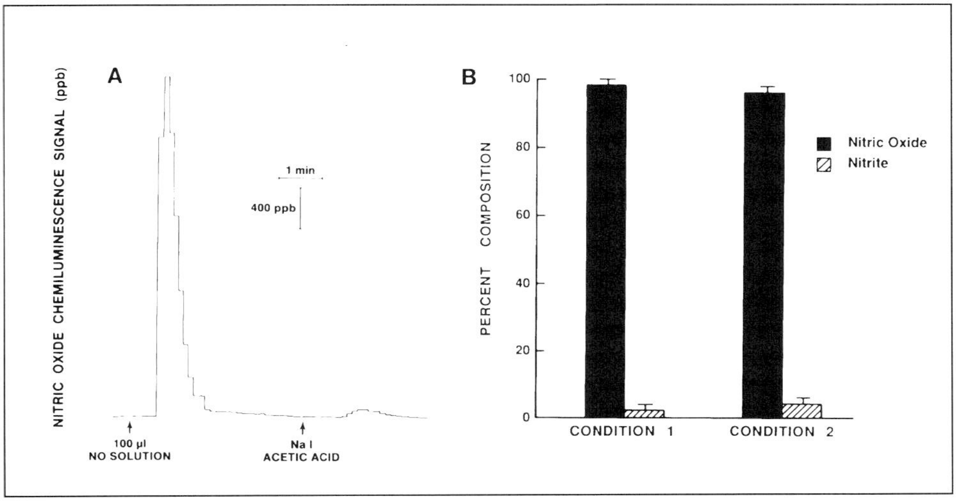

Fig. 2. Analysis of NO stock solutions. 20 ml of deoxygenated distilled water were flushed with nitrogen gas that had passed through 1M sodium dithionite to remove traces of oxygen. Aliquots of nitric oxide removed directly from a gas-tight syringe (condition 1, $n = 10$), or after passage through 30–40 cm of polyethylene tubing (condition 2, $n = 10$) were injected into the chamber, and purged nitric oxide measured by chemiluminescence. When the signal returned to baseline 1% sodium iodide in glacial acetic acid was infused into the chamber until the remaining nitrite was reduced to NO, again detected by chemiluminescence. **A:** sample recording. **B:** Distribution of NO as free NO and nitrite in stock solutions

Nitric oxide solution purity

Solutions of NO were assayed for authentic NO content by chemiluminescence of NO flushed from the solutions before and after reduction by NaI/acetic acid (Fig. 2). Stock solutions showed that greater than 95% of the nitrosyl nitrogen was removed by nitrogen before reduction showing that very little of the NO was oxidized to nitrite in the stock solution. Analysis of the solution in the syringe and in the tubing at the point immediately prior to injection into the Kreb's gave essentially identical results. After contact with oxygenated Kreb's nitric oxide is rapidly oxidized to nitrite.

Chemiluminescence measurement of NO and S-nitrosocysteine

NO was produced stoichiometrically from solutions of NO or S-nitrosocysteine by the NaI/Acetic acid reflux chamber. The response was linearly dependent on concentration over the range studied (Fig. 3).

Half life measurements

Half lives of EDRF, nitric oxide and S-nitrosocysteine were measured by interposing various lengths of tubing between the detector vessel and the endothelial cells or point of

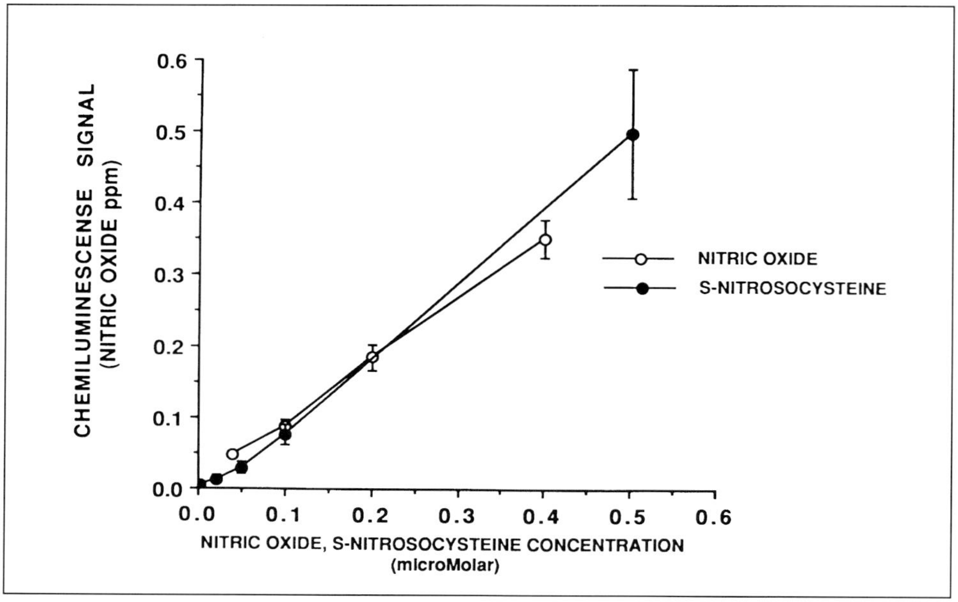

Fig. 3. Nitric oxide detection of authentic nitric oxide solutions or S-nitrosocysteine solutions. Each compound was infused into a chamber with excess 1% sodium iodide in glacial acetic acid and the released NO carried to the chemiluminescence NO analyzed by a stream of nitrogen.

injection of NO or S-nitrosocysteine. This prolonged the transit time incrementally from 3 to 30 seconds in oxygenated Kreb's before bioassay and allowed an estimation of the half life. Half lives of EDRF, nitric oxide, and S-nitrosocysteine were each approximately 30 seconds (Fig. 4).

Effects of hemoglobin, methylene blue, and superoxide dismutase

Vessels were allowed to reach a steady state of relaxation to EDRF, S-nitrosocysteine, or NO, then an infusion of hemoglobin (10^{-5}M), methylene blue (10^{-5}M), or superoxide dismutase (200 U/ml) was added at the same point in the system as the vasodilator. EDRF-, S-nitrosocysteine, and NO were indistinguishable from each other in their responses to inactivation by hemoglobin or methylene blue, and their potentiation by superoxide dismutase.

Comparison of bioassay vs NO/nitrosyl content

Varying amounts of NO or S-nitrosocysteine were infused into Kreb's solution, which superfused preconstricted detector vessels. The same solutions were alternately directed into the reflux NO detector for NO quantification. When bioassay response (% relaxation) was plotted as a function of NO detected, S-nitrosocysteine could be seen to vige much more relaxation per volume of NO released than stock solutions of NO did (Fig. 5).When the effluant from cultured BAEC was analyzed in the same manner the

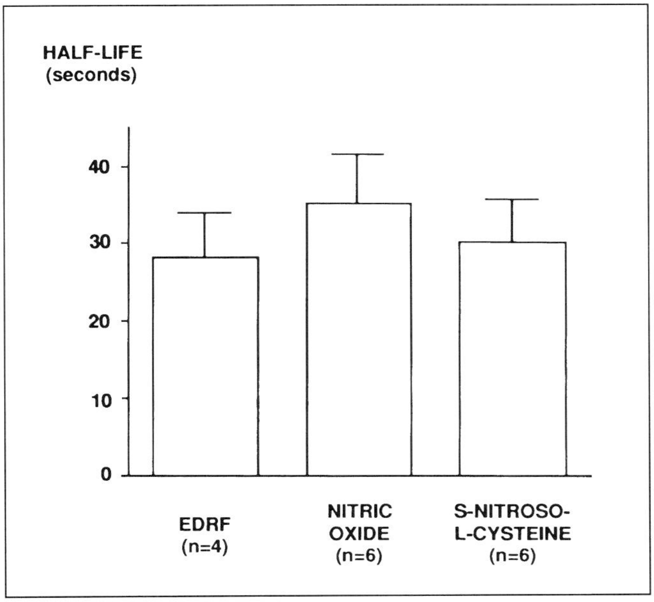

Fig. 4. Half-lives of EDRF, nitric oxide, and S-nitrosocysteine. Half-lives determined by adjusting length of intervening tubing between point of injection of drug or endothelial cell effluant into oxygenated Kreb's buffer and the detector vessel. There was a negative linear relationship between the percent relaxation and the transit time to the detector vessel ($r = -0.97 \pm 0.01$, -0.93 ± 0.02, and -0.94 ± 0.03 for EDRF, nitric oxide, and S-nitrosocysteine, respectively). Transit time to produce 50% relaxation relative to the amount at time zero was calculated from the regression equations.

relationship was essentially identical to that seen with S-nitrosocysteine, and different than that of NO.

Discussion

Much of the support for the hypothesis that EDRF is NO comes from the chemical and pharmacological similarities of the two substances. We show here that the similarity to EDRF is not a feature unique to NO. Other labile potent nitrovasodilators would likely have many similarities, and the present experiments show that the compound S-nitrosocysteine has properties very similar to EDRF. In direct comparisons with EDRF, S-nitrosocysteine resembles EDRF as well or better than NO does. Other recent studies have also found that methods that discriminate between EDRF and NO do not discriminate EDRF from S-nitrosocysteine (13, 18).

Much of the similarity between dilute solutions of S-nitrosocysteine and NO might be attributed to the spontaneous decomposition of S-nitrosocysteine to NO. S-nitrosocysteine does spontaneously decompose to form the disulfide cystine and NO. However, this reaction is second order with respect to S-nitrosocysteine, and can be shown to procede very slowly at low concentrations. Analysis of dilute solutions of S-nitrosocysteine shows

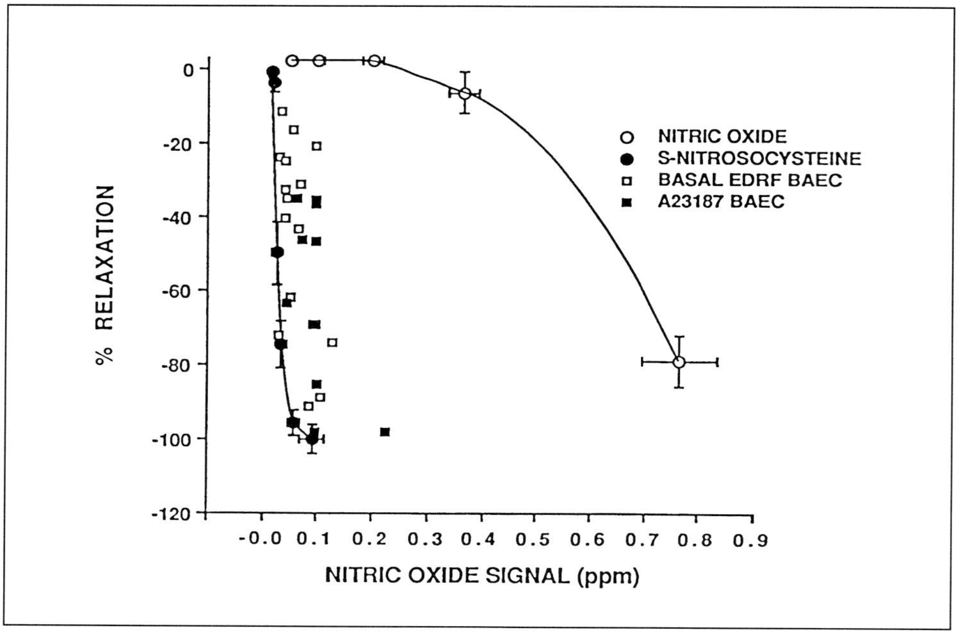

Fig. 5. Vascular response as a function of nitric oxide content. Vascular relaxation and NO content were compared for infusions of NO (○), S-nitrosocysteine (●), and EDRF. EDRF was released from bovine aortic endothelial cell (BAEC) cultures under basal flow conditions (□) or after stimulation with 10 μM calcium ionophore A23187 (■). Detector vessel relaxation was measured as described and nitric oxide signal was measured after reduction by 1% sodium iodide in glacial acetic acid. Transit time from point of injection or endothelial cells to detector vessel or NO analyzer was identical in each case.

that they do not have more than trace amounts of NO in the solution until a reducing agent (acidified sodium iodide) is added.

In the bioassay system used in these experiments S-nitrosocysteine has a greater potency than solutions of authentic NO infused at the same point in the system. If the terminal intermediate in all nitrovasodilators is NO, then NO must be at least as potent as any other nitrovasodilator. However, NO would appear to be less potent than another nitrovasodilator if it is more unstable and less survives to the completion of the bioassay. At the point where the effluant passes over the detector vessel NO is largely oxidized to nitrite (9), and differences in the reported potency of NO solutions (5, 11) may reflect varying degrees to which NO is oxidized before reaching the detector vessel. If the solutions of NO used in these experiments are tested in a muscle bath where the detector vessel is submerged, and oxidation and evaporation of NO are likely lessened, then stock NO solutions have greater potency. At the point of infusion into this system NO solutions are shown by assay to be essentially 100% NO with very little nitrite (Fig. 2). Oxidation to nitrite occurs after contact with oxygenated Kreb's buffer. The fact that EDRF and S-nitrosocysteine do not lose potency as much as NO when entering the effluant at the same point suggests a difference in their chemical identity.

It is more likely that EDRF, like S-nitrosocysteine, is a nitrovasodilator that contains NO within its structure and releases NO at or in the smooth muscle cells. There is some evidence to suggest that the primary mechanism of action of S-nitrosocysteine involves generation of NO at the surface of the smooth muscle cell. The polarity of S-nitrosocysteine would argue against simple diffusion into the smooth muscle cell. If it did act intracellularly, then other nitrosothiols which are more lipid soluble ought to be able to enter the cell more readily and be more potent. An example of a more lipid soluble nitrosothiol is S-nitroso-2-mercaptoethanol, which was studied. It is equally as potent a vasodilator and differs from S-nitrosocysteine mostly by having a much longer half-life (10). S-nitroso-D-cysteine was also prepared and studied, and it has identical properties to the L-isomer. This suggests that S-nitrosocysteine probably does not enter the smooth muscle cell via a transporter mechanism, since such transporters are usually stereospecific. It is more likely that the nitrosothiols decompose at the surface of the cell and liberate NO which enters the cell.

The possibility that endothelial-derived NO is contained in a nitrosothiol or similar compound has implications in the pathophysiology of EDRF synthesis. Several pathological conditions, including atherosclerosis (2), acute hypertension (17), ischemia with subsequent reperfusion (15), and diabetes (12), are associated with disorders of EDRF synthesis or release. In rabbits with diet-induced atherosclerosis the release of EDRF is decreased, while there is increased release of NO (measured as nitrite or other oxidized species reduced to NO by sodium iodide/acetic acid) (8). This implies that in atherosclerosis the NO in EDRF is in a form that is either less potent or is more rapidly oxidized than EDRF in normal rabbits. If EDRF is a nitrosothiol rather than free NO, then there are two steps in EDRF synthesis: 1) oxidation of the guanidino nitrogen of arginine to nitrosyl nitrogen, and 2) coupling the nitrosyl nitrogen with a thiol to form a nitrosothiol. A defect which impairs the second step, but not the first, would result in continued release of NO, but decreased EDRF activity in the bioassay. Oxidation or depletion of pertinent pools of thiols would cause a deficiency that produced just such an inhibition.

In summary, these experiments demonstrate the compound S-nitrosocysteine has properties very similar or identical to EDRF. In comparisons with a bioassay system where NO and S-nitrosocysteine have different characteristics, EDRF more closely resembles S-nitrosocysteine than NO. This suggests that the NO in EDRF is likely incorporated into a labile nitrosyl compound similar to S-nitrosocysteine.

References

1. Dusting G, Read M, Stewart A (1988) Endothelium-derived relaxing factor released from cultured cells: differentiation from nitric oxid. Clin Exp Pharmacol Physiol 15:83–92
2. Freiman PC, Mitchell, Heistad DD, Armstrong ML, Harrison DG (1986) Atherosclerosis impairs endothelium-dependent vascular relaxation to acetylcholine and thrombin in primates. Circ Res 58:783–789
3. Greenberg SS, Wilcox D, Rubanyi GM (1988) Endothelium-derived relaxing factor (EDRF) released from canine femoral artery cannot be identified as nitric oxide by electron paramagnetic resonance (EPR). Circulation 78 (Suppl II):II-182
4. Hadjiagopious C, Kaduce T, Spector A (1986) Eicosapentaenoic acid utilization by bovine aortic endothelial cells: effects of prostacyclin production. Biochim Biophys Acta 875:369–381
5. Ignarro L, Byrons R, Buga G, Wood K (1987) Endothelium-derived relaxing factor from pulmonary artery and vein posesses pharmacologic and chemical properties identical to those of nitric oxide radical. Circ Res 61:866–879
6. Kaduce T, Spector A, Bar R (1982) Linoleic acid metabolism and prostaglandin production by cultured bovine pulmonary artery endothelial cells. Arteriosclerosis 2:380–389

7. Long C, Shikano J, Berkowitz B (1987) Anion exchange resins discriminate between nitric oxide and EDRF. Eur J Pharmacol 142:317–318
8. Minor R, Myers P, Guerra R, Bates J, Harrison D (1990) Diet-induced atherosclerosis increases the release of nitrogen oxides from rabbit aorta. J Clin Invest 86:2109–2116
9. Myers P, Guerra R, Harrison D (1989) Release of NO and EDRF from cultured bovine aortic endothelial cells. Am J Physiol 256:1030–1037
10. Myers P, Minor R, Guerra R, Bates J, Harrison D (1990) Vasorelaxant properties of the endothelium-derived relaxing factor more closely resemble S-nitrosocysteine than nitric oxide. Nature 345:161–163
11. Palmer R, Ferrige A, Moncada S (1987) Nitric oxide release accounts for the biological activity of endothelium-derived relaxing factor. Nature 327:524–526
12. Pieper GM, Gross GJ (1988) Oxygen free radicals abolish endothelium-dependent relaxation in diabetic rat aorta. Am J Physiol 24:H825–H833
13. Rubanyi GM, Johns A, Harrison DG, Wilcox D (1989) Evidence that EDRF may be identical with an S-nitrosothiol and not with free nitric oxide. Circulation 80 (Suppl II):II-281
14. Shikano K, Berkowitz B (1987) Endothelium derived relaxing factor is a selective relaxant to smooth muscle. J Pharmacol Exp Ther 243:65–70
15. Van Benthuysen KM, McMurty IF, Horowitz LD (1987) Reperfusion after acute coronary occlusion in dogs impairs endothelium-dependent relaxation to acetylcholine and augments contractile reactivity in vitro. J Clin Invest 79:265–274
16. Waldman SA, Murad F (1987) Cyclin GMP synthesis and function. Pharmacol Rev 39:163–196
17. Wei EP, Kontos HA, Christman CW, DeWitt DS, Povlishock JT (1985) Superoxide generation and reversal of acetylcholine-induced cerebral arteriolar dilation after acute hypertension. Cir Res 57:781–787
18. Wei EP, Kontos HA (1990) H_2O_2 and endothelium-dependent cerebral arteriolar dilation: implications for the identity of EDRF from acetylcholine. Hypertension 16:162–169

Author's address:
James N. Bates, PhD, MD
Department of Anesthesia
University of Iowa College of Medicine
Iowa City, Iowa 52242 USA

Does EDRF/NO regulate its own release by increasing endothelial cyclic GMP? *

M. Kuhn [1] and U. Förstermann [2]

[1] Department of Clinical Pharmacology, Hannover Medical School, FRG, and
[2] Abbott Laboratories, Department 47S, Abbott Park, Illinois, USA

Summary: EDRF/NO released from bovine aortic endothelial cells was measured by transferring conditioned medium to rat fetal lung fibroblasts (RFL-6 cells). These cells contain considerable amounts of soluble guanylyl cyclase. The increase in cyclic GMP in these cells provided a sensitive bioassay for EDRF/NO activity. Bovine aortic endothelial cells released a material that markedly enhanced cyclic GMP in RFL-6 cells. The synthesis of this substance could be stimulated with bradykinin (10 nM) or Ca^{2+} ionophore A23187 (1 μM) and was completely prevented by treatment of the endothelial cells with the EDRF/NO synthesis inhibitor, N^G-nitro-L-arginine (100 μM), or incubation of the RFL-6 detector cells with the inhibitor of soluble guanylyl cyclase, methylene blue (10 μM). The release of EDRF/NO by bradykinin and A23187 was accompanied by an about two-fold increase in the cyclic GMP content in the producing endothelial cells. Incubation of bovine aortic endothelial cells with atrial natriuretic peptide (0.1 μM) or sodium nitroprusside (10 μM) enhanced their cyclic GMP content 6.5-fold and 4.1-fold, respectively. These increases in endothelial cyclic GMP levels had no effect on basal or bradykinin- and A23187-stimulated release of EDRF/NO. We conclude that cyclic GMP does not feed back on EDRF/NO formation or release in bovine aortic endothelial cells.

Key words: Cyclic GMP; soluble guanylyl cyclase; particulate guanylyl cyclase; bradykinin; Ca^{2+}-ionophore A23187; sodium nitroprusside; atrial natriuretic peptide; rat fetal lung fibroblasts

Introduction

Vascular endothelial cells release a powerful vasodilator referred to as endothelium-derived relaxing factor (EDRF) (6). The active principle of EDRF has recently been identified as nitric oxide (NO) (11, 22) and the factor directly activates the soluble isoform of guanylyl cyclase (4, 10, 20). In smooth muscle cells, the resulting increase in cyclic GMP triggers vasodilation (21) and in platelets it inhibits aggregation (1, 2, 8).

While these mechanisms of action are well characterized, little is known about the regulation of EDRF/NO production in endothelial cells. Most types of endothelial cells posses the soluble and particulate isoforms of guanylyl cyclase (7, 15). Some observations have indicated that EDRF/NO can not only activate cyclic GMP formation in neighboring target cells, but also in the producing cells themselves (18, 25). The function of endothelial cyclic GMP is not clear, but it has been suggested that it may reduce the production and/or release of EDRF/NO (3). In the present investigation, we tested whether EDRF/NO increases the levels of cyclic GMP in bovine aortic endothelial cells and whether elevated levels of cyclic GMP modulate the production and/or release of EDRF/NO.

* Supported by the Deutsche Forschungsgemeinschaft (Fo 144/1–2)

Methods and Materials

Cultured cells used in these experiments

Endothelial cells were harvested from bovine aortae using collagenase (0.025% in saline, Gibco, Karlsruhe, FRG). After washing, the cells were suspended in culture medium (v/v mixture of RPMI medium and M199 medium, both Gibco), containing 25 mM Hepes buffer, 15% (v/v) heat-inactivated fetal calf serum (Boehringer, Mannheim, FRG), 50 U/ml of penicillin, 50 μg/ml of streptomycin, and 2.5 μg/ml amphotericin-B. Endothelial cells were grown in gelatin-coated culture flasks at 37° C in 95% air and 5% CO_2 and subcultured with collagenase (0.2% in saline).

Rat fetal lung fibroblasts (RFL-6, ATCC, Rockville, Maryland, USA) were cultured in F12 Ham's nutrient mixture containing 15% heat inactivated fetal calf serum, 50 U/ml of penicillin and 50 μg/ml of streptomycin. Cells were subcultured by passaging confluent cells with a trypsin (0.05%)/EDTA (0.02%) solution (Gibco).

Experiments were performed with first passage bovine aortic endothelial cells and RFL-6 cells of passages 7–9. Both types of cells were grown to confluence in six-well plates (Nunclon delta, Nunc, Denmark, $\sim 10^6$ cells/well). Prior to experimentation, the culture media were removed and the cells were washed three times with 1 ml of phosphate buffered saline of the following composition (mM): Na^+ 149.8, K^+ 4.2, Mg^{2+} 0.5, Ca^{2+} 0.7, Cl^- 141.9, $HPO_4{}^{2-}$ 6.5, $H_2PO_4{}^-$ 1.5, glucose 5.6; pH 7.4. The cells were equilibrated in 1 ml of phosphate-buffered saline at 37° C for 30 min.

Measurement of endothelial EDRF/NO release

RFL-6 cells contain considerable amounts of soluble guanylyl cyclase (16). Therefore, the increase in cyclic GMP in these cells can be used as a measure of EDRF/NO activity (5, 12). Confluent monolayers of bovine aortic endothelial cells were pre-incubated in phosphate-buffered saline with indomethacin (30 μM) and in some experiments M&B 22,948 (0.1 mM) for 30 min. M&B 22,948 selectively inhibits cyclic GMP phosphodiesterase (17, 26). At 30 min, the medium was replaced with 1 ml of the same medium containing superoxide dismutase (20 U/ml). EDRF/NO production was stimulated with bradykinin (10 nM) or Ca^{2+}-ionophore A23187 (1 μM) during a further 1 min incubation. Then, the conditioned medium was quickly aspirated and transferred in less than 5 s to six-well plates containing RFL-6 cells. The RFL-6 cells were pre-equilibrated for 30 min in 1 ml of phosphate buffered saline containing M&B 22,948 (0.1 mM). RFL-6 cells were exposed to the bovine aortic endothelial cell-conditioned medium for 2 min. Then, the medium was removed and 1 ml of ice-cold 6% trichloroacetic acid was added to extract cyclic GMP from the RFL-6 cells. After freeze-thawing and centrifugation, supernatant fractions were extracted six times with water-saturated diethylether. Samples were frozen and lyophilized to remove all remaining ether. After reconstitution in distilled water, cyclic GMP content was measured in the supernatant using a commercially available radioimmunoassay (Amersham Buchler, Braunschweig, FRG).

Endothelial cyclic GMP levels

Bovine aortic endothelial cells were preincubated in phosphate-buffered saline containing indomethacin and, in some experiments, M&B 22,948. During the last 3 min of this incubation, cyclic GMP levels were enhanced in the M&B 22,948-treated bovine aortic endothelial cells by exposing them to atrial natriuretic peptide (0.1 μM) or sodium nitroprusside (10 μM). EDRF/NO production was then stimulated for 1 min with bradykinin (10 nM) or Ca^{2+}-ionophore A23187 (1 μM) as described. Immediately after aspirating the incubation medium (for bioassay of EDRF/NO content), 1 ml of ice-cold 6% trichloroacetic acid was added to the endothelial cells. Cyclic GMP was extracted from the endothelial cells as described and quantified by radioimmunoassay.

Drugs used

Sodium nitroprusside, bradykinin, Ca^{2+}-ionophore A23187, methylene blue and N^G-nitro-L-arginine were purchased from Sigma, Munich, FRG. Indomethacin was obtained from Merck Sharp and Dohme, Munich, FRG. Rat synthetic atriopeptin II (atrial natriuretic peptide) was from Serva, Heidelberg, FRG. M&B 22,948 (2-*o*-propoxylphenyl-8-azapurin-6-one) was supplied by May & Baker Ltd., Dagenham, UK. Superoxide dismutase was from Grünenthal, Stolberg, FRG.

Statistical analysis

Results were expressed as mean values ± S. E.. Statistical differences between mean values were determined by analysis of variance followed by Fisher's protected least-significant-difference test for comparison of different means. p values of less than 0.05 were considered significant.

Results

EDRF/NO release from bovine aortic endothelial cells

Cyclic GMP content of unstimulated RFL-6 detector cells was 2.2 ± 0.6 pmol/10^6 cells (n = 6). Exposure of RFL-6 cells to bradykinin (10 nM, 2 min) or A23187 (1 μM, 2 min) in the presence of superoxide dismutase (20 U/ml) had no effect on their cyclic GMP content. Incubation of RFL-6 cells with conditioned medium from non-stimulated (vehicle-treated) bovine aortic endothelial cells for 2 min increased the cyclic GMP content of RFL-6 cells 1.8 fold (n = 6) (cf. Fig. 1). Incubation of RFL-6 cells for 2 min with the conditioned medium of bradykinin (10 nM, 1 min)-, or A23187 (1 μM, 1 min)-stimulated endothelial cells in the presence of superoxide dismutase (20 U/ml) increased the cyclic GMP content of RFL-6 cells 9.3 fold and 9.9 fold, respectively (n = 6, each) (Fig. 1). Pretreatment of RFL-6 cells with the inhibitor of soluble guanylyl cyclase, methylene blue (10 μM, 30 min) (14), completely prevented the stimulatory effect of the conditioned medium from bradykinin- or A23187-stimulated bovine aortic endothelial cells on the cyclic GMP content of RFL-6 cells (n = 4, each) (Fig. 1). Pretreatment of bovine aortic endothelial cells with the inhibitor of EDRF/NO synthesis, N^G-nitro-L-arginine (0.1 mM, 30 min) (13), abolished EDRF/NO formation in response to bradykinin (10 nM) or A23187 (1 μM) (n = 4, each) (Fig. 1). N^G-nitro-L-arginine had no direct effect on the cyclic GMP content of RFL-6 cells (data not shown).

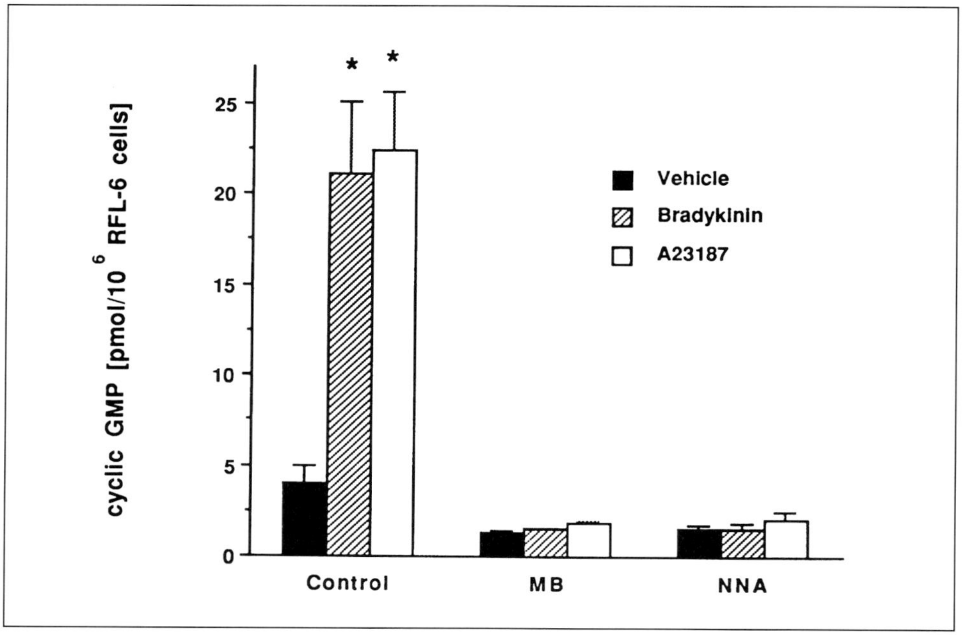

Fig. 1. EDRF/NO release from bovine aortic endothelial cells. Endothelial cell-conditioned medium was transferred onto rat fetal lung fibroblasts (RFL-6 cells). The increase in cyclic GMP in these cells was taken as a measure of EDRF/NO activity. Resting cyclic GMP content of RFL-6 cells was 2.2 ± 0.6 pmol/10^6 RFL-6 cells and was not affected by direct exposure of RFL-6 cells to bradykinin or A23187. Endothelial cells produced moderate amounts of EDRF/NO and this synthesis was markedly stimulated with bradykinin (10 nM) or A23187 (1 μM). Treatment of the RFL-6 cells with methylene blue (MB, 10 μM) or treatment of the endothelial cells with N^G-nitro-L-arginine (NNA, 0.1 mM) prevented the stimulatory effect of endothelial cell-conditioned medium. Columns represent means ± SEM of 4–6 experiments. Asterisks indicate $p < 0.05$ vs vehicle-treated control

Effect of EDRF/NO on cyclic GMP levels in the producing endothelial cells

The resting content of cyclic GMP in bovine aortic endothelial cells was 1.3 ± 0.07 pmol/10^6 cells (n = 4). Stimulation of the endothelial cells with bradykinin (10 nM) or A23187 (1 μM) (n = 4, each) had no significant effect on their cyclic GMP content. Pretreatment of endothelial cells with M&B 22,948 induced a 1.7 fold increase in cyclic GMP (n = 4). In M&B 22,948-treated endothelial cells, bradykinin and A23187 increased the cyclic GMP content 2.3 fold (n = 4, $p < 0.05$) and 2.2 fold (n = 4), respectively (Fig. 2).

Elevation of endothelial cyclic GMP levels with exogenous agents

In these experiments, the resting cyclic content of non-stimulated bovine aortic endothelial cells (controls) was 1.6 ± 0.1 pmol/10^6 cells (n = 12). The selective inhibitor of cyclic GMP phosphodiesterase, M&B 22,948, enhanced the cyclic GMP content of the endothelial cells 1.7 fold (n = 12). In the presence of M&B 22,948, atrial natriuretic pep-

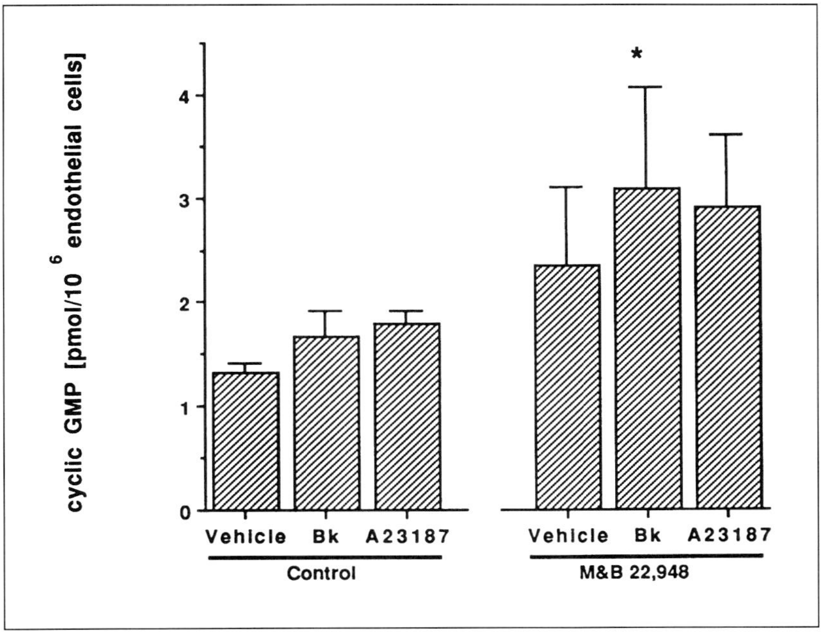

Fig. 2. Effect of stimulators of endothelial EDRF/NO formation on the levels of cyclic GMP in the bovine aortic endothelial cells themselves. The cells were stimulated with bradykinin (Bk, 10 nM) or A23187 (1 μM) in the absence and presence of the cyclic GMP phosphodiesterase inhibitor M&B 22,948. Columns represent means $\pm$ SEM of four experiments. The asterisk indicates $p<0.05$ vs vehicle-treated control

tide and sodium nitroprusside produced 6.5 fold ($n=12$) and 4.1 fold ($n=12$) increases in the cyclic GMP content of bovine aortic endothelial cells, respectively (Fig. 3).

Effect of high endothelial cyclic GMP on EDRF/NO release

The conditioned medium of non-stimulated control bovine aortic endothelial cells increased the cyclic GMP content of RFL-6 cells 2.5 fold ($n=4$). Incubation of RFL-6 cells with the conditioned medium of bradykinin- or A23187-stimulated endothelial cells enhanced their cyclic GMP content 13.0 fold ($n=4$) and 12.6 fold ($n=4$), respectively. However, neither basal nor stimulated EDRF/NO activity significantly altered when cyclic GMP levels were increased in the bovine aortic endothelial cells with M&B 22,948 and atrial natriuretic peptide or sodium nitroprusside (Fig. 4).

Discussion

EDRF/NO release from the vascular intima activates soluble guanylyl cyclase in its physiological target cells (smooth muscle cells, platelets) (9, 24). RFL-6 cells also contain considerable amounts of soluble guanylyl cyclase (16) and have proven sensitive detec-

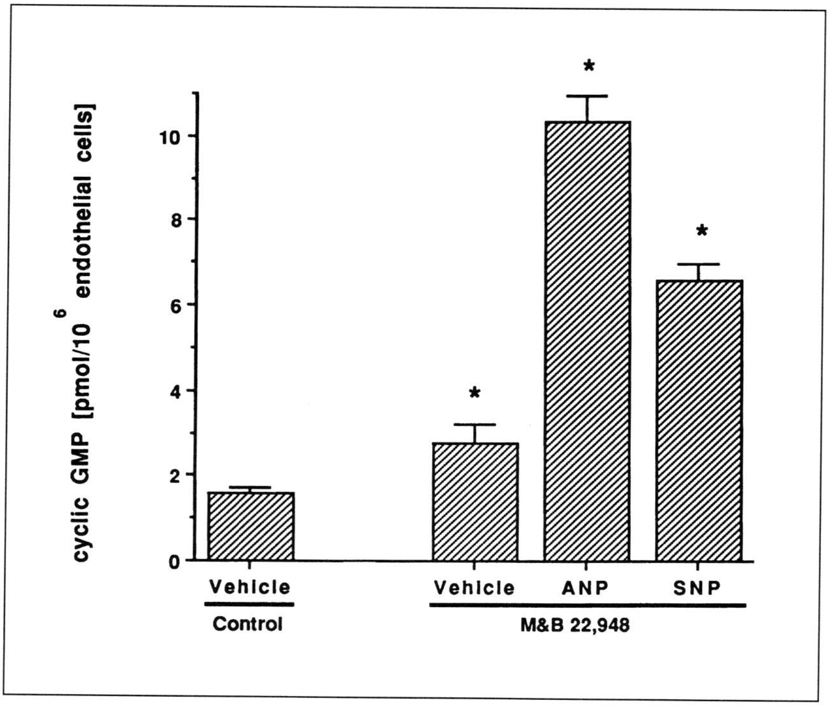

Fig. 3. Effect of the stimulators of particulate and soluble guanylyl cyclase, atrial natriuretic peptide (ANP, 0.1 μM), and sodium nitroprusside (SNP, 10 μM), on the cyclic GMP content of bovine aortic endothelial cells. Guanylyl cyclase-stimulating agents were added to the endothelial cells in the presence of the cyclic GMP phosphodiesterase inhibitor M&B 22,948 (0.1 mM). Columns represent means ± SEM of 12–18 experiments. Asterisks indicate $p < 0.05$ vs vehicle-treated control

tors of EDRF/NO activity (5, 12). Incubation of RFL-6 cells with the conditioned medium of non-stimulated bovine aortic endothelial cells increased the cyclic GMP content of RFL-6 cells. This increase was markedly enhanced when the endothelial cells were stimulated with bradykinin or Ca^{2+}-ionophore A23187. Methylene blue, which selectively inhibits soluble, but not particulate guanylyl cyclase (14), abolished the increase in cyclic GMP content of RFL-6 cells induced by the supernatant of non-stimulated as well as bradykinin- or A23187-stimulated bovine aortic endothelial cells. Similarly, pretreatment of bovine aortic endothelial cells with N^G-nitro-L-arginine, a potent inhibitor of EDRF/NO synthesis (13), completely inhibited the stimulation of RFL-6 cells by the bovine aortic endothelial cell-conditioned medium. These inhibitor experiments indicate that the material released from bovine aortic endothelial cells and detected by RFL-6 cells is EDRF/NO.

Recently, Evans et al. (3) reported that 8-bromo-cyclic GMP inhibits the release of EDRF/NO stimulated by some agonists (acetylcholine, substance P), but not others (ATP, A23187). They suggested that the potential exists for EDRF/NO to stimulate soluble guanylyl cyclase within endothelial cells and to inhibit its own release. Indeed, Martin et al. (18) found that the cyclic GMP content of porcine aortic endothelial cells was increased upon hormonal stimulation of EDRF/NO production, and also Schmidt

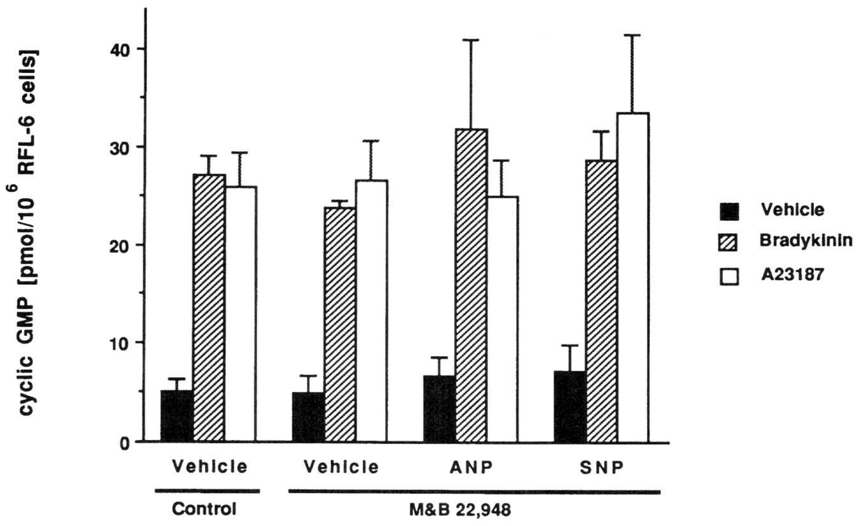

Fig. 4. Effect of cyclic GMP increases in bovine aortic endothelial cells on their production of EDRF/NO. Endothelial cell-conditioned medium was transferred to RFL-6 cells in order to assay the EDRF/NO released. The abscissa shows treatments used to stimulate cyclic GMP in the EDRF/NO-producing endothelial cells (cf. Fig. 3). The legend indicates the agents used to elicit EDRF/NO production in endothelial cells (cf. Fig. 1). Resting cyclic GMP content of RFL-6 cells was 2.08 ± 0.82 pmol/10^6 RFL-6 cells. Basal and bradykinin- or A23187-stimulated EDRF/NO production was not significantly affected by conditions that elevated cyclic GMP levels in the producing endothelial cells. Columns represent menas ± SEM from 4–6 experiments

et al. (25) reported significant increases in cyclic GMP in bovine aortic endothelial cells induced by several stimulants of EDRF/NO production. The cyclic GMP levels reached their maximum between 30 s (18) and 2 min (25). In our experiments, we selected a 1-min incubation period to study the effect of bradykinin and A23187 on the cyclic GMP content of bovine aortic endothelial cells. Although large amounts of EDRF/NO were released into the medium during this period (as detected by RFL-6 cells), endothelial cyclic GMP did not increase significantly (Fig. 2). Even in the presence of the cyclic GMP phosphodiesterase inhibitor M&B 22,948 (17, 26), only modest increases in endothelial cell cyclic GMP were observed. These results are in agreement with those of Peach et al. (23) and Glanz et al. (7) who found no significant increase in the cyclic GMP content of cultured endothelial cells in response to EDRF/NO-stimulating agents. The reason for the discrepant results obtained by different groups in different types of endothelial cells is not clear. Endothelial cells from different species may contain different amounts of soluble guanylyl cyclase, and also the culture conditions and/or passage number may play a role. It is clear, however, that our bovine aortic endothelial cells contained some soluble and particulate guanylyl cyclase because both sodium nitroprusside (which stimulates soluble guanylyl cyclase) and artrial natriuretic peptide (which stimulates particulate guanylyl cyclase) (19, 27), induced significant increases in the cyclic GMP content of these cells. However, these increases had no effect on the release of EDRF/NO.

Thus, EDRF/NO produced only a modest increase in cyclic GMP in bovine aortic endothelial cells. Marked increases in the levels of this cyclic nucleotide produced by other substances had no effect on EDRF/NO release. This suggests that even under conditions where EDRF/NO would increase endothelial cyclic GMP content, this is unlikely to represent a feed-back loop that alters the production of EDRF/NO.

References

1. Alheid U, Reichwehr I, Förstermann U (1989) Human endothelial cells inhibit platelet aggregation by separately stimulating platelet cyclic AMP and cyclic GMP. Eur J Pharmacol 164:103–110
2. Busse R, Lückhoff A, Bassenge E (1987) Endothelium-derived relaxing factor inhibits platelet aggregation. Naunyn-Schmiedeb. Arch Pharmacol 336:566–571
3. Evans HG, Smith JA, Lewis MJ (1988) Release of endothelium-derived relaxing factor is inhibited by 8-bromo-cyclic guanosine monophosphate. J Cardiovasc Pharmacol 12:672–677
4. Förstermann U, Mülsch A, Böhme E, Busse R (1986) Stimulation of soluble guanylate cyclase by an acetylcholine-induced endothelium-derived factor from rabbit and canine arteries. Circ Res 58:531–538
5. Förstermann U, Gorsky LD, Pollock JS, Schmidt HHHW, Heller M, Murad F (1990) Hormone-induced biosynthesis of EDRF/NO-like material in N1E-115 neuroblastoma cells requires calcium and calmodulin. Mol Pharmacol 38:7–13
6. Furchgott RF (1984) Role of endothelium in the responses of vascular smooth muscle to drugs. Ann Rev Pharmacol Toxicol 24:175–197
7. Ganz P, Davies JA, Leopold MA, Gimbrone Jr., Alexander RW (1986) Short- and long-term interactions of endothelium and vascular smooth muscle in coculture: effects on cyclic GMP production. Proc Natl Acad Sci USA 83:3552–3556
8. Hawkins DJ, Meyrick BO, Murray JJ (1988) Activation of guanylate cyclase and inhibition of platelet aggregation by endothelium-derived relaxing factor released from cultured cells. Biochim Biophys Acta 969:289–296
9. Holzmann S (1982) Endothelium-induced relaxation by acetylcholine is associated with larger rises in cyclic GMP in coronary arterial strips. J Cycl Nucl Res 8:409–419
10. Ignarro LJ, Harbison RG, Wood KS, Kadowitz PJ (1986) Activation of purified guanylate cyclase by endothelium-derived relaxing factor from intrapulmonary artery and vein: stimulation by acetylcholine, bradykinin and arachidonic acid. J Pharmacol Exp Ther 237:893–900
11. Ignarro LJ, Buga GM, Wood KS, Burns RE, Chaudhuri G (1987) Endothelium-derived relaxing factor produced and released from artery and vein is nitric oxide. Proc Natl Acad Sci USA 84:9265–9269
12. Ishii K, Gorsky LD, Förstermann U, Murad F (1989) Endothelium-derived relaxing factor (EDRF): the endogenous activator of soluble guanylate cyclase in various types of cells. J Appl Cardiol 4:505–512
13. Ishii K, Chang B, Kerwin JF, Huang ZJ, Murad F (1990) N^{ω}-nitro-L-arginine: a potent inhibitor of EDRF-formation. Eur J Pharmacol 176:219–223
14. Katsuki S, Arnold W, Mittal CK, Murad F (1977) Stimulation of guanylate cyclase by sodium nitroprusside, nitroglycerin and nitric oxide in various tissue preparations and comparison to the effects of sodium azide and hydroxylamine. J Cycl Nucl Res 3:23–35
15. Leitman DC, Murad F (1986) Comparison of binding and cyclic GMP accumulation by atrial natriuretic peptides in endothelial cells. Biochem Biophys Acta 885:74–79
16. Leitman DC, Agnost VL, Tuan JJ, Andressen JW, Murad F (1987) Atrial natriuretic factor and sodium nitroprusside increase cyclic GMP in cultured rat lung fibroblasts by activating different forms of guanylate cyclase. Biochem J 244:69–74
17. Lugnier C, Schoeffter P, Lebec A, Strouthou E, Stoclet JC (1989) Selective inhibition of cyclic nucleotide phosphodiesterase of human and rat aorta. Biochem Pharmacol 35:725–734

18. Martin W, White DG, Henderson AH (1988) Endothelium-derived relaxing factor and atriopeptin II elevate cyclic GMP levels in pig aortic endothelial cells. Br J Pharmacol 93:229–239
19. Mittal CK (1985) Atriopeptin II and nitrovasodilator-mediated shifts in guanosine 3′,5′-cyclic monophosphate in rat thoracic aorta: evidence for involvement of distinct guanylate cyclase pools. Eur J Pharmacol 115:127–128
20. Mülsch A, Böhme E, Busse R (1987) Stimulation of soluble guanylate cyclase by endothelium-derived relaxing factor from cultured endothelial cells. Eur J Pharmacol 135:247–250
21. Murad F (1986) Cyclic guanosine monophosphate as a mediator of vasodilation. J Clin Invest 78:1–5
22. Palmer PMJ, Ferrige AG, Moncada S (1987) Release of nitric oxide accounts for the biological activity of endothelium-derived relaxing factor. Nature 327:524–526
23. Peach MJ, Singer HA, Loeb AL (1985) Mechanisms of endothelium-dependent vascular smooth muscle relaxation. Biochem Pharmacol 34:1867–1874
24. Rapoport RM, Murad F (1983) Agonist-induced endothelium-dependent relaxation in rat thoracic aorta may be mediated through cGMP. Circ Res 52:352–357
25. Schmidt K, Mayer B, Kukovetz WR (1989) Effect of calcium on endothelium-derived relaxing factor formation and cGMP levels in endothelial cells. Eur J Pharmacol 179:157–166
26. Souness JE, Brazdil R, Diocee BK, Jordan R (1989) Role of selective cyclic GMP phosphodiesterase inhibition in the myorelaxant actions of M&B 22.948, MY-5445, vinpocetine and 1-methyl-3-isobutyl-8-(methylamino)-xanthine. Br J Pharmacol 98:725–734
27. Waldman SA, Rapoport RM, Murad F (1984) Atrial natriuretic factor selectively activates particulate guanylate cyclase and elevates cyclic GMP in rat tissues. J Biol Chem 259: 14332–14334

Author's address:

Dr. Ulrich Förstermann
Department 47 S, Building AP 9A
Abbott Laboratories
Abbott Park, Illinois 60064, USA

Molecular mechanisms of nitrovasodilator bioactivation

E. Noack [1] and M. Feelisch [2]

[1] Institute of Pharmacology, Heinrich-Heine-University, Düsseldorf, FRG;
[2] Department of Pharmacology, Schwarz Pharma AG, Monheim, FRG

Summary: All nitrovasodilators act intracellularly by a common molecular mechanism. This is characterized by the release of nitric oxide (NO). They are, thus, prodrugs or carriers of the active principle NO, responsible for endothelial controlled vasodilation. The rate of NO-formation strongly correlates with the activation of the soluble guanylate cyclase in vitro, resulting in a stimulation of cGMP synthesis. Nitrovasodilators thus are therapeutic substitutes for endogenous EDRF/NO. The pathways of bioactivation, nevertheless, differ substantially, depending on the individual chemistry of the nitrovasodilator. Besides NO, numerous other reaction products such as nitrite and nitrate anions are formed. The guanylate cyclase is only activated if NO is liberated. In the case of organic nitrates such as GTN, NO is only formed if certain thiol compounds are present as an essential cofactor. The rate of NO-formation correlates with the number of nitrate ester groups and proceeds with a simultaneous nitrite formation (with a ratio of 1 : 14 in the presence of cysteine). Nitrosamines such as molsidomine do not need thiol compounds for bioactivation. They directly liberate NO from the ring-open A-forms. This process basically depends on the presence of oxygen as electron acceptor from the sydnonimine molecule. Therefore, besides NO also superoxide radicals are formed, which may react with the generated NO under formation of nitrate ions. Organic nitrites (such as amyl nitrite) require the preceding interaction with a mercapto group to form a S-nitrosothiol intermediate, from which finally NO radicals are liberated. Nitrosothiols (like S-nitroso-acetyl-penicillamine) and sodium nitroprusside spontaneously release NO. The molecules themselves do not possess a direct enzyme activating potency. In the presence of thiol compounds organic nitrites (e.g., amyl nitrite) and nitrosothiols may act as intermediary products of NO generation.

Key words: Nitrovasodilators; organic nitrates; bioactivation mechanisms; nitric oxide (NO)

Introduction

Organic nitrovasodilators are widely and successfully used for the treatment of coronary heart disease and other related diseases. Chemically, they represent a very heterogeneous group of substances which, nevertheless, all seem to exert their pharmacodynamic action by an identical final step of bioactivation, i.e., the release of nitric oxide (NO).

NO was recently found to be the active principle of the endothelium-derived relaxing factor (EDRF), being synthesized and released from vascular endothelium in order to modulate vascular tone. Therefore, the therapeutical application of organic nitrovasodilators such as nitroglycerin, which are prodrugs of NO, has turned out to be very successful in the treatment of coronary heart disease in the past decades and, according to much of the information gained in recent years about the molecular mechanisms of bioactivation, has proved to be a very reasonable and pathophysiological oriented therapeutical concept, because it mimics the physiological role of nitric oxide/EDRF at the arterial site, and even more at the venous vessel site.

On a molecular basis NO-producing nitrovasodilators differ extensively in respect to their vasodilatory potency. This is due to the fact that penetration into the smooth muscle cell directly depends on the lipophilicity of these drugs (19), and that NO-generation following bioconversion is strongly determined by their chemical structure. The question arises whether the bioactivation pathways that finally all lead to the intracellular formation of NO and the consecutive stimulation of the target enzyme, the soluble guanylate cyclase, are always identical, and if not, whether the obtained differences may offer an explanation for the clinical observation of nitrate tolerance, which is characteristic for the classical organic nitrates on the one hand, and partly or completely missing for nitroprusside, amyl nitrite, or SIN-1 (the main metabolite of the prodrug molsidomine) on the other.

Methods

We adapted an analytical method, which is principally based on experiments of Doyle and Hoekstra (5), and which was later introduced by Haussmann and Werringloer (12), to applications in biological systems. It allows the continuous and quantitative estimation of small amounts of NO. Thus, we were able to directly measure the rate of NO liberation from a series of nitrovasodilators in vitro, and to compare it with its biological activity by using a soluble guanylate cyclase preparation from rat liver as a suitable bioassay (22). This method uses the spectral shift that is produced at 401 nm by the oxidation of oxyhemoglobin to methemoglobin at pH 7.70, taking 411 nm as an isobestic point (8). It allows the continuous measurement of NO-formation in the presence of definite concentrations of nitrovasodilators. After a short equilibration phase of some minutes the rate of methemoglobin formation and thus of NO production is constant for some time and may easily be estimated from the slope of the extinction curve.

In addition, we continuously measured the formation of other nitrogen containing reaction products such as nitrite and nitrate anions or nitrosothiols using HPLC techniques (10).

Results and discussion

Bioconversion of organic nitrates

In the following the metabolic fate of some representative nitrovasodilator species, summarized in Table 1, will be described. The results were obtained in vitro, but may be, nevertheless, also representative under in vivo conditions. If we first look at the therapeutically most often used organic nitrates, such as nitroglycerin (GTN), we may discriminate two different bioactivation pathways, one enzymatic, the other a non-enzymatic one, leading to the formation of NO as depicted in Table 2.

Table 1. Synopsis of various nitrovasodilator drugs and compounds.

Organic nitrates (GTN, ISDN,etc.)
Organic nitrites (Isopentylnitrite, etc.)
Sydnonimines nitroprusside
Furoxanes (CAS-824, etc.)
S-Nitrosothiols

Table 2. Possible pathways for NO-liberation from organic nitrates (nitroglycerin, ISDN, etc.) in vivo

1) Enzymatic denitration by cytosolic GSH-S-transferase, producing mainly inorganic nitrite;
2) Enzymatic reduction to thionitrite esters, which form NO via nitrosothiol-intermediates;
3) Nonenzymatic formation of NO in the presence of cysteine, especially favored in the presence of higher tissue concentrations.

Both, the enzymatic and the non-enzymatic pathways may be competing with each other in vivo. Numerous early studies (4, 17) already confirmed that organic nitrates are metabolized to some extent by a GSH-dependent enzyme system which, therefore, was named nitrate ester reductase or glutathione polyolnitrate oxidoreductase. It catalyzes the degradation of organic nitrates to inorganic nitrite, requiring the oxidation of two moles of GSH for the liberation of one mole nitrite. It was only about 15 years ago that it became obvious that nitrate ester reductase is one of the various activities possessed by the multifunctional enzyme system, the glutathione-S-transferases (EC 2.5.1.18) which are present at high concentrations in the cytosol (28). In contrast, little is known at the moment about the precise significance of other enzymatic degradation pathways like the reductive denitration by NADPH in the presence of cytochrome P-450 (27) or by the NADPH-dependent microsomal monooxygenase system at low substrate concentrations (30).

Non-enzymatic degradation of organic nitrates in vitro

In our in vitro experiments, we observed that organic nitrates, especially in the presence of higher concentrations, are rapidly non-enzymatically degradated if certain SH-containing compounds such as cysteine or N-acetyl-cysteine are present. Typical reaction products are NO, nitrite, and nitrate, from which only NO is bioactive. Figure 1 shows a typical experiment, in which the rate of NO-liberation from nitroglycerin (GTN) was continuously recorded and quantified in the presence and absence of cysteine.

The rate of NO liberation is directly dependent on the drug concentration used (Fig. 2), so that NO liberation from different organic nitrates may be compared at a definite drug concentration.

The NO generation increases with the number of nitrate ester substitutes (24–26) in the molecular, GTN being more active than ISDN, and ISDN being more potent than isosorbide-5-mononitrate. This difference in biological activity can easily be demonstrated at the isolated guanylate cyclase as well (Fig. 3).

We performed comparable experiments with all available nitrate esters and observed a very close correlation between the rate of NO liberation from these compounds on the one hand, and the concentration for half-maximal activation of the guanylate cyclase on the other (8), as shown in Fig. 4.

If conditions are chosen with drug concentrations that produce a just half-maximal activation of the guanylate cyclase, the rate of NO-liberation was observed to be constant (Fig. 4).

This strongly indicates that NO is the essential product of the bioactivation mechanism, which ultimately promotes the pharmacological action of organic nitrates. Nevertheless, besides NO, also nitrite anions are generated in a constant ratio. Therefore, it may be assumed that during degradation a common intermediate compound is

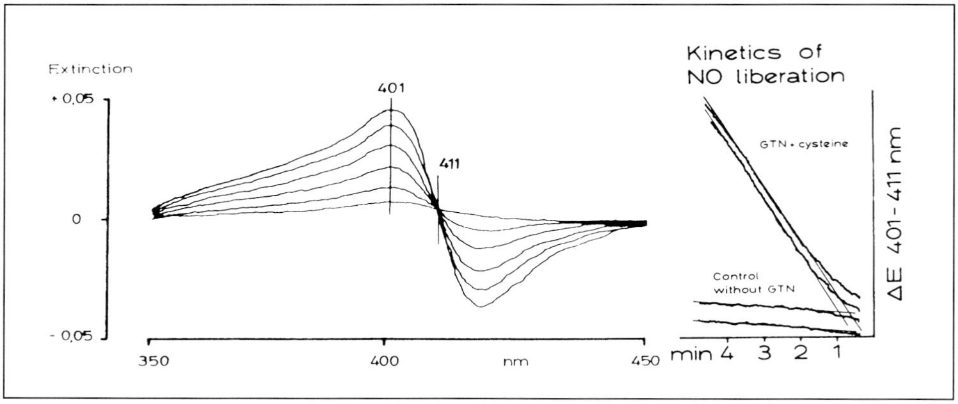

Fig. 1. Spectral shift of the extinction curve at 402 nm in the presence of rising concentrations of NO and methemoglobin, respectively (left). Kinetics of NO generation from GTN in the first 4 min of incubation (right). Control in the presence of cysteine only

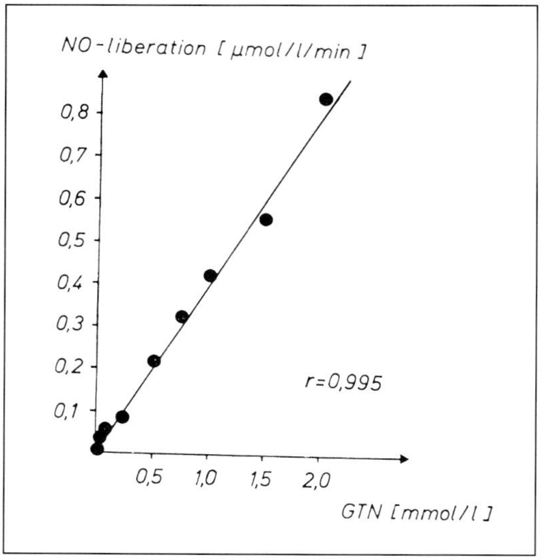

Fig. 2. Correlation between thiol-induced (5 mM L-cysteine) NO generation and the concentration of GTN in the incubation medium. 2.5 μM oxyhemoglobin; 37° C, pH 7.70; mean values ± SEM, n=3–5 [according to (8)]

transiently formed, from which NO, as well as nitrite anions originate. This is the reason that in the past nitrite anions have erroneously been taken for essential intermediates of nitrate bioactivation and were believed to be a prerequisite for the pharmacological response (14). We assume that a reductive denitration of organic nitrates may take place by a nucleophilic attack of thiolate anions on the nitrogen atom of the nitric acid esters. These thiolate anions originate from the tissue sulphydryl-containing compounds such as cysteine if the pH-value of the medium is near or above the pKs-value of the thiols.

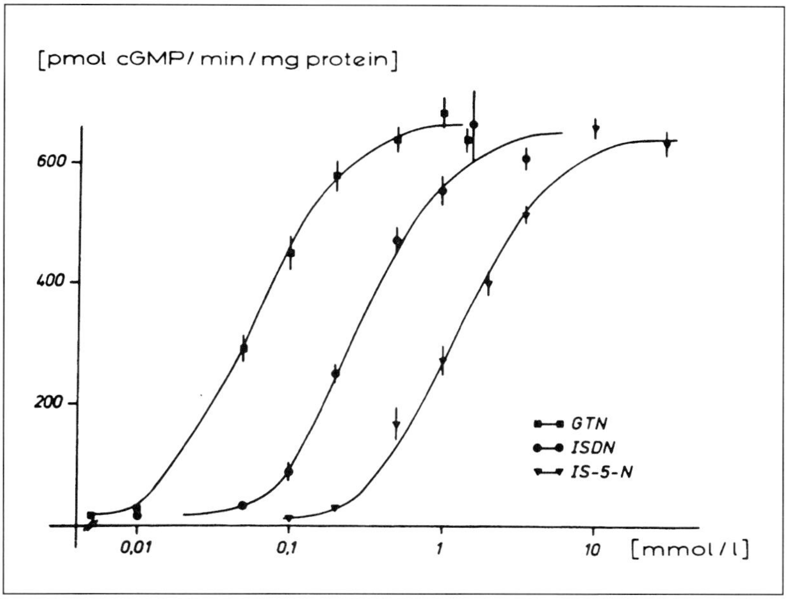

Fig. 3. Activation of isolated soluble guanylate cyclase by rising concentrations of three organic nitrates (GTN, ISDN, IS-5-N)

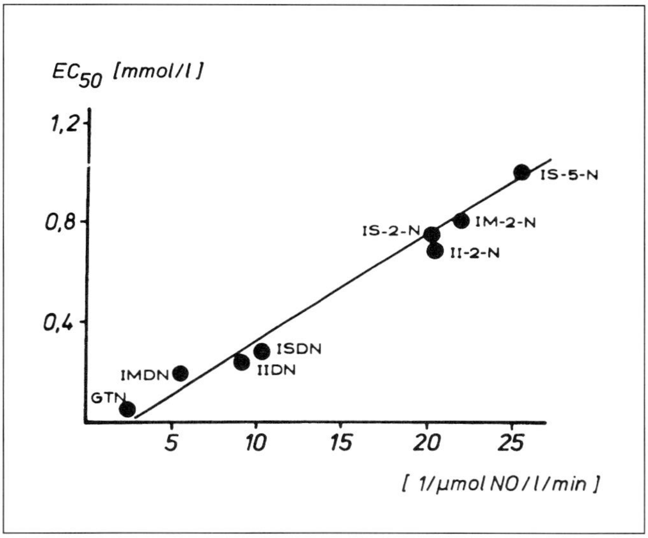

Fig. 4. Inverse correlation between half-maximal activation of guanylate cyclase activity (EC_{50}) and velocity of NO generation in vitro under identical experimental conditions.

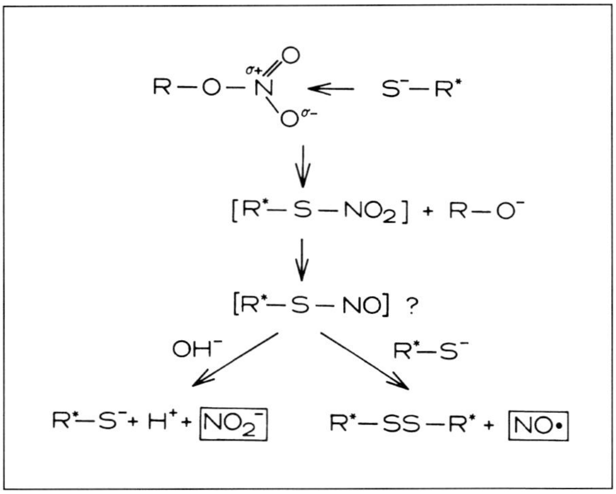

Fig. 5. Hypothetical bioactivation pathway of organic nitrates, involving the interaction of special sulfhydryl containing compounds, e.g., cysteine, and leading to the generation of NO

These may thus have a co-catalytic function, probably as a consequence of the thiolate ions reacting with an electrophilic nitrogen to produce the unstable intermediate compounds. The intermediate product which results from this transesterification reaction and which is highly unstable in aqueous solution is supposed to be a thiolate ester or sulphenyl nitrate ($RS{-}NO_2$), which then after reduction will rapidly degradate to NO and nitrite, as shown in Fig. 5, by a non-enzymatic attack of a second molecule of R*-SH to release inorganic nitrite, NO, and thiol disulphide.

There is a great deal of experimental evidence that there are several cysteine molecules in the close environment of the active center of the soluble guanylate cyclase itself, which might be at least partly essential for enzyme activation. They could play a similar role in the bioactivation pathway in vivo, as we demonstrated for in vitro conditions. Thus, the non-enzymatic bioactivation pattern demonstrated may reflect one biochemical reaction pathway which could take place at the active enzyme site in vivo.

For a series of SH-containing compounds tested in our laboratory there was a clear correlation between the pKs-values of the thiol compound and the formation rate of nitrite or NO formation from organic nitrates in vitro (6).

In summary, we believe that this non-enzymatic pathway of organic nitrate bioactivation plays an important if not the dominant role in vivo. The significance of the non-enzymatic or enzymatic pathway will certainly depend on the local enzymatic outfit, the intracellular concentrations, and availability of thiol compounds, and thus, also, on the type of vascular tissue.

Bioactivation pathway of isopentyl nitrite

In contrast, those nitrovasodilators which are chemically different from the organic nitrates do not need special thiol-containing compounds in order to generate NO for guanylate cyclase activation. This holds true for isopentyl nitrite (amyl nitrite), nitroprusside, and also SIN-1.

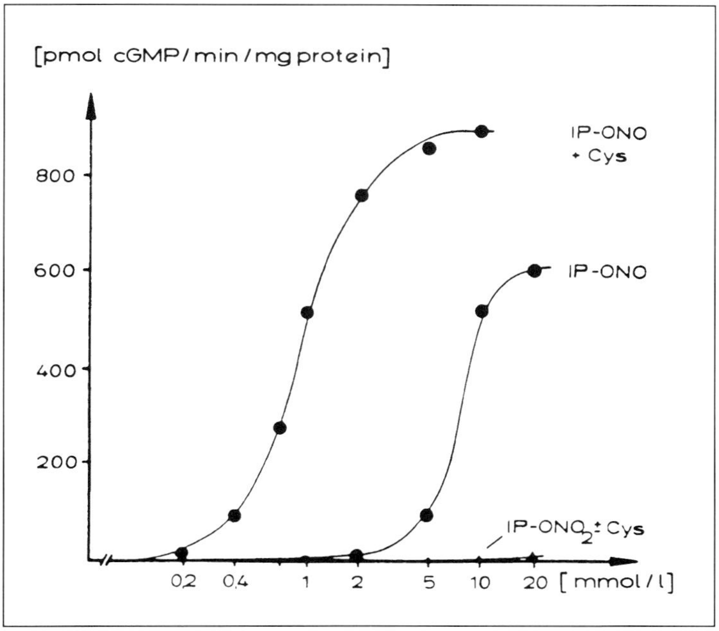

Fig. 6. Isolated soluble guanylate cyclase: concentration-response-curve for isopentyl-nitrite and -nitrate in the presence and absence of 5 mM L-cysteine

We found that isopentyl nitrite spontaneously releases NO in aqueous solution and activates the guanylate cyclase in contrast to the corresponding nitric acid ester isopentyl nitrate (Fig. 6).

Nevertheless, if cysteine is present, it further extensively destabilizes isopentyl nitrite (according to our HPLC results) by formation of cysteine-S-nitrosothiol, from which NO is generated, resulting in a leftward shift of the concentration-response curve (EC_{50}-values: 7.8 mM and 0.96 mM, respectively).

Sydnonimines degrade in the absence of thiol compounds

Another therapeutically important family of nitrovasodilators concerns the sydnonimines such as molsidomine. By including compounds with quite different structures, we recently were able to clarify the molecular processes of bioactivation (10, 21). Figure 7 shows a series of representative compounds that we tested.

It had been postulated that in the case of the sydnonimines hyponitrous acid, NOH, acts as an essential intermediate of bioactivation. This is contradicted by the results of Bohn and Schönafinger (2), who were not able to detect any NOH formation by chemical methods, and by our finding that the SIN-1A derivative C78-0652 also activates guanylate cyclase, although it is unable to undergo β-elimination of nitrous acid (see Fig. 7 for chemical structure) due to the fact that no hydrogen atom is left at the carbon atom in α-position because it is permethylated. After the release of NO, 4-amino-3-

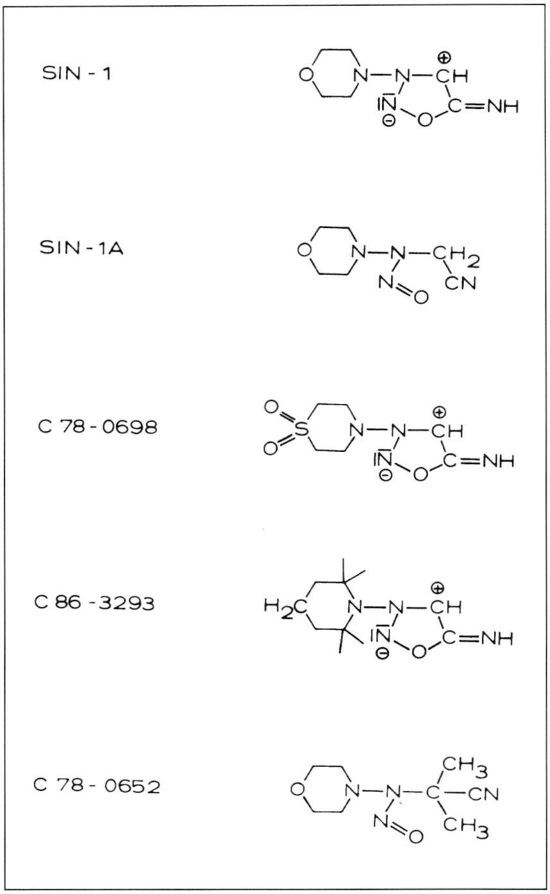

Fig. 7. Chemical structures of various sydnonimine derivatives

cyano-morpholine is left as a biological inactive reaction product of the bioactivation cascade.

The activation of the enzyme, however, is directly dependent on the rate of NO liberation. Table 3 shows the quite different NO liberation rates of these compounds.

They correlate very well with the extent of enzyme activation, as presented by the EC_{50} values obtained at the isolated guanylate cyclase. On a molecular basis the sydnonimine derivatives and especially SIN-1 proved to be substantially more active than the organic nitrates such as GTN or ISDN (see Table 3). In contrast to the latter, guanylate cyclase activation was independent from the presence of special thiol-containing compounds such as cysteine (9). The addition of 5 mM L-cysteine even slightly shifted the dose-reponse curve of SIN-1 to the right, as shown in Fig. 8.

Measuring the initial rate of NO formation, we also observed that the stimulatory potency of the sydnonimines at the guanylate cyclase is very well correlated with the kinetics of NO generation, but not with the formation of the ring-open A-forms, which

Table 3. Comparison between velocity of NO-liberation and activation of isolated soluble guanylate cyclase by various sydnonimines and organic nitrates

Compound	NO-liberation (µmol/l/min)	EC_{50} (µmol/l)
SIN-1	2.30	1.23
SIN-1A	9.69	0.36
C 86-3293	0.13	460.00
C 78-0698	3.81	0.62
GTN	0.42	79.00
ISDN	0.10	290.00
IS-5-N	0.04	940.00

Sydnonimines (1 mM) were incubated in the presence of 50 mM phosphate buffer at 37° C. In the case of organic nitrates, (1 mM) 5 mM L-cysteine was additionally added. NO-liberation was estimated at pH 7.70, enzyme activation at pH 7.40.

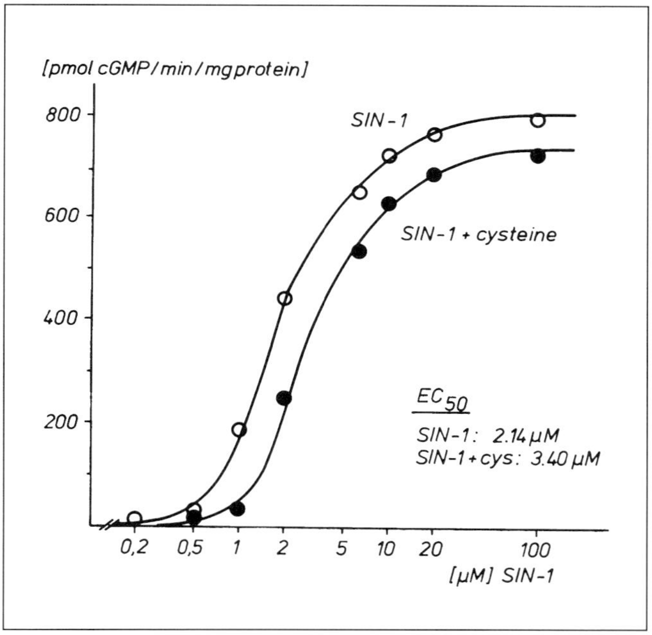

Fig. 8. Influence of cysteine (5 mM) on the activation pattern of SIN-1 on isolated soluble guanylate cyclase

are essential intermediates of the bioactivation process. This result, therefore, clearly contradicts the opinion that the ring-open structure itself is the activating principle at the enzyme site. Against this hypothesis are also our findings, depicted in Fig. 9, that small amounts of oxy-hemoglobin (10 µM), but not of met-hemoglobin, shift the dose-response-curve of SIN-1 at the isolated guanylate cyclase to the right.

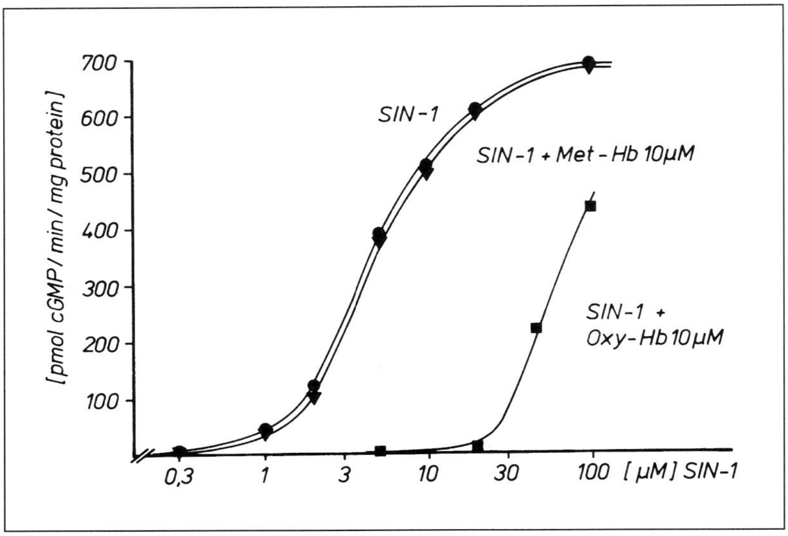

Fig. 9. Isolated guanylate cyclase: activation by SIN-1 in the absence and presence of oxy- and methemoglobin

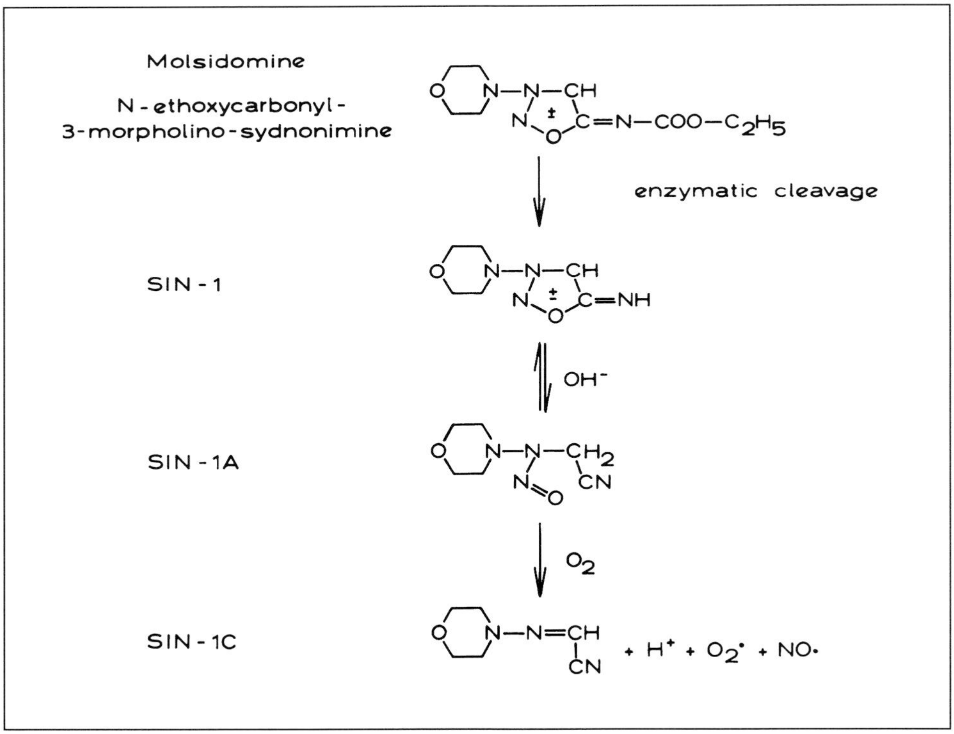

Fig. 10. Metabolic bioactivation pathway of molsidomine and related sydnonimines

This is due to the fact that oxyhemoglobin exerts a strong scavenger function for NO. The bioactivation pathway of molsidomine thus comprises the following steps (Fig. 10).

It is interesting to note that the liberation of NO from the ring-open structure SIN-1A only takes place in the presence of oxygen (2). Obviously, already minute amounts of oxygen molecules in the incubation medium are sufficient to start the reaction sequence of bioactivation, in which an electron is transferred from the nitrogen atom of the sydnonimine to molecular oxygen. It is assumed that an oxidative activation of the morpholino nitrogen of SIN-1A results in the formation of a cation radical, which then facilitates the release of NO.

S-nitrosothiols are not direct activators of guanylate cyclase

Finally, we have studied whether S-nitrosothiols are direct activators of the guanylate cyclase, or whether they activate the target enzyme indirectly by the release of NO, as all other known nitrovasodilators do. Especially from the work of Ignarro's group (14) it became obvious that nitrosothiols may be active themselves. We synthesized a series of nitrosothiols which, in general, are difficult to handle due to chemical instability. We measured the individual NO liberation rates and found a strong inverse correlation between the rate of NO liberation and the chemical stability of the compounds. Since the least stable compound showed the highest activity, NO and not the nitrosothiol should be the ultimate activator at the enzyme site.

In the presence of thiolate anions S-nitrosothiol compounds like S-nitroso-N-acetylpenicillamine (SNAP) can be further destabilized, producing higher rates of NO. At a given pH of 7.70, equimolar concentrations of cysteamine yield higher concentrations of thiolate anions than cysteine. Therefore, cysteamine was also more active in producing nitric oxide from nitrosothiols. This was, for example, the case with SNAP, confirming our suggestion that thiolate anions may be active as nucleophilic agents in this kind of reaction (Table 4).

The following diagram (Fig. 11) summarizes the bioactivation pathways, leading to the formation of NO and guanylate cyclase activation.

From our results it is obvious that nitrovasodilators have very different pathways leading to the formation of the active principle NO. Only the bioactivation of such organic nitrates as nitroglycerin is basically dependent on the presence of highly specific thiols such as cysteine. In the presence of all other sulfhydryl-containing compounds organic nitrates are also more or less rapidly degraded, however, without the formation of any bioactive compound (7). In contrast, all other available nitrovasodilators react with any available thiol in order to liberate NO, or they also directly release NO in the absence of these cofactors for enzyme stimulation.

Table 4. Effect of different thiols on the rate of NO-release from S-nitroso-N-acetylpenicillamine (SNAP)

Compound	NO-formation rate (μmol/l/min)
SNAP	1.38
SNAP + cysteine	7.73
SNAP + cysteamine	11.28

0.1 mM SNAP, 5 mM thiols; pH 7.70 and 37° C; n = 2).

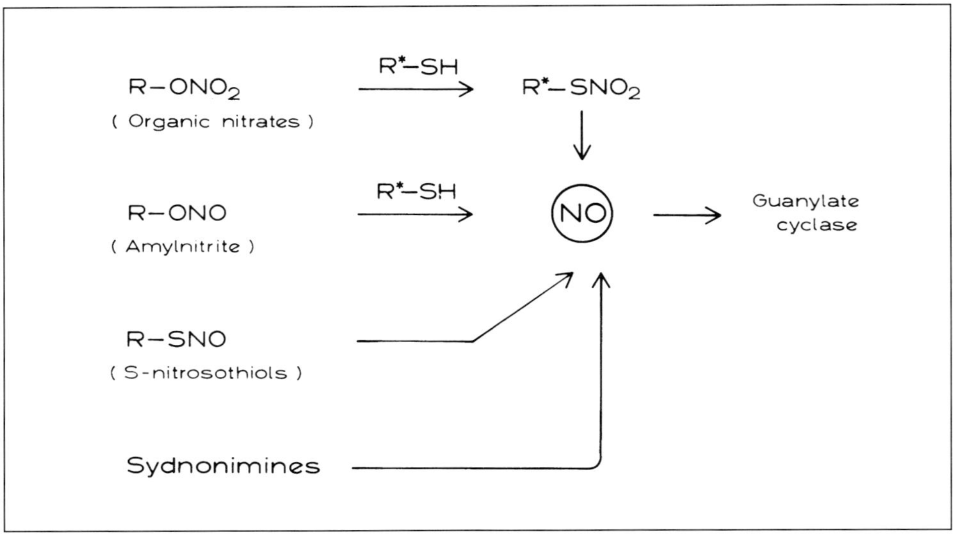

Fig. 11. Bioactivation pathways of different nitrovasodilators resulting in the generation of NO

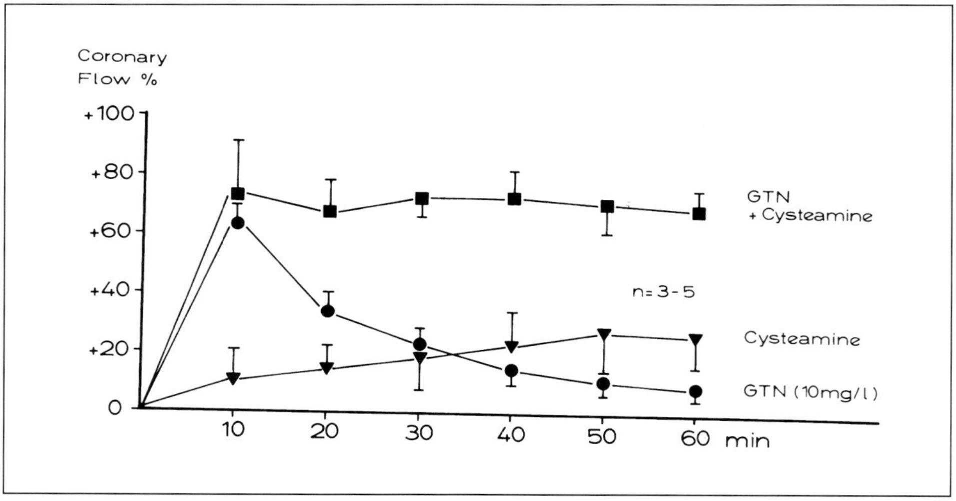

Fig. 12. Working heart model: increase of coronary flow by a rapidly tolerance-promoting GTN concentration (10 mg/l) in the presence and absence of cysteamine (50 μmol/l)

Differences of bioactivation may explain nitrate tolerance

These substantial differences of the bioactivation mechanisms may give an explanation for the finding that especially organic nitrates tend to develop nitrate tolerance at the vascular site in contrast to other vasodilators, although in all cases NO liberation represents the ultimate activation step for GC stimulation and cGMP formation (20).

There is much evidence that nitrate tolerance is favored by an intracellular depletion of sulphydryl-containing compounds. According to our experience the working heart model allows to study nitrate tolerance in an acute experiment. After adding 10 mg nitroglycerin per liter to the coronary perfusate, desensitization starts already after 10 min. With small concentrations of the thiol cysteamine, we prevented vascular tolerance, as shown in Fig. 12.

Nevertheless, the clinical situation may be different. This would explain why in the past interventions with thiols such as cysteine have lead to controversial results (1, 11, 15, 16, 23, 29). Interestingly, it was recently demonstrated that S-nitrosocaptopril, a novel vasodilator which carries its own SH-group in its molecule, is resistant to nitrate tolerance (3). In addition, it was shown in a new model of tolerance in the rat that there exists a stereospecificity concerning the effect of N-acetyl-cysteine for the prevention of nitrate tolerance (18). Most likely, nitroglycerin-induced tolerance affects multiple sites in the organic nitrate bioconversion cascade (13, 20), impairing their biotransformation, so that a desensitization of soluble guanylate cyclase or any inhibitory step distal to cGMP formation is unlikely to be involved in the mechanisms of nitrate tolerance development.

Acknowledgements. This work was supported in part by the Deutsche Forschungsgemeinschaft (SFB 242, Coronary Heart Disease, Teilprojekt C3 Noack, Düsseldorf, FRG)

References

1. Abdollah A, Moffat JA, Armstrong PW (1987) N-acetylcysteine does not modify nitroglycerin-induced tolerance in canine vascular rings. J Cardiovasc Pharmacol 9:445–450
2. Bohn H, Schönafinger K (1989) Oxygen and oxidation promote the release of nitric oxide from sydnonimines. J Cardiovasc Pharmacol 14 (Suppl 11):S6–S12
3. Cooke JP, Andon N, DelDuca D, Dzau V, Loscalzo J (1989) S-nitrosocaptopril: a novel vasodilator resistant to nitrate tolerance. Circulation 80 (Suppl) II–559
4. Crandall LA (1932) The fate of glyceryl trinitrate in the tolerant and non-tolerant animal. J Pharmacol Exptl Therapeut 48:127–140
5. Doyle MP, Hoekstra JW (1981) Oxidation of nitrogen oxides by bound dioxygen in hemoproteins. J Inorg Biochem 14:351–358
6. Feelisch M (1988) Experimentelle Untersuchungen zum intrazellulären Wirkungsmechanismus der Nitrovasodilatatoren und der endothelabhängigen Gefäßregulation. Beweis für die Bildung von Stickoxid (NO) als gemeinsamem, intermediärem Wirkungsvermittler. Thesis, Düsseldorf
7. Feelisch M, Noack (1987) Molecular prerequisites of thiol-containing compounds like cysteine for their stimulatory action on the degradation of organic nitrates and activation of soluble guanylate cyclase. N S Arch Pharmacol 335 Suppl:46
8. Feelisch M, Noack E (1987) Correlation between nitric oxide formation during degradation of organic nitrates and activation of guanylate cyclase. Eur J Pharmacol 139:19–30
9. Feelisch M, Noack E (1987) Nitric oxide (NO) formation from nitrovasodilators occurs independently of hemoglobin or non-heme iron. Eur J Pharmacol 142:465–469
10. Feelisch M, Ostrowski J, Noack E (1989) On the mechanism of NO release from sydnonimines. J Cardiovasc Pharmacol 14 (Suppl. 11):S13–S22
11. Gruetter CA, Lemke SM (1986) Effects of sulfhydryl reagents on nitroglycerin-induce relaxation of bovine coronary artery. Can J Physiol Pharmacol 64:1395–1401
12. Haussmann HJ, Werringloer J (1985) Nitric oxide and nitrite formation during the degradation of N-nitrosamines. Nauny-Schmiedeberg's Arch Pharmacol 329 (Suppl R21):84
13. Henry PJ, Horowitz JD, Louis WJ (1989) Nitroglycerin-induced tolerance affects multiple sites in the organic nitrate bioconversion cascade. J Pharmacol Exp Ther 248:762–768

14. Ignarro LJ, Kadowitz PJ, Baricos WH (1981) Evidence that regulation of hepatic guanylate cyclase activity involves interactions between catalytic site SH-groups and both substrate and activator. Arch Biochem Biophys 208:75–86
15. May DC, Popma JJ, Black WH, Schaefer S, Lee HR, Levine BD, Hillis LD (1987) In vivo induction and reversal of nitroglycerin tolerance in human coronary arteries. N Engl J Med 317:805–809
16. Moffat JA, Armstrong PW, Marks GS (1982) Investigations into the role of sulfhydryl groups in the mechanism of action of the nitrates. Can J Physiol Pharmacol 60:1261–1266
17. Needleman P, Krantz JC (1965) The biotransformation of nitroglycerin. Biochem Pharmacol 14:1225–1230
18. Newman CM, Warren JB, Taylor GW, Boobis AR, Davies DS (1990) Rapid tolerance to the hypotensive effects of glyceryl trinitrate in the rat: prevention by N-acetyl-L- but not N-acetyl-D-cysteine. Br J Pharmacol 99:825–829
19. Noack E (1984) Investigations on structure-activity relationship in organic nitrates. Meth and Find Exptl Clin Pharmacol 6:583–586
20. Noack E (1990) Mechanisms of nitrate tolerance – influence of the metabolic activation pathways. Z Kardiol 79:Suppl 2
21. Noack E, Feelisch M (1989) Molecular aspects underlying the vasodilator action of molsidomine. J Cardiovasc Pharmacol 14 (Suppl 11):S1–S5
22. Noack E, Schröder H, Feelisch M (1986) Continuous determination of nitric oxide formation during non-enzymatic degradation of organic nitrates and its correlation to guanylate cyclase activation. N S Arch Pharmacol 332 Suppl:125
23. Packer M, Lee WH, Kessler PD, Gottlieb SS, Medina N, Yushak M (1987) Prevention and reversal of nitrate tolerance in patients with congestive heart failure. N Engl J Med 317:799–804
24. Schröder H, Noack E (1986) Neue Ergebnisse zur thiolabhängigen Aktivierung der Guanylatcyklase durch organische Nitrate. Z Kardiol 75, Suppl 3:20–24
25. Schröder H, Noack E (1987) Structure-activity relationship of organic nitrates for activation of guanylate cyclase. Arch int pharmacodyn Ther 290:225–246
26. Schröder H, Noack E, Müller R (1985) Evidence for a correlation between nitric oxide formation by cleavage of organic nitrates and activation of guanylate cyclase. J Mol Cell Cardiol 17:931–934
27. Servent D, Delaforge M, Ducrocq C, Mansuy D, Lenfant M (1989) Nitric oxide formation during microsomal hepatic denitration of glyceryl trinitrate: involvement of cytochrome P-450. Biochem Biophys Res Commun 163:1210–1216
28. Taylor T, Taylor IW, Chasseaud LF, Bonn R (1987) Pharmacokinetics and metabolism of organic nitrate vasodilators. Progress in Drug metabolism 10:207–336
29. Torresi J, Horowitz JD, Dusting GJ (1985) Prevention and reversal of tolerance to nitroglycerine with N-acetylcysteine. J Cardiovasc Pharmacol 7:777–783
30. Wolf J, Werringloer J (1988) Metabolic degradation of glyceryl trinitrate. N S Arch Pharmacol 337 (Suppl):34

Author's address:

Prof. Dr. med. Eike Noack
Institute of Pharmacology
Heinrich-Heine-University
Moorenstr. 5; Geb. 22.21
D-4000 Düsseldorf 1, FRG

Angiogenesis in the adult heart

W. Schaper

Max-Planck-Institute, Department of Experimental Cardiology, Bad Nauheim, FRG

Summary: We have studied the development of the collateral circulation in the heart in response to gradual and progressive coronary artery occlusion. When the coronary stenosis becomes critical, tissue ischemia occurs, which we believe leads to the production (and probably to release from storage sites) of tissue hormones (mitogens) that lead to mitosis of endothelial and smooth muscle cells. We have identified from hearts several known mitogens (aFGF, bFGF), non-mitogenic angiogenic factors (TGF-β), a new anti-mitogen, and a new myocyte-derived growth factor (structures of the last two not yet elucidated). An important principle in the development of collaterals is the remodeling of pre-existing small vessels into the much larger vascular structure. To accomodate new cells old structures have to be removed by controlled proteolysis (tPA, uPA, elastase).

Key words: Collateral circulation; growth factors

Introduction

Angiogenesis is a term that was reserved for the ingrowth of capillaries into tissue during embryonic development. The organ to be invaded "induces" capillaries by secretion of growth factors (18). Tumor tissue is also capable of inducing capillaries to invade cancer tissue by ingrowth of endothelial cells from neighboring normal tissue (6).

Angiogenesis is also known to occur in the adult heart in response to coronary stenosis and occlusion, in fact, experimental studies in myocardial angiogenesis began earlier (31) than studies in experimental tumor angiogenesis (8). Since compensatory vascular growth in the heart consists mainly of enlargement of preexisting vascular structures by addition of new cells (endothelium, smooth muscle, and fibroblasts) rather than by sprouting of new capillaries, the term "non-sprouting angiogenesis" was adopted for the growth of collateral vessels in the heart (proposal made by Folkman at the Anaheim-conference of the AHA, 1987). The study of growth adaptation of the collateral circulation appears to be of value, because our knowledge of the developmental biology of the vascular supply of organs is still very rudimentary. Studies on vascular growth in the adult heart have also a direct clinical significance because it is imaginable that drug design in the future may concentrate on the angiogenic signal arising in transiently ischemic myocardium for the development of new medicines for the treatment of ischemic heart disease.

Ischemia is a potent mitogen

Experiments from our group in the late 1960s and early 1970s (27, 26, 29, 30) had already shown that progressive stenosis of a coronary artery in the canine heart and porcine heart leads to mitosis of endothelial and smooth muscle cells. Epicardial vessels in the canine heart increased from an initial diameter of 40 µm to a final (average) diameter of 800 µm. Mitoses could be observed with the light and electron microscopes, mainly in the canine model, somewhat less frequently in the porcine model. In the pig heart the entire vasculature of the region at risk of infarction participates with growth and enlargement, especially the capillaries (5, 9, 22, 28, 33). Only very few visible collateral connections exist close to the tip of the posterior papillary muscle (in the case of the right coronary artery that supplies part of the posterior papillary muscle (31).

Since cell division is always preceded by DNA-synthesis, the mitotic activity is more conveniently studied by incorporation of one of the four bases of DNA carrying a radioactive label (i.e., 3-H-thymidine). Quantitative labelling studies have shown that the growth response to progressive coronary occlusion (3 days from onset of stenosis to complete occlusion) started with a wave of endothelial mitosis, followed by smooth muscle mitosis (15). The labeling index of endothelium rose from immeasurably low (below 1 per 1000 cells) to 8 per 100, and the labeling index of smooth muscle cells rose from below 1 per 1000 to 2.4 per 100. In the porcine heart the situation was different in that we found measurable cell-labeling already in the normal heart (we always studied young land race pigs), but progressive stenosis drastically increased DNA-synthesis; labeling of interstitial fibroblasts increased by a factor of 11 times, capillary label increased by a factor of 3 times, label in small resistance vessels increased by a factor of 90 times control, and even ischemic cardiac myocytes incorporated thymidine (5). Smooth muscle growth is conspicuously sparse in the pig heart for reasons that are largely unknown. We speculate that, since all these vessels are endomurally located, the tangential wall tension is also borne by the cardiac myocytes that are in close proximity to the enlarged microvessels.

Labeling studies have also shown (27) that the time from onset of stimulation to completion of mitosis is about 22 h. This is relatively long (2) and explains why the growth of collaterals is not an effective response in acute and unannounced coronary occlusion: the tolerance of myocytes toward ischemia is counted in minutes (30–40) rather than hours. Our studies were the first to show a mitotic response of adult vascular cells in vivo and under clinically relevant conditions. Leading textbooks of that time, the 1960s, claimed that smooth muscle cells were terminally differentiated and incapable of division.

Physical vs chemical signals

It was not immediately clear to us that the existence of mitosis necessitated the presence of a peptide growth factor. Mechanical factors dominated the hypotheses explaining vascular growth, mainly in stenosed/occluded arteries in the limb circulation (34). The blood velocity or viscous drag (32) and tangential wall stress (25) seemed to be likely candidates to initiate mitosis. Two observations produced a wing away from mechanical factors and toward biochemical transmitters:

1) the finding that labelled vascular cells are also found (although at much lesser density) in veins (14, 15) accompanying densely labelled arteries in the canine model, and
2) the observation that monocytes invaded transforming arterioles and seemed to play an important part in the growth-remodeling of the enlarging artery (24).

The labeling of veins near growing arteries strongly suggests a biochemical transmitter: a tissue-source (ischemic myocardium?) produces a peptide growth factor which diffuses toward the nearest vessels and reaches both arteries and veins. However, not all labelled arteries are accompanied by labelled veins, and when they are, they are often not in the vicinity of ischemic cardiac myocytes. Another unexplained observation with regard to large epicardial collaterals is the fact that the part that enlarges by growth is situated on the border of two perfusion territories extending also into the normal region. It is difficult to see how biochemical transmitters originating from the ischemic myocardium will reach these vessels. Furthermore, it is unknown (and probably uncertain, even almost improbable) whether dog myocardium in the direct vicinity of growing epicardial collaterals will experience marked ischemia. A close spatial and temporal relationship between ischemia, transmitter production, and vascular growth exists only in the microvascular adaptation that occurs in the subendo- and midmyocardium in the porcine and human heart. It is conceivable that chronically increased flow in epicardial vessels leads to endothelial stimulation with production of a smooth muscle mitogen by endothelial cells.

Mitogenic peptides can also be carried into the regions of vascular growth. We have observed the adherence of monocytes and platelets onto growing epicardial collaterals (24), and invading monocytes are known to produce a host of growth factors (12) that may act as mitogens for endothelium and smooth muscle in addition to the mitogens that we believe are produced by ischemic cardiac myocytes and by endothelium itself. Activated monocytes produce interleukin I and 6, interferon alpha, tumor necrosis factor alpha (TNFa, a known angiogenesis factor), colony stimulating factor (CSF, G, M, GM), PDGF, FGF, TGF-β, and other non-peptide vasoactive factors. Platelets are the richest known sources for platelet-derived growth factor (PDGF) (10), transforming growth factor (TGF-β) (20), and platelet-derived endothelial growth factor (PDECGF) (39). These peptides are either potent mitogens (PDGF, PDECGF) or known angiogenic factors or both. Platelets adhere to defects in the endothelial cover of growing collaterals which occurs not infrequently and which is the basic observation for our injury-repair hypothesis that we formulated years ago (26). This hypothesis is still valid, but the processes involved are now called "remodeling". Meanwhile, mechanical forces have resumed a new role in (patho)physiological regulation: transmitters were identified for flow-dependent vasodilation, and stretch-reactive ion channels were identified. However, so far no mitogenic activity was reported from these systems.

We believe that biochemical *and* physical factors must act in concert to achieve the specialized structure (i.e., an artery); function will finally model structure.

Angiogenesis factors are present in myocardium

Recently, we isolated heparin-binding growth factors (mitogens) from normal, bovine and porcine hearts (16, 17). Amino-acid sequence analysis of these endothelial-cell mitogens showed a very high degree of sequence homology with two of the family of heparin-binding growth factors (HBGF), i.e., acidic and basic fibroblast growth factor[1] (aFGF and b-FGF), which had previously been isolated from bovine brain (35, 36) and kidney (19). The base sequence of the two FGF genes showed the absence of an important element necessary for a secreted hormone: a hydrophobic signal sequence of amino acids that enables the hormone to traverse the cell membrane (1). Although it remains principally unclear how such a hormone will reach a cell-membrane receptor, FGF was nevertheless detected in the *extra*cellular matrix (7). Storage in the matrix prevents the hormone from occupying a cell surface receptor, and it is hypothesized that proteolysis (i.e., by activated endothelial cells secreting plasminogen activator) must occur for hormone release.

---

[1] Fibroblast growth factor is a misnomer that originated from the test system first used (fibroblasts). FGF is a mitogen for almost all cell types that have maintained the ability to divide under culture conditions.

Another hypothesis assumes that the hormone-receptor interaction occurs intracellularly (21). Still another hypothesis speculated that death of a cell releases FGF, which then stimulates surviving neighbor cells (Schaper, unpublished).

We have shown that normal pig myocardium does not transcribe the aFGF gene, but progressive coronary stenosis and occlusion does (37). The transcript is found in growing collateral vessels (by in situ hybridization using a labeled FGF cRNA homologous to a sequence of 100 bases of the human gene).

This finding points to another interesting question: what stimulates the vascular cell to upregulate its gene expression to produce an autocrine mitogen?

It was clear to us for quite some time that a signal must arise from ischemic cardiac myocytes for the stimulation of vascular growth. Alternatively, a non-myocyte cell (but with a similar sensitivity for oxygen shortage), i.e., a nerve ending or a pericyte (4) can also be imagined to produce a primary transmitter. Activities in our lab to prove the existence of such a primary transmitter were successful, but the structure of this myocyte-derived growth factor is not yet known.

We have also provided evidence that TGF-β is present in the normal heart and in collateralized regions of the heart (Wünsch et al. 1990, submitted). Gene transcription for TGF-β was significantly increased in collateralized regions. Our data do not provide evidence for a role of basic FGF or TNFa in the process of collateralization, but we found the mRNA for vascular endothelial growth factor (VGEF) in a cDNA library of normal porcine heart (Sharma et al., unpublished).

Remodeling is as important as growth

The addition of new cells to an existing arterial structure does not necessarily lead to a larger vessel. On the contrary, subendothelial cell proliferation, a recognized condition for atherosclerosis, reduces the luminal cross-section. Remodeling – the controlled and graded destruction of the existing structure – makes vascular enlargement possible. First, the internal elastic lamina is cut (probably by leucocyte elastase), the matrix glue between smooth muscle cells is lysed, and even some smooth muscle cells undergo necrosis to make way for the new cells in a much larger artery. It is quite obvious that proteolytic enzymes like urokinase-type plasminogen-activator play an important role in remodeling (13). Since arterioles are often surrounded by cardiac myocytes, these have to be destroyed to accomodate the larger arterial structure; this proceeds by a perivascular inflammation (23).

Strategies for future research

The isolation of growth factor peptides that are present in tissue in only very small amounts requires too much biological material and is therefore impracticable in experimental situations where the yield of tissue-of-interest is small. Research related to the interplay of different growth factors in in-vivo models is difficult to envisage on the protein level, even when antibodies are available as research tools. The extreme dilution of the antigen may reduce the value of immunohistochemistry. A gene level approach is usually tried when a minimum of amino acid information is available. However, a gene-level approach without any previous information from the protein level was recently developed using substractive cloning (3, 11, 38). This approach is ideally suited for the collateralized heart where a transformed region exists that differs in only few mRNA species from a normal region of the same heart. By subtracting the reverse transcribed mRNA of the transformed region from the mRNA of the normal region, unhybridized single-stranded cDNA is further cloned. Since the difference between the two regions is only a few hundred clones, the direct sequencing of these clones is not a forbiddingly difficult task. We are presently working on this problem.

References

1. Abraham J, Mergia A, Whang J, Tumolo A, Friedman J, Hjerrild K, Gospodarowicz D, Fiddes J (1986) Nucleotide sequence of a bovine clone encoding the angiogenic protein, basic fibroblast growth factor. Science 233:545–548
2. Alberts B, Bray D, Lewis J, Raff M, Roberts K, Watson J (eds) Molecular Biology of the Cell: Differentiated Cells and the Maintenance of Tissues. Garland Publishing Inc., New York London 1989, pp 952–997
3. Belyavsky AV, Rajewsky TK (1989) PCR-based library construction: general cDNA libraries at the level of a few cells. Nucl Acids Res 21:2919–2932
4. Borgers M, Schaper J, Schaper W (1971) Adenosine producing sites in the mammalian heart – a cytochemical study. J Mol Cell Cardiol 3:287–296
5. DeBrabander M, Schaper W, Verheyen F (1973) Regenerative changes in the porcine heart after gradual and chronic coronary artery occlusion. Aschoffs Arch 149:170–185
6. Folkman J, Klagsbrun M (1987) Angiogenic factors. Science 235:442–447
7. Folkman J, Klagsbrun M (1987) A family of angiogenic peptides. Nature 329:671–672
8. Folkman J, Merler E, Abernathy C, Williams G (1971) Isolation of a tumor factor responsible for angiogenesis. J Exp Med 133:275
9. Görge G, Schmidt T, Ito B, Pantely G, Schaper W (1989) Microvascular and collateral adaptation in swine hearts following progressive coronary artery stenosis. Basic Res Cardiol 84: 524–535
10. Heldin C, Westermark B (1988) Platelet-derived growth factor and its relation to oncogenes. ISI Atlas of Science: Immunology 44–48
11. Hla T, Maciag T (1990) Isolation of immediate-early differentiation mRNAs by enzymatic amplification of substracted cDNA from human endothelial cells. Basic Res Cardiol 167: 637–643
12. Löms Z-H, HW (1989) The biology of the monocyte system. Eur J Cell Biol 49:1–12
13. Montesano RP, Möhle-Steinlein S, Risau U, Wagner W, Orci EL (1990) Increased proteolytic activity is responsible for the aberrant morphogenetic behavior of endothelial cells expressing the middle t-oncogene. Cell 62:435–445
14. Pasyk S, Flameng W, Wüsten B, Schaper W (1976) Influence of tachycardia on regional myocardial flow in chronic experimental coronary occlusion. Basic Res Cardiol 71:243–251
15. Pasyk S, Schaper W, Schaper J, Pasyk K, Miskiewicz G, Steinseifer B (1982) DNA synthesis in coronary collaterals after coronary artery occlusion in conscious dog. Am J Physiol 242: H1031–H1037
16. Quinkler W, Lüthe N, Maasberg M, Lottspeich F, Schaper W (1988) Acidic fibroblast growth factor (a-FGF) is present in bovine, canine, and porcine heart. Z Kardiol 77 (Suppl I):214 (abstr)
17. Quinkler W, Maasberg M, Bernotat-Danielowski S, Lüthe N, Sharma H, Schaper W (1989) Isolation of heparin binding growth factors from bovine, porcine, and canine hearts. Eur J Biochem 181:67–73
18. Risau W, Ekblom P (1986) Growth factors and the embryonic kidney. In: Serrero G (ed) Progress in clinical and biological research, hormonal control of embryonic and cellular differentiation. Liss, New York
19. Risau W, Ekblom P (1986) Production of heparin-binding angiogenesis factor by the embryonic kidney. J Cell Biol 103:1101–1107
20. Roberts A, Anzano M, Lam L, Smith J, Sporn M (1981) New class of transforming growth factors: potentiated by epidermal growth factor isolation from neoplastic tissues. Proc Natl Acad Sci USA 78:5339–5343

21. Rogelj S, Weinberg R, Fanning P, Klagsbrun M (1988) Basic fibroblast growth factor fused to a signal peptide transforms cells. Nature 331:173–175
22. Roth D, White F, Bloor C (1988) Altered minimal coronary resistance to antegrade reflow after chronic coronary artery occlusion in swine. Circ Res 63:330–339
23. Schaper J, Borgers M, Xhonneux R, Schaper W (1973) Cortisone influences developing collaterals, Part 1 (A morphologic study). Virchows Arch (Pathol Anat) 361:263–282
24. Schaper J, Koenig R, Franz D, Schaper W (1976) The endothelial surface of growing coronary collateral arteries. Intimal margination and diapedesis of monocytes A combined SEM and TEM study. Virchows Arch (Pathol Anat) 370:193–205
25. Schaper W (1967) Tangential wall stress as a molding force in the development of collateral vessels in the canine heart. Experientia (Basel) 23:595–598
26. Schaper W (1971) The Collateral Circulation of the Heart. 1971 North-Holland Publishing Company. Amsterdam
27. Schaper W, DeBrabander M, Lewi P (1971) DNA-synthesis and mitoses in coronary collateral vessels of the dog. Circ Res 28:671–679
28. Schaper W, Flameng W, Snoeckx L, Jageneau A (1971) Der Einfluß körperlichen Trainings auf den Kollateralkreislauf des Herzens. Verh Dt Ges Kreislaufforschg 37:112–121
29. Schaper W, Schaper J (1969) DNA-synthesis in developing coronary collateral vessels. Scientific Exhibit. Circulation 40:126 (abstract)
30. Schaper W, Schaper J, Xhonneux R et al. (1969) The morphology of intercoronary anastomoses in chronic coronary artery occlusion. Cardiovasc Res 3:315–323
31. Schaper W, Vandesteene R (1967) The rate of growth of interarterial anastomoses in chronic coronary artery occlusion. Life Sci 6:1673
32. Scheel K, Fitzgerald E, Martin R, Larsen R (1979) The possible role of mechanical stresses on coronary collateral development during gradual coronary occlusion – a simulation study. In: Schaper W (ed) The pathophysiology of myocardial perfusion. Elsevier/North-Holland Biomedical Press. Amsterdam, New York, Oxford 489–518
33. Schmidt T, Renczes R, Schaper J, Stämmler G, Möbs A, Schaper W (1988) Kollateralentwicklung im ischämischen Myokard des Schweines. Z Kardiol 77 (Suppl I):106 (abstr)
34. Schoop W, Jahn W (1961) Entwicklungsstadien arterieller Kollateralen und ihre begriffliche Definition. Z Kreislaufforsch 50:249
35. Schreiber, Kenney, Kowalski, Thomas, Gimenez-Gallego, Rios-Candelore, DiSalvo, Barritault, Courty, Courtois, Moenner, Loret, Burgess, Mehlmann, Friesel, Johnson, Maciag T (1985) A unique family of endothelial cell polypeptide mitogens: the antigenic and receptor cross-reactivity of bovine endothelial cell growth factor, brain-derived acidic fibroblast growth factor, and eye-derived growth factor-II. J Cell Biol 101:1623–1626
36. Schreiber A, Kenney J, Kowalski W, Friesel R, Mehlman T, Maciag T (1985) Interaction of endothelial cell growth factor with heparin: Characterization by receptor and antibody recognition. Proc Natl Acad Sci USA 82:6138–6142
37. Sharma H, Wünsch M, Kandolf R, Schaper W (1989) Angiogenesis by slow coronary artery occlusion in the pig heart: Expression of different growth factors mRNAs. J Mol Cell Cardiol 21 (Suppl III):24 (abstr)
38. Timblin CB, Kuehl JW (1990) Application for PCR technology to substractive cDNA cloning: identification of genes expressed specifically in murine plasmocytoma cells. Nucl Acids Res 31:1587–1593
39. Usuki K, Heldin N, Miyazono K, Ishikawa F, Takaku F, Westermark B, Heldin C (1989) Production of platelet-derived endothelial cell growth factor by normal and transformed human cells in culture. Proc Natl Acad Sci USA 86:7427–7431

Author's address:
Prof. Dr. W. Schaper
Max-Planck-Institute
Department of Experimental Cardiology
Benekestraße 2
W-6350 Bad Nauheim, FRG

The endothelium in control of blood flow in vivo

Endothelium and blood flow mediated vasomotion in the conscious dog

M. Bigaud and S. F. Vatner

Departments of Medicine, Harvard Medical School, Brigham & Women's Hospital, Boston, and the New England Regional Primate Research Center, Southborough, Massachusetts, USA

Summary: Numerous in vitro studies have demonstrated the important role of the vascular endothelium on the vasoactivity of vascular smooth muscle. Experimentation, particularly in conscious animals, is required to study the integrated role of endothelium in the regulation of vascular tone. This article reviews some of the evidence demonstrating endothelium mediated vasodilation and inhibition of vasoconstriction by the endothelium in the chronically instrumented conscious animal. Furthermore, a role for endothelial cells has been shown in the mechanism of blood flow-mediated vasodilation. Finally, the endothelium, through elaboration of constricting factors, e.g., endothelin, can also induce potent vasoconstriction. In the conscious animal endothelin elicits markedly differing degrees of vasoconstriction among the various regional vascular beds.

Key words: Endothelium; endothelium-derived-relaxing factor; endothelin

Introduction

It has been recognized for some time that vascular endothelial cells, which serve as an interface between the blood and vascular system, are not only a passive diffusion barrier, but also play a key role in the regulation of hemostasis and thrombosis, and exert active control over vascular tone (2, 8, 21, 27). Since the discovery of prostacyclin (PGI_2) (39), endothelium-derived relaxing factors (EDRF) (17, 40, 43), endothelium-derived contractile factors (EDCF) (10), and endothelin (EDT) (59), the most insight into mechanisms of endothelium-mediated vascular responses has been gained from in vitro experiments (16, 53). However, experiments have also been conducted in vivo to assess the importance of this endothelium-mediated regulation of vascular tone in the whole organism (28, 44, 60, 62). Such experimentation is especially important since vessels often do not respond in an identical manner when they are studied in vitro or in vivo (13, 61).

This article reviews several of the investigations that have examined endothelium-mediated vasoactivity in conscious dogs, in which vascular resistances and reflex control of the circulation have not been altered by the presence of general anesthetic and/or recent surgery (1, 55). Dogs were chronically instrumented with Doppler ultrasonic flow transducers for measurement of blood flow, miniature ultrasonic dimension transducers for measurement of external vascular diameter, and hydraulic occluders, localized distally to the site of diameter measurement (Fig. 1), for restriction or occlusion of blood flow in either the iliac (62) or coronary circulation (23). The main advantage of using the hindlimb vessels, compared to the coronary vessels, is the ability to control or restrict blood flow without severely affecting oxygen delivery to the regional skeletal muscles, and also the responsiveness of the large vessels in the hindlimb circulation are affected less by

Supported in part by US Public Health Service Grant HL 38070, HL 33107 and RR 00168

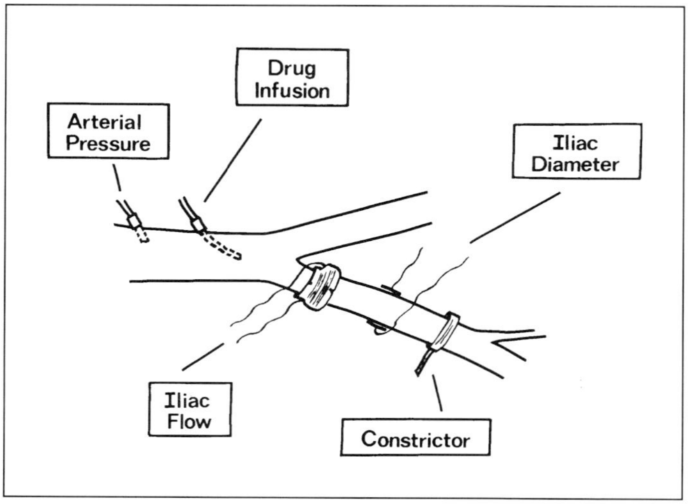

Fig. 1. Diagram of the method used to assess the responsiveness of the iliac artery. Dogs were studied in the conscious state after they fully recovered from the surgical intervention (2 weeks). Similar methods were used for the study of the responsiveness of coronary arteries [From (64), reprinted with permission.]

changes in metabolic requirements than in the coronary circulation (35). However, in either case, the changes in local flow reflect changes occurring at the level of the small resistance vessels, whereas changes in large vessel diameter are more representative of vascular wall reactivity at the site of the dimension transducers (56). Using these methods it is possible to study in vivo the influence of blood flow changes, and of endothelium, simultaneously on the reactivity of large and small vessels.

Results and discussion

Endothelium-mediated vasodilation

The historical paradox that existed between the results of in vitro and in vivo studies on the role of acetylcholine was due to the fact that the fragile monocellular layer of the endothelium was easily destroyed by the manipulation of the isolated vessel preparations. Furchgott and Zawadzki (1980) demonstrated that it was possible to keep the endothelium functional, and that a gentle rubbing of the lumen of the vessels was sufficient to destroy it (17). It was then possible to compare the effects of drugs on vascular tissues with and without endothelium in vitro, experiments which are more difficult to perform in vivo. In the intact animal, there is always the question of extent of denudation of endothelium and also of potential damage to the other vascular structures due to the process of endothelial denudation. A commonly employed technique, using the inflation of a balloon positioned within the vessel (62), enables successful denudation of the vessel from its endothelium. Using these techniques, it was possible to demonstrate, in vivo, the mediation of cholinergic vasodilation by the endothelium (63), and to study the influence of the endothelium on the vasoactivity of agents that induce dilation or constriction of

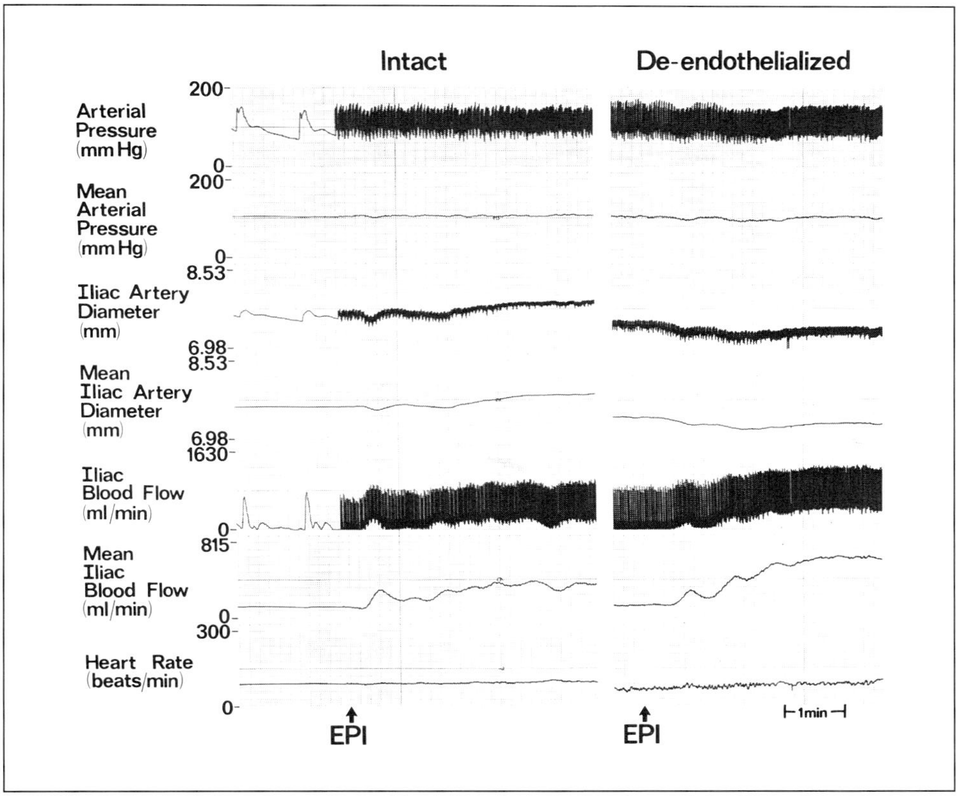

Fig. 2. Representative example of the hemodynamic and vascular responses provoked by the infusion of epinephrine (EPI) in a conscious dog with intact iliac arteries (intact), and in the same dog after removal of endothelium (de-endothelialized). Clearly, removal of the endothelium unmasked the vasoconstrictor effect of EPI [From (60), reprinted with permission.]

large arteries (Fig. 3). For example, the direct endothelium-independent nature of the vasodilation induced by nitroglycerin, well demonstrated in vitro (20), was confirmed in vivo (62) (Fig. 3). Since the effect of nitroglycerin was unaltered by the destruction of the endothelium, this demonstrates that the vascular smooth muscle is not affected adversely by the mechanical abrasion, which resulted in endothelial removal.

Figures 2 and 3 demonstrate that the direct vasoconstrictor response induced by epinephrine is unmasked by destruction of the endothelium. These observations indicate that endothelium-mediated vasodilation competes actively with drug-induced vasoconstriction, a concept which is supported by the fact that the vasoconstrictor effects of norepinephrine and phenylephrine are markedly potentiated by destruction of the endothelium, both in vivo (60) and in vitro (18). Thus, in intact vessels release of EDRF in response to these vasoconstrictors attenuates the efficacy of the vasoconstriction. The most commonly advanced hypothesis to explain this phenomenon is a tonic or spontaneous release of EDRF opposing a non-specific dilator component to all vasoconstrictor stimuli (36). However, other factors may be involved in vivo, e.g., ab-

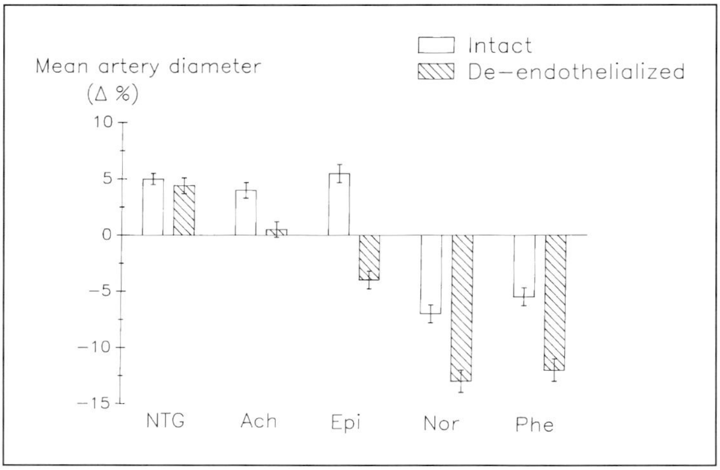

Fig. 3. The effects of nitroglycerin (NTG), acetylcholine (ACH), epinephrine (EPI), norepinephrine (NOR), and phenylephrine (PHE) are compared when the iliac artery was intact (open bars) and after removal of the endothelium (dashed bars). [Redrawn from data contained in (60).]

sence of natural diffusion barrier, absence of local PGI_2 release, and/or accumulation of mediators released by stimulated platelets. The recent identification of an EDRF compound (40, 43), and the synthesis of specific inhibitors of its biosynthesis pathway (42, 45), will enable further elucidation of these potential mechanisms.

Blood-flow-mediated vasodilation

The phenomenon of flow-induced caliber was described in 1933 (49), and now it is well recognized that changes in blood flow or shear stress can modify the diameter of large arteries (25, 31, 46). A clear example of this phenomenon has been demonstrated in the conscious dog, during the postischemic reactive hyperemia provoked by the release of a temporary coronary occlusion (Fig. 4a) (23). Typically following the release of a brief period of coronary artery occlusion there is an immediate increase in coronary blood flow above control levels (reactive hyperemia). We observed that the reactive hyperemia is followed by an increase in diameter of the large vessel, and was termed "reactive dilation" (23). The reactive dilation is completely abolished by restricting blood flow to control levels upon release of the occlusion (Fig. 4b), indicating that the mechanism involved increases in blood flow. This reactive dilation has also been shown to be mediated by the endothelium (44).

Using the same technique of restricting the blood flow with the use of an hydraulic occluder, it has been possible to demonstrate that this flow dependent vasodilation can explain the in vivo vasodilator effect of several agents (Fig. 5) (57, 62). For example, the dilation induced by isoproterenol, nitroglycerin and acetylcholine is only partially mediated by an increase in flow, whereas the vasodilation induced by epinephrine is primarily blood-flow mediated. Thus, blood-flow-dependent vasomotion is an endothelium-mediated process which requires the integrity of the vascular endothelium, with increasing evidence suggesting that EDRF is responsible for this phenomenon (24, 44, 48).

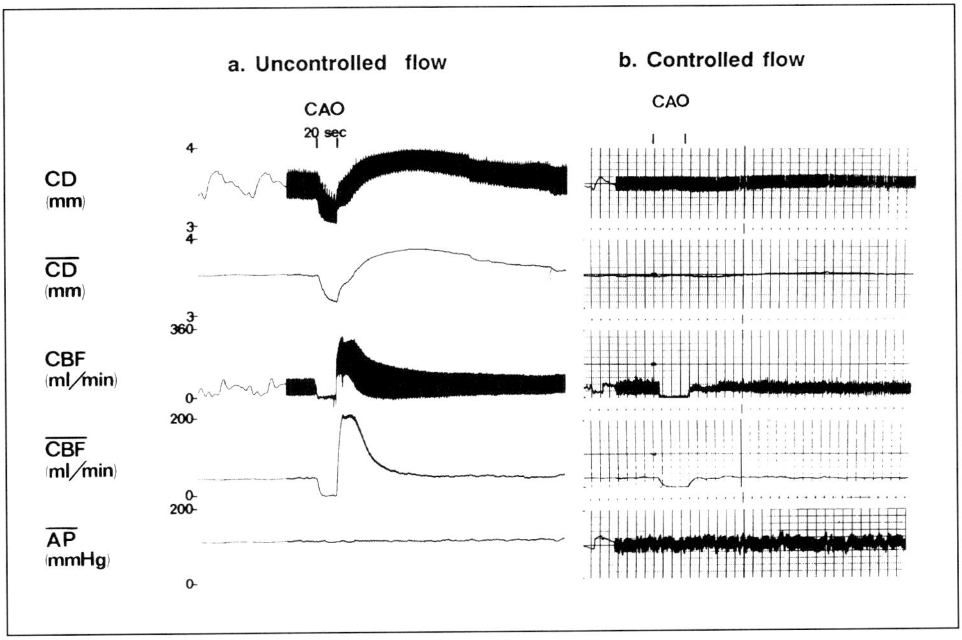

Fig. 4 a, b. A representative example of the effect of a brief (20 s) coronary occlusion (CAO) of the left circumflex coronary artery is shown in the first panel (**a**). The CAO was performed proximal to the measurement of phasic and mean coronary dimensions (CD) and blood flow (CBF). After release of CAO, CBF increased markedly (typical reactive hyperemia), whereas CD increased more slowly. CD reached a peak approximatively 60 s after reperfusion, at a time when coronary blood flow had already returned to control. Arterial pressure (AP) was not affected by the CAO and its release. The second panel (**b**) represents a similar experiment except that the coronary flow was held constant upon the release of the occlusion. In this condition, the blood flow-induced reactive coronary dilation was no longer observed. [From (23) reprinted with permission.]

Endothelium-mediated vasoconstriction

Endothelium-dependent vasoconstriction has been observed in response to various chemical and physical stimuli in in vitro preparations (54). Although the exact nature of all the mediators involved in this phenomenon is still unknown, several different factors have been detected thus far (33). One of these agents was recently identified and called endothelin (EDT) (59). EDT is a 21-amino acid vasoconstrictor peptide which was initially described as being released from cultured endothelial cells (37); it was then recently found to be secreted from in vitro vascular preparations (6), and is now considered to be a circulating agent. Increased plasma concentrations of endothelin are associated with pathological states such as essential hypertension (50), myocardial infarction (38), subarachnoid hemorrhage (30), acute renal failure (14, 50), and cardiogenic and endotoxin shock (9, 41). Three isoforms of EDT have even been found to coexist in human plasma (26). EDT-1 is the peptide originally isolated from porcine endothelial cells, and has been studied most intensively thus far.

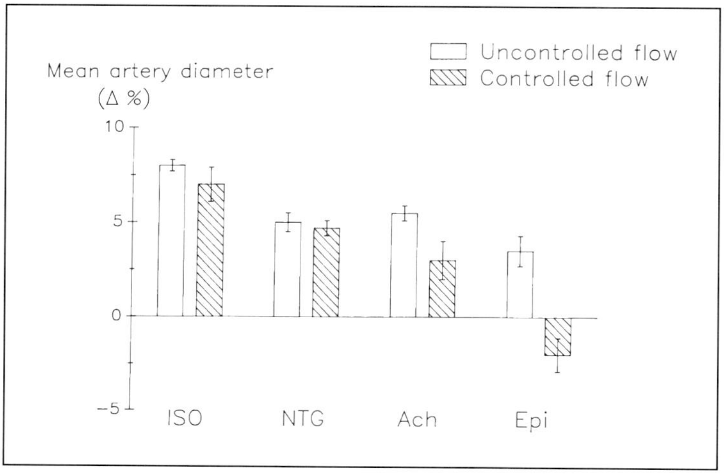

Fig. 5. The effects of isoproterenol (ISO), nitroglycerin (NTG), acetylcholine (ACH) and epinephrine (EPI) are compared when arterial blood flow was allowed to increase (open bars) and when it was held constant (dashed bars). The dilation with ACH was attenuated, and that with EPI was abolished, by holding blood flow constant. [Redrawn from data contained in (64).]

EDT-1 is an extremely potent vasoconstrictor in a variety of isolated vessel preparations from several species (7, 12, 59). However, its integrated cardiovascular effects appear complex since it has been shown in both anesthetized and conscious animals that intravenous bolus injections of EDT-1 induces a biphasic response characterized by an initial transient depressor phase followed by an intense and prolonged pressor phase (3, 4, 19, 47, 58). A representative example of the cardiovascular response elicited by the intravenous bolus injection of EDT-1 in a conscious dog is illustrated by Fig. 6. Typically, bolus i.v. injection of endothelin in an intact conscious animal induces an initial vasodilation, occurring during the first minute of the response, at a time when arterial pressure tends to decrease. The vasodilation is particularly marked and prolonged in the celiac bed, with less intense vasodilation in the coronary, renal, and mesenteric beds. A vasopressor phase occurs within the first 2 min of the response, and is characterized by persistent hypertension, accompanied by systemic vasoconstriction, particularly intense in the mesenteric and renal beds. One hour is usually required for all the hemodynamic parameters to return to control values.

The vasoconstrictor effect of EDT-1 has been studied extensively using in vitro preparations. EDT-1 induces contraction of vascular smooth muscle cells by binding to specific membrane receptors, stimulation of phosphatidylinositol turnover and activation of protein kinase C (29). From experiments in conscious dogs, it appears that the vasoconstrictor effect of EDT is characterized by significant regional differences, with the renal and mesenteric beds affected more than the coronary and celiac beds (Fig. 6). The reasons for this vascular selectivity are still unknown (differences in receptor density or sensitivity, local competing mechanisms), but this phenomenon suggests that some beds, particularly the coronary and cerebral beds, are in some way protected against the effects of EDT.

Less is known about EDT-1-induced vasodilation and, since no direct vasodilator effect of EDT has been observed in vitro, it is now believed that it could be the result of induction of an endogenous vasodilator. Atrial natriuretic peptides (ANP) (15, 51), PGI_2

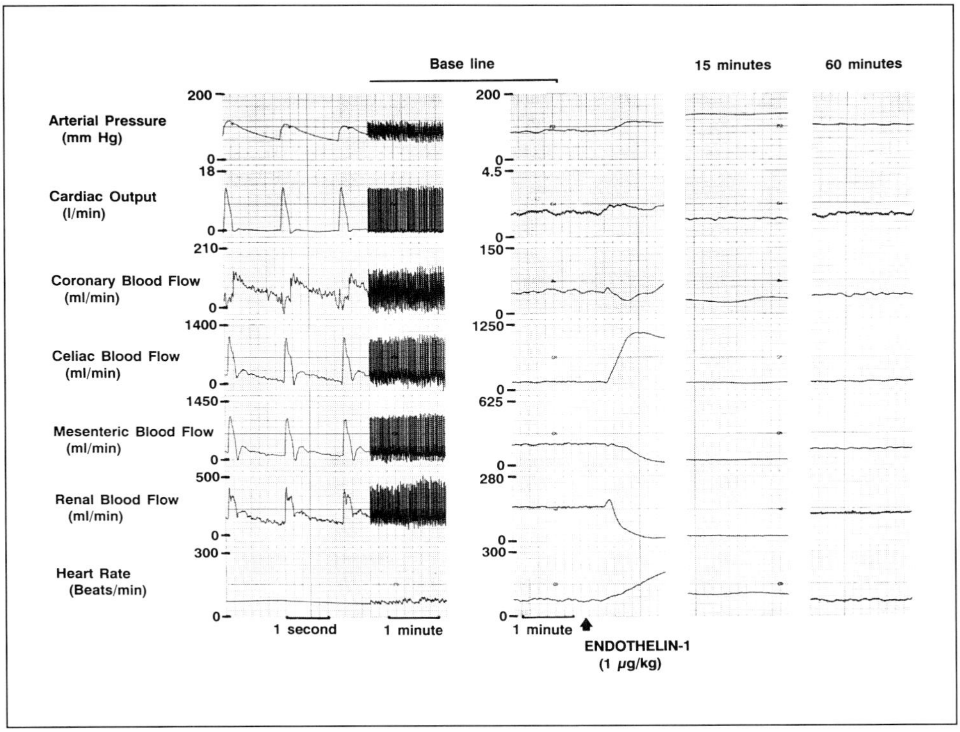

Fig. 6. Representative example of the systemic and peripheral hemodynamic changes induced by the i.v. injection of endothelin-1 (1 μg/kg) in a conscious dog. Increases in blood flow occurred initially in the systemic, coronary, renal, and celiac beds at a time when arterial pressure was not increased. Arterial pressure then rose dramatically, accompanied by marked decreases in regional blood flows except in the celiac bed, where it remained elevated for approximatively 15 min. These hemodynamic changes then waned gradually within 1 h.

and EDRF (11) are possible candidates, but it still remains to be shown that these substances are involved in the EDT-induced systemic and regional vasodilation in vivo. Recent work has demonstrated an inhibitory interaction between EDT-1 and EDRF in vitro (6, 34), supporting the hypothesis that a biological equilibrium may well exist between these two endothelium-derived vasoactive factors.

Concluding remarks

The important role of the endothelium in mediating vascular reactivity in response to both vasodilator or vasoconstrictor stimuli, physical and/or humoral, can be demonstrated in intact, conscious animals. Pathologic stimuli, such as atherosclerosis, hypercholesterolemia and, particularly, hypertension have been suggested to result in a loss or alteration of endothelial vascular function, and a concomitant impairment of endothelium mediated vasodilation (5, 22, 32) which may predispose to vasospasm (52). In the case of endothelin, while its effects have been clearly demonstrated both in vitro and in vivo, it still remains to be established whether it parallels EDRF as a regulator under physiological or pathophysiological conditions. However, both for EDRF as well as other endothelial derived vasoactive agents, careful longitudinal, physiological measurements coupled with histopathological studies remain to be performed to understand the extent to which these agents participate in integrative regulation of vascular smooth muscle tone in vivo.

References

1. Altura BT, Altura BM (1975) Pentobarbital and contraction of vascular smooth muscle. Am J Physiol 229:1635–1640
2. Bassenge E, Busse R (1988) Endothelial modulation of coronary tone. Prog Cardiovasc Dis 30:349–380
3. Bigaud M, Kohin S, Scicli AG, Vatner SF (1990) Cardiovascular effects of endothelin in conscious dogs. FASEB J 4:A1080, abstr 4724
4. Bigaud M, Kohin S, Scicli AG, Vatner SF (1990) Effects of endothelin on regional blood flow distribution and vascular conductances in conscious dogs. Submitted for publication
5. Bossaller C, Yamamoto H, Lichtlen PR, Henry PD (1987) Impaired cholinergic vasodilation in the cholesterol-fed rabbit in vivo. Bas Res Cardiol 82:396–404
6. Boulanger C, Lüscher TF (1990) Release of endothelin from porcine aorta. Inhibition by endothelium-derived nitric oxide. J Clin Invest 85:587–590
7. Brain SD, Crossman DC, Buckley TL, Williams TJ (1989) Endothelin-1: demonstration of potent effects on the microcirculation of humans and other species. J Cardiovasc Pharmacol 13 (suppl 5):S147–149
8. Busse R, Trogisch G, Bassenge E (1985) The role of endothelium in the control of vascular tone. Basic Res Cardiol 80:475–490
9. Cernacek P, Duncan JS (1989) Immunoreactive endothelin in human plasma: marked elevations in patients in cardiogenic shock. Biochem Biophys Res Commun 161:562–567
10. De Mey JG, Vanhoutte PM (1983) Anoxia and endothelium dependent reactivity of the canine femoral artery. J Physiol (Lond) 335:65–74
11. De Nucci G, Thomas R, D'Orleans-Juste P, Antunes E, Walder C, Warner TD, Vane JR (1988) Pressor effects of circulating endothelin are limited by its removal in the pulmonary circulation and by the release of prostacyclin and endothelium-derived relaxing factor. Proc Natl Acad Sci 85:9797–9800
12. D'Orleans-Juste P, Finet M, De Nucci G, Vane JR (1989) Pharmacology of endothelin-1 in isolated vessels: Effect of nicardipine, methylene blue, hemoglobin and gossypol. J Cardiovasc Pharmacol 13 (suppl 5):S19–S22
13. Feigl EO (1983) Coronary physiology. Physiol Rev 63:1–205
14. Firth JD, Ratcliffe PJ, Raine AEG, Ledingham JGG (1988) Endothelin: an important factor in acute renal failure? The Lancet, November 19:1179–1182
15. Fukuda Y, Hirata Y, Yoshimi H, Kojima T, Kobayashi Y, Yanagisawa M, Masaki T (1988) Endothelin is a potent secretagogue for atrial natriuretic peptide in cultured rat atrial myocytes. Biochem Biophys Res Commun 135:167–172
16. Furchgott RF (1983) Role of endothelium in responses of vascular smooth muscle. Circ Res 53:557–573
17. Furchgott RF, Zawadzki JV (1980) The obligatory role of endothelial cells in the relaxation of arterial smooth muscle by acetylcholine. Nature 288:373–376
18. Godfraind T, Eglème C, Al Osachie I (1986) Role of endothelium in the contractile response of rat aorta to α-adrenoceptor agonists. Clin Sci 68 (suppl 10):65s–71s
19. Goetz KL, Wang BC, Madwed JB, Zhu JL, Leadley Jr RJ (1988) Cardiovascular, renal and endocrine responses to intravenous endothelin in conscious dogs. Am J Physiol 225:R1064–1068
20. Gruetter CA, Gruetter DY, Lyon JE, Kadowitz PJ, Ignarro JL (1981) Relationship between cyclic guanosine 3′:5′-monophosphate formation and relaxation of coronary arterial smooth muscle by glyceryl trinitrate, nitroprusside, nitrate and nitric oxide: effects of methylene blue and methemoglobin. J Pharmacol Exp Ther 219:181–186

21. Gryglewski RJ, Botting RM, Vane JR (1988) Mediators produced by the endothelial cell. Hypertension 12:530–548
22. Harrison DG, Freiman PC, Mitchell GG (1986) Atherosclerosis significantly impairs vasoactive responses to a variety of humoral agents. Blood Vess 23:73–77
23. Hintze TH, Vatner SF (1984) Reactive dilation of large coronary arteries in conscious dogs. Circ Res 54:50–57
24. Holtz J, Förstermann U, Pohl U et al. (1984) Flow-dependent, endothelium-mediated dilation of epicardial coronary arteries in conscious dogs: effects of cyclooxygenase inhibition. J Cardiovasc Pharmacol 6:1161–1169
25. Ingebrigsten R, Leraand S (1970) Dilation of a medium-sized artery immediately after local changes of blood pressure and flow as measured by ultrasonic technique. Acta Physiol Scand 79:552–558
26. Inoue A, Yanagisawa M, Kimura S, Kasuya Y, Miyauchi T, Goto K, Masaki T (1989) The human endothelin family: three structurally and pharmacologically distinct isopeptides by three separate genes. Proc Natl Acad Sci 86:2863–2867
27. Jaffe EA (1987) Physiologic functions of normal endothelial cells. Ann N Y Acad Sci 454:279–291
28. Kaiser L, Sparks HV (1986) Mediation of flow dependent arterial dilation by endothelial cells. Circ Shock 18:109–114
29. Le Monnier de Gouville AG, Lippton HL, Cavero I, Summer WR, Hyman AL (1989) Endothelin – a new family of endothelium-derived peptides with widespread biological properties. Life Sci 45:1499–1513
30. Levesque H, Sevrain L, Freger, P, Tadie M, Courtois HH, Creissard P (1990) Raised plasma endothelin in aneurysmal subarachnoid haemorrhage. The Lancet, February 3:290
31. Lie M, Sejersted OM, Kiil F (1970) Local regulation of vascular cross section during changes in femoral arterial blood flow in dogs. Circ Res 27:727–737
32. Ludmer PL, Selwyn AP, Shook TL, Wayne RR, Mudge GH, Alexander RW, Ganz P (1986) Paradoxical vasoconstriction induced by acetylcholine in atherosclerotic coronary arteries. N Engl J Med 315:1046–1051
33. Lüscher TF (1990) The endothelium. Target and promoter of hypertension? Hypertension 15:482–485
34. Lüscher TF, Yang Z, Tschudi M, von Segesser L, Stulz P, Boulanger C, Siebenmann R, Turina M, Bühler FR (1990) Interaction between endothelin-1 and endothelium-derived relaxing factor in human arteries and veins. Circ Res 66:1088–1094
35. Macho P, Vatner SF (1981) Effects of nitroglycerin and nitroprusside on large and small coronary vessels in conscious dogs. Circulation 64:1101–1107
36. Martin W, Furchgott RF, Villani GM, Jothianandan D (1986) Depression of contractile responses in rat aorta by spontaneously released endothelium-derived relaxing factor. J Pharmacol Exp Ther 237:529–537
37. Masaki T (1989) The discovery, the present state and the future prospects of endothelin. J Cardiovasc Pharmacol 13(suppl 5):S1–S4
38. Miyauchi T, Yanagisawa M, Tomizawa T, Sugishita Y, Suzuki N, Fujino M, Ajisaka R, Goto K, Masaki T (1989) Increased plasma concentrations of endothelin-1 and big endothelin-1 in acute myocardial infarction. The Lancet, July 1:53–54
39. Moncada S, Gryglewski RJ, Bunting S, Vane JR (1976) An enzyme isolated from arteries transforms prostaglandin endoperoxidases to an unstable substances that inhibits platelet aggregation. Nature 263:663–665
40. Moncada S, Palmer RM, Higgs EA (1989) Biosynthesis of nitric oxide from L-arginine. A pathway for the regulation of cell function and communication. Biochem Pharmacol 38:1709–1715
41. Morel DR, Lacroix JS, Hemsen A, Steinig DA, Pittet JF, Lundberg JM (1989) Increased plasma and pulmonary lymph levels of endothelin during endotoxin shock. Eur J Pharmacol 167:427–428
42. Mülsch A, Busse R (1990) NG-nitro-L-arginine (N5-[imino(nitroamino)methyl]-L-ornithine) impairs endothelium-dependent dilations by inhibiting cytosolic nitric oxide synthesis from L-arginine. Naunyn Schmiedebergs Arch Pharmacol 341:143–147
43. Palmer RMJ, Ferrige AG, Moncada S (1987) Nitric oxide release accounts for the biological activity of endothelium-derived relaxing factor. Nature 327:524–526

44. Pohl U, Holtz J, Busse R, Bassenge E (1986) Crucial role of endothelium in the vasodilator responses to increased flow in vivo. Hypertension 8:37–44
45. Rees DD, Palmer RM, Hodson HF, Moncada S (1989) A specific inhibitor of nitric oxide formation from L-arginine attenuates endothelium-dependant relaxation. Br J Pharmacol 96:418–424
46. Rodbard S (1975) Vascular caliber. Cardiology 60:4–49
47. Rohmeiss P, Photiadis J, Rohmeiss S, Unger T (1990) Hemodynamic actions of intravenous endothelin in rats: comparison with sodium nitroprusside and methoxamine. Am J Physiol 258:H337–H346
48. Rubanyi GM, Romero JC, Vanhoutte PM (1986) Flow-induced release of endothelium derived relaxant factor. Am J Physiol 250:H1145–H1149
49. Schretzenmayr A (1933) Über kreislaufregulatorische Vorgänge an den großen Arterien bei der Muskelarbeit. Pflügers Arch Ges Physiol 232:743–748
50. Shichiri M, Hirata Y, Ando K, Emori T, Ohta K, Kimoto S, Ogura M, Inoue A, Marumo F (1990) Plasma endothelin levels in hypertension and chronic renal failure. Hypertension 15:493–496
51. Stasch JP, Hirth-Dietrich C, Kazda S, Neuser D (1989) Endothelin stimulates release of atrial natriuretic peptides in vitro and in vivo. Life Sci 45:869–875
52. Tomoike H, Egashira K, Yamamoto Y, Nakamura M (1989) Enhanced responsiveness smooth muscle, impaired endothelium-dependent relaxation and the genesis of coronary spasm. Am J Cardiol 63:33E–39E
53. Vanhoutte PM, Rubanyi GM, Miller VM, Houston DS (1986) Modulation of vascular smooth muscle contraction by the endothelium. Annu Rev Physiol 48:307–320
54. Vanhoutte PM (1987) Endothelium-dependent contractions in arteries and veins. Blood Vess 24:141–144
55. Vatner SF, Braunwald E (1975) Cardiovascular control mechanisms in the conscious state. New Engl J Med 293:970–976
56. Vatner SF, Pagani M, Manders WT, Pasipoularides AD (1980) Alpha adrenergic vasoconstriction and nitroglycerin vasodilation of large coronary arteries in the conscious dog. J Clin Invest 65:5–14
57. Vatner DE, Knight DR, Homcy CJ, Vatner SF, Young MA (1986) Subtypes of beta adrenergic receptors in bovine coronary arteries. Circ Res 59:463–473
58. Wright CE, Fozard JR (1988) Regional vasodilation is prominent feature of haemodynamic response to endothelin in anaesthetized, spontaneously hypertensive rats. Eur J Pharmacol 155:201–203
59. Yanagisawa M, Kurihara H, Kimura S, Tomobe Y, Kobayashi M, Mitsui Y, Yazaki Y, Goto K, Masaki T (1988) A novel potent vasoconstrictor peptide produced by vascular endothelial cells. Nature 332:411–415
60. Young MA, Vatner SF (1986) Enhanced adrenergic constriction of iliac artery with removal of endothelium in conscious dogs. Am J Physiol 250:H892–H897
61. Young MA, Vatner SF (1986) Brief review: regulation of large coronary arteries. Circ Res 59:579–596
62. Young MA, Vatner SF (1987) Blood flow, and endothelium-mediated vasomotion of iliac arteries in conscious dogs. Circ Res 61 (suppl II):88–93
63. Young MA, Vatner SF (1987) Autonomic control of large coronary arteries and resistance vessels. Prog Cardiovasc Dis 15:211–234
64. Young MA, Vatner SF (1988) Endothelium, blood flow and vascular responses in arteries of conscious dogs. In: Vanhoutte PM (ed) Relaxing and contracting factors. Humana Press, 88:347–360

Author's address:
Stephen F. Vatner, M.D.
New England Regional Primate Research Center
One Pine Hill Drive
Southborough, MA 01772

Endothelium-mediated regulation of coronary tone

E. Bassenge

Lehrstuhl für Angewandte Physiologie der Universität Freiburg, FRG

Summary: To what extent endothelial autacoids like endothelium-derived relaxant factor/nitric oxide (EDRF/NO), in addition to neural-humoral factors, are involved in the regulation of myocardial perfusion, is presently not known. Therefore, we investigated in conscious, chronically instrumented dogs the effect of stereospecific inhibitors (N^G-monomethyl-L-arginine (L-NMMA), N^G-nitro-L-arginine (L-NNA), N^G-monomethylester-L-arginine (L-NAME)) of nitric oxide-synthesis and -release on epicardial coronary tone (and coronary diameter) and myocardial perfusion. A hydraulic coronary cuff was used, to produce reactive hyperemia and to keep the myocardial perfusion constant over short periods. 40 mg/kg L-NNA i.v. caused a long-lasting increase in mean arterial blood pressure from 94 ± 8 to 129 ± 11 mmHg and a simultaneous decrease in coronary diameter by 2.8 ± 0.3%. Heart rate dropped from 87 to 58 min^{-1}, but the double product of heart rate and blood pressure dropped by only 8 ± 2% ($p = 0.05$). The maximal coronary conductance during peak reactive hyperemia (after 20 s ischemia) indicating complete coronary dilation was diminished by 48% after L-NNA.

The severe drop in resting myocardial perfusion and O_2-supply, and nearly unchanged rate pressure product and thus myocardial metabolic rate following the inhibition of nitric oxide formation demonstrate a substantial contribution of EDRF/NO to the regulation of myocardial perfusion.

Key words: Endothelial nitric oxide (NO) formation; inhibitors of NO-formation; vasomotor control; endothelial impairment

Introduction

Until 1980, when Furchgott (11) made his pioneering observation of an agonist-induced, receptor-mediated (acetylcholine stimulated) autacoid release from a functionally intact endothelial lining, the key role of an endothelium-dependent control mechanism of vascular tone and, hence, tissue perfusion was not recognized. Nobody had anticipated that the tiny endothelial lining is so metabolically active in producing powerful local hormones that diffuse into the adjacent vasculature and cause decisive changes in vascular tone and organ perfusion rates. An impairment of endothelium-dependent control mechanisms becomes particularly important under pathophysiological conditions, when endothelial function is impaired due to atheromatosis, diabetes, hypertension, balloon catheter treatments, immunological diseases, and also heart transplantation.

This report presents new data on the significance of endothelial endothelium-derived relaxant factor (EDRF)/nitric oxide (NO) for the adjustment of myocardial perfusion and vascular tone (both in large epicardial arteries and in coronary resistance vessels) obtained in conscious, chronically instrumented dogs.

In addition, this brief article summarizes findings of several investigators on the physiological and pathophysiological aspects of endothelial autacoid release in the regulation of large conduit artery tone with special emphasis on endothelium-derived ERDF/NO-release in the coronary bed. This NO release significantly affects arteriolar tone and thereby the control mechanism of myocardial perfusion and function. Furthermore, it has been shown that EDRF/NO inhibits platelet adhesion and aggregation, thereby improving blood fluidity and suppressing thrombotic events with a concomitant release of vasoconstrictor compounds. Especially under pathophysiological conditions an impaired endothelial NO-production and release decisively affects vascular tone in atheromatotic large coronary arteries, resulting in a limitation of adequate myocardial blood supply (for review see (4)).

Methods

The experiments were carried out in mongrel dogs (weight: 23–28 kg). Under pentobarbital anesthesia (25 mg/kg) they were instrumented to chronically measure coronary blood flow, aortic pressure, and epicardial coronary artery diameters using ultrasonic transit time crystals, which were attached to the left circumflex and descending coronary arteries. Aortic pressure was registered using a Statham P23 pressure transducer; coronary flow was measured with a Gould SP 2202 flowmeter. Zero flow was established with a pneumatic cuff distal to the flow probe, a microcatheter was inserted through a small side branch into the left circumflex coronary artery proximal to the flow probe. Heart rate was derived from the arterial pressure signal. Phasic and mean tracings of all variables were recorded on a Beckman Dynograph and readings of the variables were averaged over 30 s. Acetylcholine (ACh) was used to elicit endothelium-dependent dilator responses, papaverin and nitroglycerin were used to elicit endothelium-independent dilator responses. The NO-mediated dilator activity was suppressed using the L-arginine-analogue L-nitro-arginine (L-NNA; 20–40 mg/kg i.v.) or L-mono-methyl-arginine (L-NMMA; infused intracoronarily over 10 min at a dosage of 5 mg/kg). All experiments were carried out under resting conditions. During the experiments the dogs were trained to lie quietly on a table.

Origin and control mechanisms of endothelium-dependent NO/EDRF production

NO is formed in the arginine-containing cytosol of endothelial cells by a Ca^{2+}-calmodulin- (7) and NADPH-dependent oxidative conversion of the guanidino-terminal nitrogen of L-arginine (21). A receptor-dependent stimulation probably initiates EDRF/NO release. A second Ca^{2+}-independent NO formation probably accounts for the continuous basal NO release (22). How this basal release is stimulated by mechanical shear stress (acting as viscous drag upon the endothelial lining) during flow-dependent dilation following augmented perfusion rates, is not yet exactly known (3). Shear stress-induced hyperpolarization (which would favor NO release) has been demonstrated in cultured cells (25), which could explain this phenomenon. Also, shear stress-induced increases in intracellular Ca^{2+} (2) that would also tend to increase NO release have been observed in this context.

cGMP-mediated mechanisms as general biological signals in different cell systems

NO/EDRF is the principal of three physiological compounds known to stimulate soluble guanylate cyclase (sGC) in a variety of cell systems (vascular smooth muscle, platelets, macrophages, leukocytes, nerve cells) which elicit a rise in intracellular cGMP. This rise may be associated with protein phosphorylation of certain key enzymes, which are not yet identified and which probably initiate a variety of cellular events.

Table 1.

sGC Activation elicits: in VSM → vasodilation		(Ignarro et al. 1990; Murad 1989)
in platelets → inhibition of platelet	activation adhesion aggregation	(Moncada 1989; Busse et al. 1987)
in nerve cells of the peripheral nerves → suppression of NE-effects	(cGMP-involvement unknown)	(Cohen and Weisbrod 1988; Tesfamarian et al. 1987)
→ inhibitory transmitter of non-adrenergic noncholinergic innervation		(Bult et al. 1990)
in central nervous system → NO as intracellular messenger	(transmitter)	(Garthwaite et al. 1988)
→ NO-release results in central inhibition of spontaneously active pressor neurons. Consequently, suppression of NO-release by L-NMMA results in sympathetic stimulation		(Sakuma et al. 1990)
in leukocytes → cGMP-mediated metabolic changes exerting microbiocidal actions		(McCall et al. 1989)

EDRF effects on general hemodynamics

When the continuous basal release of EDRF from the endothelial lining is offset an increase in vascular tone (see Table 2) and resistance to flow can be observed in a variety of peripheral vascular beds (1, 8, 12, 26, 27, 29, 31, 32). EDRF-actions can be suppressed by binding and inactivating EDRF using hemoglobin (Hb) (31, 32) or by stopping its release by providing biological inert analogues such as L-mono-methyl-arginine (L-NMMA) to endothelial cells instead of the biologically active precursor substance for NO generation, namely, L-arginine. Blocking EDRF actions by Hb has been shown to cause coronary constriction in isolated perfused hearts and to reduce myocardial perfusion, and, when coronary flow is experimentally kept constant, to increase coronary inert analogue L-NMMA (1, 27, 28) identical findings were obtained.

Similar results have been found with a number of other peripheral beds (cerebral, mesenteric, renal, muscle, hindquarters) (12, 26–28) or in the systemic circulation as shown in Table 2 and by other authors (8).

When L-NMMA or a similar analogue, nitro-L-arginine (L-NNA), was administered into the systemic circulation, there was an immediate increase in peripheral resistance

Table 2. Effect of suppressing endothelial NO formation by L-nitro-arginine (40 mg/kg) on coronary hemodynamics and coronary tone in resting conscious dogs. Mean arterial pressure (MAP), heart rate (HR), coronary diameter (CD), endothelium-dependent dilation (EDD) to ACh [% difference coronary diameter (Δ CD)], flow-dependent dilation (FDD) during reactive hyperemia following 20 s ischemia [% difference coronary diameter (Δ CD)], coronary flow (CF) per 100 g × min^{-1}, coronary vascular resistance (CVR). Data of experiments in 5 dogs ± SEM

	HR [min^{-1}]	MAP [mmHg]	Resting CD [mm]	EDD [% Δ CD] (1 µg ACh)	FDD [% Δ CD] (RH, 20 s)	CF $\left[\frac{ml}{min \times 100\,g}\right]$	CVR [% of control]
Control	87 ± 5	96 ± 8	3.25 ± 0.05	4.35 ± 0.62	5.60 ± 0.51	58 ± 8	100
L-NNA	58 ± 6*	129 ± 11*	3.05 ± 0.05*	2.23 ± 0.31*	2.51 ± 0.69*	34 ± 7*	228 ± 14*

* Significantly different from control $p < 0.02$, L-NNA (40 mg/kg/20 min)

and arterial blood pressure as presented in Table 2 and by others (8, 29). Even when L-NMMA was chronically supplied orally to rats in the drinking water, there was a lasting elevation of peripheral resistance and arterial blood pressure (12). Thus, continuous release of EDRF/NO from the endothelial cell lining may be an important regulator of blood pressure. If NO release is suddenly suppressed, significant hypertension originates, which surprisingly, is not easily counterregulated by a number of other biological compensatory mechnisms.

To what extent the impaired endothelial function and NO release is the cause for the induction of hypertension of the effect of the hypertension-induced endothelial damage has not yet been analyzed in detail. Experimental hypertension in rats is associated with a substantial reduction in endothelium-mediated vasomotor responses (19) and in hypertensive patients endothelium-dependent regulation of peripheral blood flow (forearm) is likewise reduced (17).

An increase in peripheral vascular tone and resistance can also be detected by suppressing the effects of locally released NO acting as a neurotransmitter compound in the central nervous system (30). A continuous NO-release in the paracisternal area is apparently capable of suppressing spontaneous central sympathetic activity. Inhibition of this NO-release by intracisternal application of L-NMMA, therefore, results in the suppression of this central inhibitor effect. Consequently, sympathetic activity has been reported to immediately increase after intracisternal L-NMMA application, augmenting peripheral vascular tone and resistance. In favor of this concept is the fact that intracisternal application of the real precursor, L-arginine, reverses this enhancement of sympathetic activity, leading to the cessation of this centrally mediated vasoconstriction. Such an L-NMMA-induced augmentation of sympathetic tone would also tend to limit adequate myocardial oxygen supply.

Endothelium-dependent modulation of tone in coronary arterioles

When biological inert arginine analogues such as L-NNA are supplied to beating isolated heart preparations there is an immediate increase in arteriolar tone (1, 8, 28), which can lower myocardial perfusion under experimental conditions to even less than 50% (28). Under this experimental condition there is increased lactate release from the partially ischemic heart, indicating that an enhanced metabolic stimulation and release of vasodilator catabolites in this preparation does not adequately compensate for the sup-

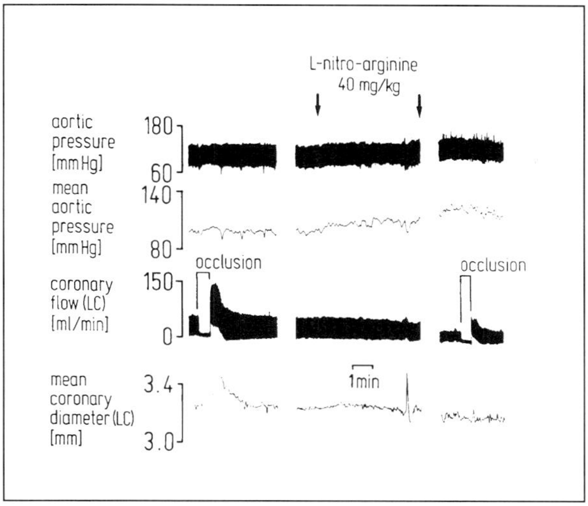

Fig. 1. Reduction in coronary blood flow, myocardial perfusion and reactive hyperemia (20 s ischemia) following suppression of endothelial NO formation by L-nitro-arginine (40 mg/kg). Tracings of a typical experiment in a conscious, instrumented dog. Coronary blood flow is reduced to 61% of resting control value. In spite of a substantial increase in aortic and coronary perfusion pressure there is a tendency for reduction of left circumflex diameter.

pressed endothelium-dependent continuous dilator activity in response to EDRF (28). This finding demonstrates that endothelium-dependent control of coronary tone may probably be as important as local metabolic regulation, and may under pathophysiologial conditions with impaired endothelial function be responsible for an inappropriate regulation of myocardial perfusion.

An increase in coronary resistance and a simultaneous reduction in reactive hyperemia by suppressing the continuous EDRF-mediated coronary dilator effect was also observed in chronically instrumented conscious dog preparations (with reflex reactions left intact) after administration of L-NNA as a suppressor of EDRF-formation, as presented in Table 2 and Fig. 1. Similar results using L-NMMA were obtained by Chu et al. (8).

Endothelium-dependent modulation of tone in epicardial coronary arteries

Suppression of EDRF-release in large coronary arteries by L-NMMA or by L-NNA in chronically instrumented conscious dogs leads to a substantial increase in tone marked by a significant diameter reduction even in the presence of an increased arterial perfusion pressure and distending pressure, as shown in Table 2. Similar results have been obtained by Chu et al. (8).

When L-NMMA is administered intracoronarily in chronically instrumented conscious dogs at a concentration of 5 mg/kg there is a substantial suppression of the endothelium-dependent dilator response to intracoronary ACh (1 μg), as demonstrated in Fig. 2. This dilator response is reestablished, when L-arginine is administered intracoronarily (30 mg/kg). Similarly the flow-dependent dilation (FDD) is suppressed under L-NMMA, a response which is also dependent on an unimpaired endothelial func-

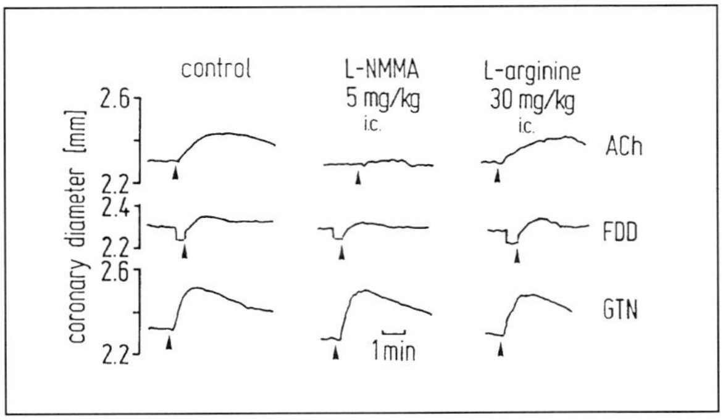

Fig. 2. Reduction in endothelium-mediated dilator responses to acetylcholine (ACh) and during flow-dependent dilation (FDD) following the intracoronary administration of L-mono-methyl-arginine (L-NMMA; 5 mg/kg). Tracings from a typical experiment. Dilator responses are reestablished following the nitracoronary administration of L-arginine (30 mg/kg). Endothelium-independent vasomotor responses following nitroglycerin administration are not affected by L-NMMA. Arrows indicate time of i.c. administration/release of occlusion for FDD responses.

tion and EDRF/NO release, whereas the endothelium-independent dilator response to nitroglycerin is not affected. After i.c. administration of L-arginine the FDD response is reestablished (Fig. 1). How much of this L-NMMA-induced suppression of FDD response during intracoronary L-NMMA cannot be exactly quantified under these in vivo conditions.

These findings demonstrate that also large coronary conductance arteries are under the control of a continuous basal EDRF-release which tends to augment coronary conductance and to counterbalance the continuous myogenic constrictor impulses (28), which – mainly in the arteriolar section – reduce conductivity and myocardial perfusion.

A loss of endothelium-mediated dilator function becomes particularly important under pathophysiological conditions, like with hypercholesterolemia, atheromatosis, hypertension, diabetes, and also, following balloon catheter interventions and other sources of functional endothelial impairment (10, 14, 15, 17, 18, 34, 36, 37, for review see (4)). A number of factors and circulating agonists, which have been shown to induce in the presence of an intact endothelial lining endothelium-dependent coronary dilation, have been shown to lose their ability to dilate or may instead even initiate constrictor responses. Thus, exogenous Ach intracoronarily injected causes dose-dependent dilation in patients without atheromatosis and risk factors; however, in the presence of CAD dose-dependent constrictor responses are observed (18, 35). In patients with heart transplantation the subsequent immunization processes likewise lead to endothelial impairment; thus, it is not surprising that in these patients upon intracoronary ACh test injections, exclusively coronary constrictions are observed in the transplanted vessels (24). Likely, such reactions can be used to test endothelial integrity and function, which also seems to deteriorate with age. There has recently been indications that the endothelial dilator function decreases with age (37).

References

1. Amezcua JL, Palmer RMJ, DeSouza BM, Moncada S (1989) Nitric oxide synthesized from L-arginine regulates vascular tone in the coronary circulation of the rabbit. Br J Pharmacol 97:1019–1024
2. Ando J, Komatsuda T, Kamiya A (1988) Cytoplasmic calcium response to fluid shear stress in cultured vascular endothelial cells. In Vitro Cell Develop Biol 24:871
3. Bassenge E, Münzel T (1988) Consideration of conduit and resistance vessels in regulation of blood flow. Am J Cardiol 62:40E–44E
4. Bassenge E, Heusch G (1990) Regulation of coronary blood flow: nervous, hormonal and endothelial factors. Rev Physiol Biochem Pharmacol 116:77–165
5. Bult H, Boeckxstaens, GE, Pelckmans PA, Jordaens FH, Van Maercke YM, Hermann AG (1990) Nitric oxide as an inhibitory non-adrenergic non-cholinergic neurotransmitter. Nature 345:346–347
6. Busse R, Lückhoff A, Bassenge E (1987) Endothelium-derived relaxant factor inhibits platelet activation. Naunyn-Schmiedebergs Arch Pharmacol 336:566–571
7. Busse R, Mülsch A (1990) Calcium-dependent nitric oxide synthesis in endothelial cytosol is mediated by calmodulin. FEBS Letters 265:133–136
8. Chu A, Chambers DE, Lin CC, Kuehl WD, Cobb FR (1990) Nitric oxide modulates epicardial coronary basal vasomotor tone in awake dogs. Am J Physiol 258:H1250–H1254
9. Cohen RA, Weisbrod RM (1988) Endothelium inhibits norepinephrine release from adrenergic nerves of rabbit carotide artery. Am J Physiol 254:H871–H878
10. Fischell TA, Nellessen U, Johnson DE, Ginsburg R (1989) Endothelium-dependent arterial vasoconstriction after balloon angioplasty. Circulation 79:899–910
11. Furchgott RF, Zawadzki JV (1980) The obligatory role of endothelial cells in the relaxation of arterial smooth muscle by acetylcholine. Nature 288:373–376
12. Gardiner SM, Compton AM, Bennett T, Palmer RMJ, Moncada S (1990) Control of regional blood flow by endothelium-derived nitric oxide. Hypertension 15:486–492
13. Garthwaite J, Charles SL, Chess-Williams R (1988) Endothelium-derived relaxing factor release on activation of NMDA receptors suggests role as intercellular messenger in the brain. Nature 336:385–388
14. Harrison DG, Armstrong ML, Freiman PC, Heistad DD (1987) Restoration of endothelium-dependent relaxation by dietary treatment of atherosclerosis. J Clin Invest 80:1808–1811
15. Harrison DG, Freiman PC, Armstrong ML, Marcus ML, Heistad DD (1987) Alterations of vascular reactivity in atherosclerosis. Circ Res 61(Suppl. II):II-74-II-80
16. Ignarro LJ (1989) Biological actions and properties of endothelium-derived nitric oxide formed and released from artery and vein. Circ Res 65:1–21
17. Linder L, Kiowski W, Bühler FR, Lüscher TF (1990) Indirect evidence for the release of endothelium-derived relaxing factor in the human forearm circulation in vivo: blunted response in essential hypertension. Circulation 81:1762–1767
18. Ludmer PL, Selwyn AP, Shook TL, Wayne RR, Mudge GH, Alexander RW, Ganz P (1986) Paradoxical vasoconstriction induced by acetylcholine in atherosclerotic coronary arteries. N Engl J Med 315:1046–1051
19. Lüscher T, Raji L, Vanhoutte PM (1987) Endothelium-dependent vascular responses in normotensive and hypertensive Dahl rats. Hypertension 9:157–163
20. McCall TB, Boughton-Smith NK, Palmer RMJ, Whittle BJR, Moncada S (1989) Synthesis of nitric oxide from L-arginine by neutrophils: release and interaction with superoxide anion. Biochem J 261:293–296
21. Moncada S, Palmer RMJ, Higgs EA (1989) Biosynthesis of nitric oxide from L-arginine – A pathway for the regulation of cell function and communication. Biochem Pharmacol 38:1709–1715
22. Mülsch A, Bassenge E, Busse R (1989) Nitric oxide synthesis in endothelial cytosol: evidence for a calcium-dependent and a calcium-independent mechanism. Naunyn-Schmiedebergs Arch Pharmacol 340:767–770

23. Murad F (1989) Modulation of the guanylate cyclase-cGMP system by vasodilators and the role of free radicals as second messengers. In: Catravas JD, Gillis CN, Ryan US (eds) Vascular endothelium: receptors and transduction mechanisms. Plenum Press, New York-London 1989, pp 157–164
24. Nellessen U, Lee TC, Fischell TA, Ginsburg R, Masuyama T, Alderman EL, Schroeder JS (1988) Effects of acetylcholine on epicardial coronary arteries after cardiac transplantation without angiographic evidence of fixed graft narrowing. Am J Cardiol 62:1093–1097
25. Olesen SP, Clapham DE, Davies PF (1988) Haemodynamic shear stress activates a K^+ current in vascular endothelial cells. Nature 331:168–170
26. Pohl U, Herlan K, Huang A, Bassenge E (1990) EDRF-mediated, shear-induced dilation antagonizes myogenic vasoconstriction. FASEB J 4:A555
27. Pohl U, Herlan K, Huang A, Bassenge E (1990 [in press]) EDRF-mediated, shear-induced dilation opposes myogenic vasoconstriction. Am J Physiol
28. Pohl U, Lamontagne D, Bassenge E, Busse R (1990 [abstract]) EDRF augments coronary conductivity through attenuation of myogenic autoregulation. Pflügers Arch 415(Suppl. 1):R62
29. Rees DD, Palmer RM, Moncada S (1989) Role of endothelium-derived nitric oxide in the regulation of blood pressure. Proc Natl Acad Sci USA 86:3375–3378
30. Sakuma I, Togashi H, Yoshioka M, Kobayashi T, Saito H, Yasuda H, Gross SS, Levi R (1990) Effects of intravenous and intracisternal administration of NG-monomethyl-L-arginine on renal sympathetic nerve activity in anaesthetized rats. In: Moncada S, Higgs EA (eds) Nitric oxide from L-arginine: a bioregulatory system. Elsevier, Amsterdam 1990, pp 481–482
31. Stewart DJ, Holtz J, Pohl U, Bassenge E (1987) Balance between endothelium-mediated dilator and direct constrictor actions of serotonin on resistance vessels in the isolated rabbit heart. Eur J Pharmacol 143:131–134
32. Stewart DJ, Münzel T, Bassenge E (1987) Reversal of acetylcholine-induced coronary resistance vessel dilation by hemoglobin. Eur J Pharmacol 136:239–242
33. Tesfamariam B, Weisbrod RM, Cohen RA (1987) Endothelium inhibits responses of rabbit carotid artery to adrenergic nerve stimulation. Am J Physiol 253:H792–H798
34. Verbeuren TJ, Jordaens FH, Zonnekeyn LL, Van Hove CE, Herman AG (1986) Effect of hypercholesterolemia on vascular reactivity in the rabbit. I. Endothelium-dependent and endothelium-independent contractions and relaxations in isolated arteries of control and hypercholesterolemic rabbits. Circ Res 58:552–564
35. Zeiher AM, Drexler H, Wollschläger H, Saurbier B, Just H (1989) Coronary vasomotion in response to sympathetic stimulation in humans – importance of the functional integrity of the endothelium. J Am Coll Cardiol 14:1181–1190
36. Zeiher AM, Drexler H, Wollschläger H, Just H (1989 (abstract)) Preserved flow mediated vasodilation despite acetylcholine-induced vasoconstriction in atherosclerotic coronary arteries in man. J Am Coll Cardiol 13(Suppl. A):132A
37. Zeiher AM, Drexler H, Wollschläger H (1990) (abstract) Endothelium-dependent dilation of the coronary resistance vasculature declines with increasing age in normal humans. Circulation 82 (Suppl III):III–443

Author's address:

Prof. Dr. med. E. Bassenge
Lehrstuhl für Angew. Physiologie
der Universität
Hermann-Herder-Str. 7
W-7800 Freiburg i. Brsg., FRG

Role of EDRF and endothelin in coronary vasomotor control

D. J. Stewart

The McGill Unit for the Prevention of Cardiovascular Disease, McGill University, and the Royal Victoria Hospital, Montreal, Canada

Summary: It has recently been recognized that the endothelium plays a crucial role in the regulation of coronary vasomotor tone through the elaboration of potent endothelium-derived vasoactive factors. The properties of endothelium-derived relaxing factor (EDRF) and the constrictor peptide, endothelin-1 (ET) are briefly reviewed. Data is summarized which supports an important physiological role of EDRF in the control of coronary vascular resistance. Although ET is possibly the most potent constrictor of coronary arteries yet described, its role in physiological regulation of coronary vasomotor tone is less certain. Interactions between EDRF and ET in the coronary circulation are highlighted and a schema of regulation of release of endothelium-derived vasoactive factors is proposed.

Key words: endothelium-derived relaxing factor (EDRF); endothelin-1; coronary vasomotor tone; coronary resistance vessels; myocardial ischemia; free radicals; hemoglobin

Among the many important functions of the remarkable layer of cells which lines the inner surface of all blood vessels is the elaboration and release of a variety of potent vasoactive factors. It is only in the last decade that a true appreciation of the extent to which the endothelium contributes to vascular tone has emerged. The now classic observations of Furchgott (8) led to the discovery of the endothelium-derived relaxing factor (EDRF), which has recently been identified as nitric oxide (NO) (7, 12, 25) or a closely related precursor compound (23). More recently, Yanagisawa and coworkers have purified a constricting factor, termed endothelin (ET), from endothelial cell-conditioned media (39). This 21-residue peptide has potent vasoconstrictor effects in the coronary circulation, however, its role in the physiological regulation of coronary tone is unknown. It is very likely that other endothelium-derived factors may, to a greater or lesser extent, also influence coronary smooth muscle tone, including prostaglandins (dilator and constrictor), the endothelium-derived hyperpolarizing factor (EDHF) (3, 15), and possibly other endothelium-derived constricting factors (7). The purpose of the present text is to present an overview of the significance of endothelium-dependent vasomotion in the coronary bed, concentrating on the actions of EDRF and ET. Important interactions between these opposing endothelium-dependent vasoactive mechanisms in the coronary bed will be discussed, and novel concepts concerning the regulation of vasoactive factor production by the endothelium will be presented.

Supported by grants from the Medical Research Council of Canada, the Canadian Heart Foundation and les Fonds de Recherches en Santé du Quebec.

Large coronary arteries from many species, including man, demonstrate substantial endothelium-dependent vasodilation (1, 7, 9). There has been much interest in elucidating the possible contribution of a disorder of EDRF release or response to the vasospasm which can complicate coronary artery disease (37). The interactions between EDRF, platelets, and the vessel wall are discussed elsewhere and further underline the critical role of the endothelium in maintaining an appropriate state of large coronary artery tone and blood fluidity. However, until recently the importance of the endothelium with regard to the control of resistance vessel tone was uncertain. It is technically much more difficult to study small arteries and arterioles in vitro, and the endothelial layer in these smaller vessels is much more adherent than in larger arteries, therefore, complicating endothelial removal. These problems are multiplied when studying the intact isolated perfused heart. Methods of damaging or removing the endothelium from the microcirculation can cause a disruption in other important endothelial functions, such as its permeability or barrier properties, and lead to a rapid deterioration of the preparation.

We made use of the strong inhibitory effects of reduced haemoglobin on EDRF-mediated responses to provide some of the first evidence for an important role of EDRF in the coronary microcirculation. In the Langendorff isolated rabbit heart, perfused at constant flow with a buffered physiological saline solution, acetylcholine and serotonin are potent vasodilating agents (32, 34), resulting in maximal decreases in coronary vascular resistance, not different from those in response to papaverine (Fig. 1). In large arteries, relaxation in response to acetylcholine (8) and serotonin (5) is endothelium-dependent, and mediated by EDRF. EDRF has a very high affinity for the ferrous group of haemoglobin (19), which can readily bind and inactivate it. In large arteries, haemoglobin effectively reverses the dilation seen in response to endothelium-dependent agents. Therefore, the ability of haemoglobin to inhibit the response to agents characterized as endothelium-dependent dilatators in large arteries was tested in the intact microcirculation of the isolated perfused heart. As shown in Fig. 1, during exposure to haemoglobin there was a selective and reversible loss of dilation to acetylcholine, while the response to the endothelium-independent dilator papaverine was not reduced. As well, the balance between dilator and constrictor actions of serotonin was altered by haemoglobin, resulting in a net increase in coronary vascular resistance. Therefore, these results are consistent with substantial EDRF-mediated, endothelium-dependent dilation in the small arteries and arterioles of the coronary resistance bed.

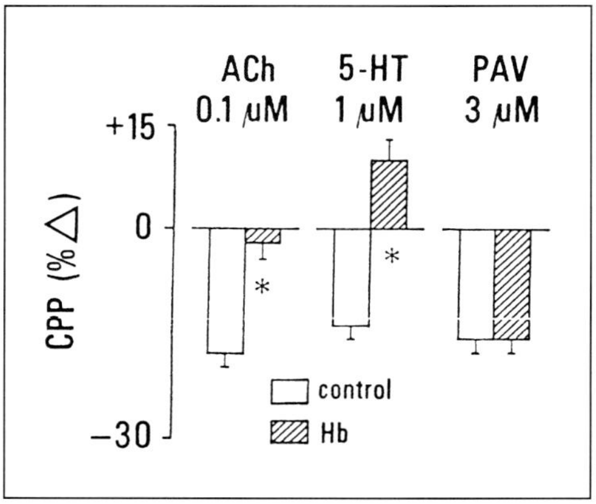

Fig. 1. Resistance vessel responses to acetylcholine (ACh), serotonin (5-HT), and papaverine (PAV) in the isolated perfused rabbit heart expressed as percent change in coronary perfusion pressure (CPP) at constant flow. Open bars represent control responses, whereas hatched bars indicate responses during infusion of haemoglobin (6 μM). [Modified from (32).]

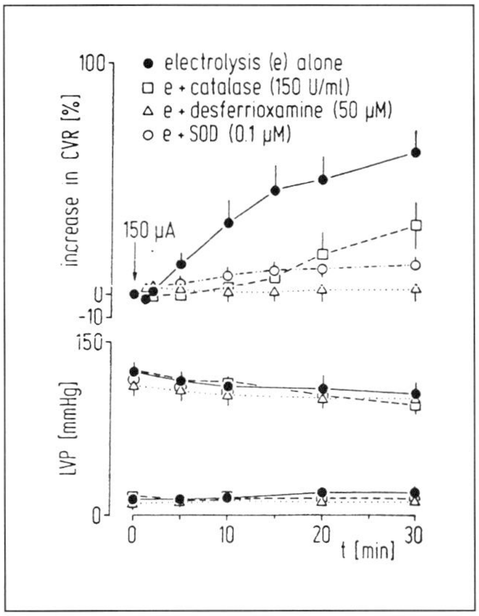

Fig. 2. The effect of electrolysis (150 μA) on coronary vascular resistance (CVR) and left ventricular pressure (LVP) in the isolated, perfused rabbit heart. [From (35).]

These findings have important implications with respect to the physiological regulation of resistance vessel tone in the coronary microcirculation and suggest that EDRF may play a crucial role in the control of blood flow distribution within and between vascular beds. There are also implications with respect to disease states characterized by disordered vascular tone. If EDRF contributes importantly to basal resistance vessel tone, then under conditions of damage to the microvascular endothelium, a loss of this basal dilatory influence may result in increased coronary vascular resistance and therefore reduced perfusion. There is currently considerable interest concerning the role of oxygen-derived free radicals in the pathophysiological consequences of ischemia and reperfusion (20). In addition, it has been known for some time that EDRF is highly susceptible to oxidation/reduction reactions and is readily inactivated by superoxide anion (29). However, it is not clear to what extent a disorder of endothelium-dependent dilation might contribute to the circulatory abnormalities induced by exposure to oxygen-derived free radicals. Therefore, using a modification of the isolated Langendorff-perfused heart model described above, we studied the direct effects of oxygen-derived free radicals on endothelium-dependent response in the coronary resistance bed (35). Reactive oxygen products were generated by passing a small current (150 μA) between a stainless anode and a platinum cathode. This results in the generation of superoxide anion and hydrogen peroxide, as well as the release of ferric iron from the anode (13). By virtue of the iron catalyzed "Haber-Weiss" reaction the hydroxyl radical will be formed secondarily (10). Figure 2 shows the effect of threshold levels of hydrolysis on coronary vasomotor and myocardial function in the isolated rabbit heart. Although electrical generation of reactive oxygen products at these low rates had only a minor effect on myocardial contractile function, there was a substantial and progressive rise in coronary vascular resistance, which could be blocked by scavenging free radicals or altering their production. To a large extent this increase in coronary vascular resistance was due to an increase in resistance vessel tone (rather than vascular damage and edema) since the vasodilator actions of direct acting agents (i.e., papaverine and adenosine) were preserved and even

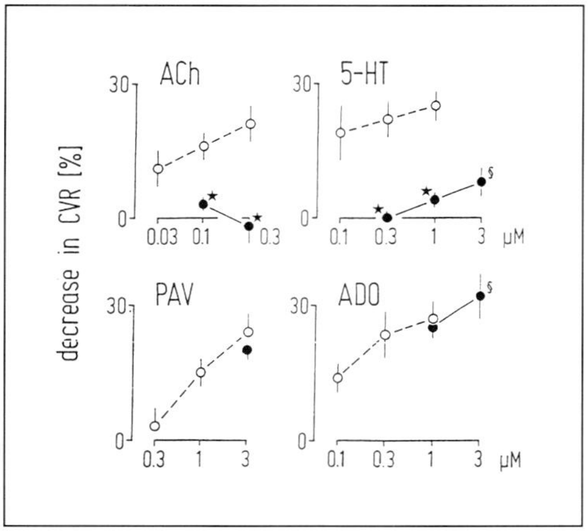

Fig. 3. The effect of electrolysis on vasodilator responses to acetylcholine (ACh), serotonin (5-HT), papaverine (PAV) and adenosine (ADO) expressed as percent decrease in coronary vascular resistance (CVR) in isolated rabbit hearts. Open symbols show control responses and closed symbols indicate responses during electrical generation of free radicals. [From (35).]

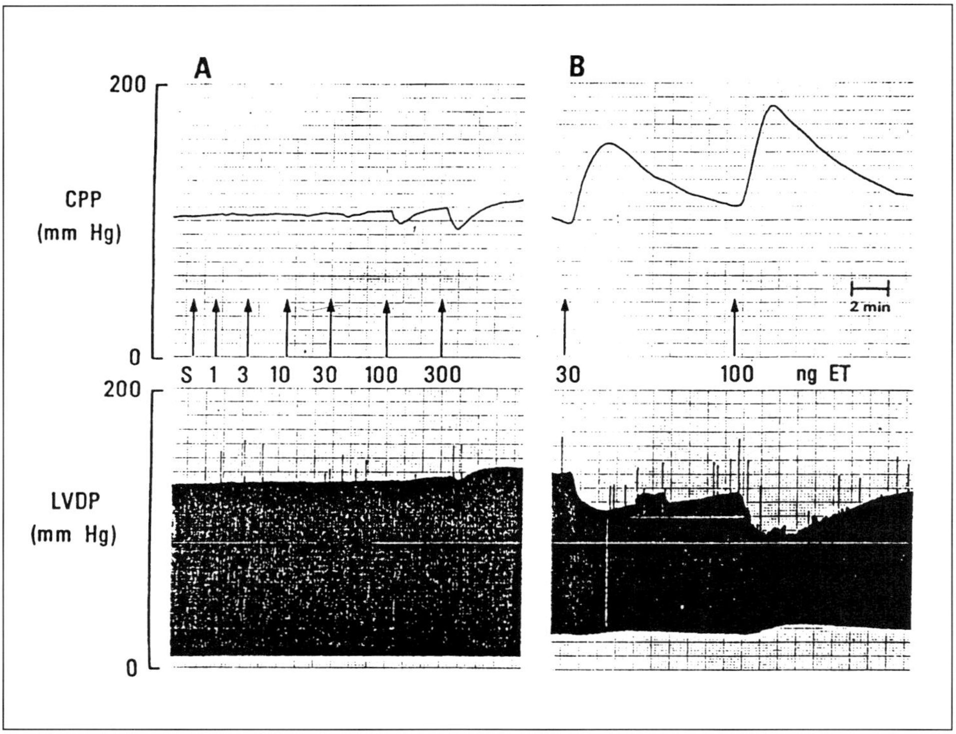

Fig. 4. Representative tracings of coronary perfusion pressure (CPP) and left ventricular developed pressure (LVDP) during constant flow perfusion. Arrows show bolus injection of 0.3 ml saline (S) or increasing doses of endothelin (ET) into the coronary circulation. Panel A shows control responses and panel B shows responses following embolization of 0.5 ml of air. [Modified from (30).]

potentiated (Fig. 3). However, responses to endothelium-dependent dilators were drastically reduced or even eliminated by exposure to free radicals. These findings point to the selective abolition of EDRF-mediated coronary resistance vessel dilation at levels of oxygen radical generation which were only threshold for altering myocardial function. Thus, in pathophysiological states where the generation of reactive oxygen products is enhanced (i.e., ischemia and reperfusion), one might anticipate an early loss of coronary endothelium-dependent dilation in the resistance bed which may further compromise perfusion and thus contribute to myocardial damage. In addition, the marked increases in basal coronary vascular resistance associated with a selective defect in endothelium-dependent dilation suggests an important contribution of EDRF to basal resistance vessel tone in the coronary bed.

Recently, direct techniques of measuring EDRF production have been developed (25) and applied to the perfused heart (14). It is now generally accepted that EDRF is chemically indistinguishable from nitric oxide (NO) (12, 25), and may be NO itself or a closely related precursor compound (23). Chemical methods of detection of NO production have shown measurable release from into the coronary circulation of the isolated perfused rabbit heart (14), confirming the earlier more indirect data. From the elucidation of the synthetic pathway for EDRF (NO) within the endothelial cytosol (26) has come the development of competitive antagonists of NO synthesis, the substituted analogues of L-arginine. Tools such as N-monomethyl L-arginine (28) or L-nitro-arginine (24) provide more versatile and selective inhibitors of EDRF synthesis, suitable for studies in vitro and in vivo, and a recent report supports an important basal role of EDRF in the physiological regulation of resistance vessel tone in isolated guinea pig hearts (36).

What then of the importance of the potent endothelium-derived constricting peptide, ET, in the regulation of coronary vasomotor tone? Much less is currently known about its production under physiological conditions. Endothelial cells in culture produce large amounts of ET-1 (39) which, when administered to the coronary circulation in vitro or in vivo, has profound effects on large and small coronary artery tone (17). In their original report, Yanagisawa and co-workers tested the constrictor activity of ET-1 using the porcine coronary artery as a bioassay (39). They showed that this novel endothelium-derived peptide was several fold more potent than angiotensin II, and possibly the most potent coronary vasoconstrictor yet identified. Similar results have been obtained using human tissue (4, 11, 18). We have recently shown that ET is a potent vasoconstrictor of human internal mammary artery and saphenous vein, tissues used in coronary artery revascularization surgery. In Fig. 4 it can be seen that ET is a much more potent contractile agent than norepinephrine in the human internal mammary artery, raising the possibility that ET may contribute to abnormal states of vasoconstriction in man. However, EDRF (NO) was readily able to reverse ET-induced contraction, suggesting that there may be a regulatory interaction between these opposing systems of endothelium-dependent vasomotion.

In the coronary circulation of the isolated rabbit heart we have studied the ability of native endothelium to modify the effect of exogenous ET on vascular and myocardial function (31). As can be seen in panel A of Fig. 5, in the control state, there was very little increase in coronary vascular resistance even following large doses of ET and in some cases a dose-dependent dilation could be observed. However, after the native endothelial layer had been altered by microembolization of air (panel B), the same doses of ET now produced extreme vasoconstriction, resulting in a marked deterioration of myocardial contractile function. There are a number of mechanisms by which an intact endothelial layer could dramatically alter the response to circulating ET. Pohl and co-workers in Freiburg have shown that the endothelium may present a tight barrier to diffusion of ET

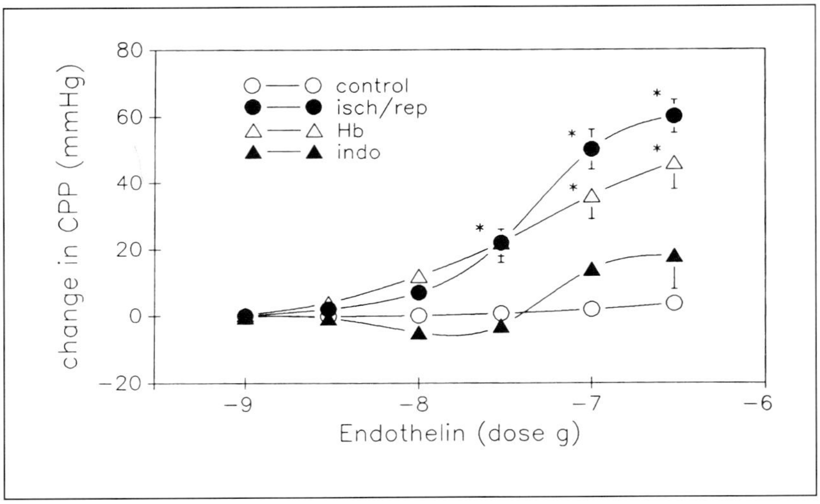

Fig. 5. Effect of endothelin on coronary perfusion pressure (CPP) in the isolated, constant-flow perfused rabbit heart under control conditions (open circles) and following ischemia and reperfusion (isch/rep, closed circles), or exposure to haemoglobin (Hb 6 μM, open triangles) or indomethacin (indo 6 μM, closed triangles). * = $p < 0.05$. [Modified from (30).]

(27), so that when administered intraluminally ET cannot reach the underlying smooth muscle layers. It is possible therefore that air damage to the coronary microvascular resulted in an alteration in the permeability properties of the endothelium allowing better access of intraluminal ET to the vascular media. However, the specific inhibition of endothelium-dependent dilation with ferrous haemoglobin (Fig. 6) also produced a significant potentiation of ET-induced vasoconstriction, supporting a role for EDRF in the modulation of coronary microvascular responsiveness to ET. Thus, in the coronary bed, there appears to be a regulatory interaction between endothelium-dependent mechanisms of dilation and constriction which serves to maintain myocardial perfusion and prevent extreme vasoconstriction. Such a regulatory mechanism has obvious physiological advantages.

We have also shown that ischemia and reperfusion in the rabbit heart produced a marked potentiation of coronary vasoconstrictor responses to ET (Fig. 6) (30). Thus, local damage may upset the protective action of normal endothelium and increase the vulnerability of the coronary bed to the potent contractile actions of circulating ET, predisposing to further compromise myocardial perfusion. It must be kept in mind, however, hat ET is a product of the endothelium, and therefore can be released locally by the coronary vasculature. At present, the importance of local endothelin production in the coronary bed under physiological and pathophysiological conditions is uncertain. Several groups have demonstrated substantial increases in plasma ET levels following myocardial infarction in man (21, 22, 40). Figure 7 summarizes results from our laboratory (16). Plasma levels of ET were consistently elevated in the early hours following onset of myocardial infarction, even in patients with entirely uncomplicated infarctions. The peak in plasma ET preceded by many hours the peak in creatinine phosphokinase, the classical clinical marker of myocardial damage. These results are

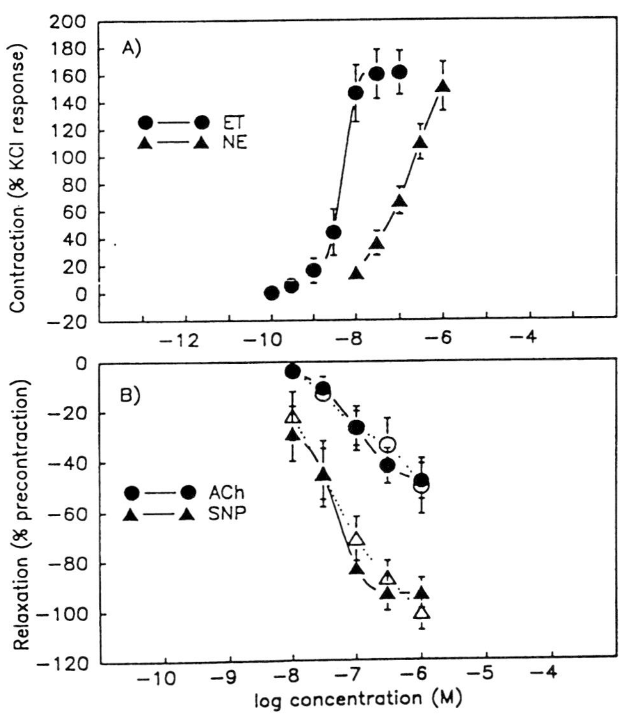

Fig. 6. Contraction of isolated rings of human internal mammary artery to endothelin (ET) and norepinephrine (NE) is presented as a percent of the response to 30 mM KCl (Panel A). Relaxation in response to acetylcholine (ACh) and sodium nitroprusside (SNP) of internal mammary artery rings preconstricted with ET (solid symbols) or NE (open symbols) (Panel B).

consistent with preliminary laboratory work using animal models of myocardial infarction (38), and suggest the release of considerable amounts of ET by the coronary bed during ischemia. Indeed, the concentrations of ET within the vessel wall at the site of its production and release may be orders of magnitude greater than the circulating levels found in plasma, and well within the range for its potent biological actions. Locally produced endothelin may ultimately increase infarct size by jeopardising perfusion to potentially viable myocardium. When infused in high concentration into the coronary circulation in vivo, ET can induce severe cardiac ischemia (6) leading to catastrophic myocardial dysfunction and death.

Therefore, under physiological conditions it is imperative that the release of endothelium-derived vasoactive factors be regulated in a coordinated manner. The excess production of ET for example, as may occur in ischemic injury, could compromise myocardial perfusion. Very little is known at present about the potential mechanisms which may operate to regulate the synthetic activity of normal endothelium. In situ, the endothelium

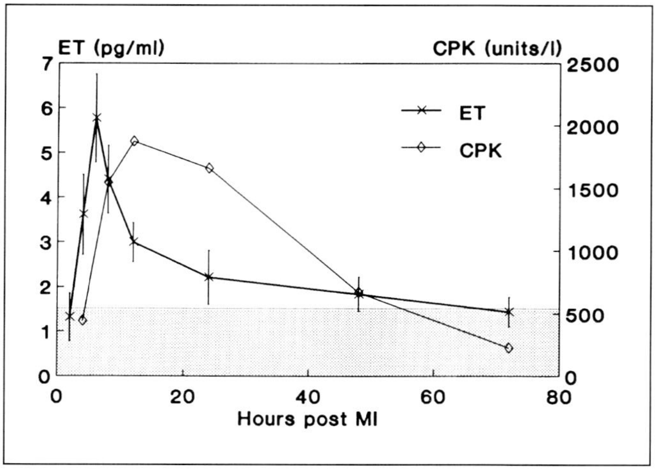

Fig. 7. Serial plasma levels of endothelin (ET, lefthand ordinate) and creatinine phosphokinase (CPK, righthand ordinate) are shown for 16 patients from 2 to 72 h following uncomplicated, acute myocardial infarction (MI).

demonstrates considerable basal release of EDRF, while the release of ET from intact vascular tissue may be less than that from endothelial cells culture. It has recently been suggested that EDRF (NO) may in fact inhibit thrombin-stimulated production of ET by a cyclic GMP-dependent mechanism (2) in strips of porcine aorta. However, this mechanism did not alter basal release of ET from aortic strips. We have suggested that basal ET release in intact vessels may be reduced by an inhibitory interaction between endothelial cells and cells of the vascular media, particularly smooth muscle cells. We have tested this hypothesis using co-culture of endothelial and smooth muscle cells (33). When cultured alone, endothelial cells released large amounts of ET into the media in a constitutive manner. However, in co-culture with smooth muscle, the release of ET was markedly reduced, by greater than 80% of control values. Furthermore, this inhibitory activity could be transferred in media conditioned by prior exposure to smooth muscle cells, indicating the release of an inhibitory factor by smooth muscle (33). The chemical nature and biological activity of the putative smooth-muscle derived inhibitory factor is now under investigation. It is possible that this represents a novel system for the regulation of endothelial cell function in the vessel wall. It has been long recognized that the endothelium can markedly alter the functional state of the underlying smooth muscle by virtue of the release of endothelium-derived vasoactive factors. We now propose that vascular smooth muscle may "feedback" on the endothelium by the action of its own regulatory factor(s).

In the decade following the landmark observations of Furchgott, much has been learned about the role of the endothelium in the control of coronary vasomotor tone. Far from being a pharmacological curiosity, endothelium-dependent vasomotion appears to be a fundamental mechanism of physiological regulation of conductance and resistance coronary vessel tone. Communication between endothelial and smooth muscle cells is vital to the ability of the vessel wall to adapt to changing rheological conditions. At present, EDRF and ET represent two of the best characterized endothelial-derived vasoactive factors, and abundant evidence is accumulating supporting their crucial roles in various physiological and/or pathophysiological processes. In the future we may learn that additional factors produced by the endothelium, and perhaps other cells of the vessel wall as well, may play an equally important part in the complex local mechanisms which optimize vascular tone at all levels of the coronary bed in response to the ever changing hemodynamic conditions and myocardial needs.

References

1. Bassenge E, Busse R (1988) Endothelial modulation of coronary tone. Prog Cardiovasc Dis 30:349–380
2. Boulanger C, Lüscher TF (1990) Release of endothelin from the porcine aorta. Inhibition by endothelium-derived nitric oxide. J Clin Invest 85:587–590
3. Busse R, Fichtner H, Lückhoff A, Kohlhardt M (1988) Hyperpolarization and increased free calcium in acetylcholine-stimulated endothelial cells. Am J Physiol 255:H965–H969
4. Chester AH, Dashwood MR, Clarke JG, Larkin SW, Davies GJ, Tadjkarimi S, Maseri A, Yacoub MH (1989) Influence of endothelin on human coronary arteries and localization of its binding sites. Am J Cardiol 63:1395–1398
5. Cocks TM, Angus JA (1983) Endothelium-dependent relaxation of coronary arteries by noradrenaline and serotonin. Nature 305:627
6. Ezra D, Goldstein RE, Czaja JF, Feuerstein GZ (1989) Lethal ischemia due to intracoronary endothelin in pigs. Am J Physiol 257:H339–H343
7. Furchgott RF, Vanhoutte PM (1989) Endothelium-derived relaxing and contracting factors. FASEB J 3:2007–2018
8. Furchgott RF, Zawadzski JV (1980) The obligatory role of endothelial cells in the relaxation of arterial smooth muscle to acetylcholine. Nature 288:373–376
9. Griffith TM, Lewis MJ, Newby AC, Henderson AH (1988) Endothelium-derived relaxing factor. J Am Coll Cardiol 12:797–806
10. Halliwell B, Gutteridge JMC (1986) Iron and free radical reactions: two aspects of antioxidant protection. TIBS 11:372–375
11. Hughes AD, Thom SAM, Woodall N, Schachter M, Hair WM, Martin GN, Sever PS (1989) Human vascular responses to endothelin-1: observations in vivo and in vitro. J Cardiovasc Pharmacol 13 (Suppl 5):S225–S228
12. Ignarro LJ, Buga GM, Byrns RE, Wood KS, Chaudhuri G (199) Endothelium-derived relaxing factor and nitric oxide possess identical pharmacologic properties as relaxants of bovine arterial and venous smooth muscle. J Pharmacol Exp Ther 246:218–226
13. Jackson CV, Mickelson JK, Pope TK, Rao PS, Lucchesi BR (1987) O_2 free radical-mediated myocardial and vascular dysfunction. Am J Physiol 251:H1225–H1231
14. Kelm M, Schrader J (1988) Nitric oxide release from the isolated guinea pig heart. Eur J Pharmacol 155:317–321
15. Komori K, Lorenz RR, Vanhoutte PM (1988) Nitric oxide, Ach, and electrical and mechanical properties of canine arterial smooth muscle. Am J Physiol 255:H207–H212
16. Kubac G, Cernacek P, Mohamed F, Stewart DJ (1990) Plasma endothelin (ET) is elevated in the early hours following myocardial infarction (MI): possible diagnostic and prognostic implications. 13th Scientific Meeting of the International Society of Hypertension June 24–29 (abstract)
17. Lüscher TF, Richard V, Tschudi M, Yang Z, Boulanger C (1990) Endothelial control of vascular tone in large and small coronary arteries. J Am Coll Cardiol 15:519–527

18. Lüscher TF, Yang Z, Tschudi M, Segesser L von, Stulz P, Boulanger C, Siebenmann R, Turina M, Bühler FR (1990) Interaction between endothelin-1 and endothelium-derived relaxing factor in human arteries and veins. Circ Res 66:1088–1094
19. Martin W, Villani GM, Jothiananda D, Furchgott RF (1985) Selective blockade of endothelium-dependent and glyceryl trinitrate-induced relaxation by hemoglobin and methylene blue in rabbit aorta. J Pharmacol Exp Ther 232:708–716
20. McCord JM (1985) Oxygen-derived free radicals in postischemic tissue injury. N Engl J Med 312:159–163
21. Miyauchi T, Yanagisawa M, Tomizawa T, Sughishita Y, Suzuki N, Fujino M, Ajisaka R, Goto K, Masaki T (1989) Increased plasma concentrations of endothelin-1 and big endothelin-1 in acute myocardial infarction. Lancet 2:53–54
22. Moghtader S, Belichard P, Calderone A, Rouleau JL, Stewart DJ (1990) Endothelin-induced coronary vasoconstriction is enhanced by experimental heart failure in dogs. FASEB J 4:A960 (abstract)
23. Myers PR, Guerra R Jr, Harrison DG (1989) Release of NO and EDRF from cultured bovine aortic endothelial cells. Am J Physiol 256:H1030–H1037
24. Mülsch A, Busse R (1990) N^G-nitro-L-arginine (N^5-[imino(nitroamino)methyl]-L–ornithine) impairs endothelium-dependent dilations by inhibiting cytosolic nitric oxide synthesis from L-arginine. Naunyn Schmiedebergs Arch Pharmacol 341:143–147
25. Palmer RMJ, Ferrige AG, Moncada S (1987) Nitric oxide release accounts for the biological activity of endothelium-derived relaxing factor. Nature 327:524–526
26. Palmer RMJ, Moncada S (1989) A novel citrulline-forming enzyme implicated in the formation of nitric oxide by vascular endothelial cells. Biochem Biophys Res Commun 158:348–352
27. Pohl U, Busse R (1989) Differential vascular sensitivity to luminally and adventitially applied endothelin-1. J Cardiovasc Pharmacol 13 (Suppl 5):S188–S190
28. Rees DD, Palmer RMJ, Hodson HF, Moncada S (1989) A specific inhibitor of nitric oxide formation from L-arginine attenuates endothelium-dependent relaxation. Br J Pharmacol 96:418–424
29. Rubanyi GM, Vanhoutte PM (1986) Superoxide anions and hyperoxia inactivate endothelium-derived relaxing factor. Am J Physiol 250:H822–H827
30. Stewart DJ, Baffour R (1990) Ischemia-reperfusion potentiates endothelin-induced constriction in the coronary resistance bed. In: Rubanyi GM, Vanhoutte PM (eds) Endothelium-derived vasoactive factors. Basel: Karger
31. Stewart DJ, Baffour R (1990) Functional state of the endothelium determines the response to endothelin in the coronary circulation. Cardiovasc Res 24:7–12
32. Stewart DJ, Holtz J, Pohl U, Bassenge E (1987) Balance between endothelium-mediated dilating and direct constricting actions of serotonin on resistance vessels in the isolated rabbit heart. Eur J Pharmacol 143:131–134
33. Stewart DJ, Langleben D, Danes D, Cernacek P, Cianflone K (1990) Endothelin (ET) release is markedly reduced in co-culture: evidence for a transferable inhibitor. FASEB J 4:A1081–A1081 (Abstract)
34. Stewart DJ, Münzel T, Bassenge E (1987) Reversal of acetylcholine-induced coronary resistance vessel dilation by hemoglobin. Eur J Pharmacol 136:239–242
35. Stewart DJ, Pohl U, Bassenge E (1988) Free radicals inhibit endothelium-dependent dilation in the coronary resistance bed. Am J Physiol 255:H765–H769
36. Thomas G, Farhat M, Myers AK, Ramwell PW (1990) Effect of Nα-benzoyl-L-arginine ethyl ester on coronary perfusion pressure in isolated guinea pig heart. Eur J Pharmacol 178:251–254
37. Vita JA, Treasure CB, Nabel EG, McLenachan JM, Fish RD, Yeung AC, Vekshtein VI, Selwyn AP, Ganz P (1990) Coronary vasomotor response to acetylcholine relates to risk factors for coronary artery disease. Circulation 81:491–497
38. Watanabe T, Suzuki N, Shimamoto N, Fujino M, Imada A (1990) Endothelin in myocardial infarction. Nature 344:144–144
39. Yanagisawa M, Kurihara H, Kimura S, Tomobe Y, Kobayashi M, Mitsui Y, Yazaki Y, Goto K, Masaki T (1988) A novel potent vasoconstrictor peptide produce by vascular endothelial cells. Nature 332:411–415

40. Yasuda M, Kohno M, Tahara A, Itagane H, Toda I, Akioka K, Teragaki M, Oku H, Takeuchi K, Takeda T (1990) Circulating immunoreactive endothelin in ischemic heart disease. Am Heart J 119:801–806

Author's address:
D. J. Stewart
Royal Victoria Hospital
Rm M4.76
687 Pine Avenue West
Montreal, Canada, H3A 1A1

Blood flow and optimal vascular topography: role of the endothelium

T. M. Griffith, D. H. Edwards [1], M. D. Randall

[1] Department of Radiology and Cardiology, University of Wales College of Medicine, Heath Park, Cardiff, UK

Summary: We have used x-ray microangiography to investigate the influence of EDRF and endothelin-1 on arterial diameters (70–800 µm) at bifurcations in the isolated rabbit ear and the "optimality" of its branching geometry. The median value of the junction exponent x (which is given by $d_0^x = d_1^x + d_2^x$, where d_0, d_1 and d_2 are parent and daughter artery diameters respectively) was close to 3 at different flow rates in unconstricted preparations. When $x = 3$, branching geometry is optimal in that i) power losses and intravascular volume are both minimised, and ii) fractal considerations suggest that the total surface area for metabolic exchange is maximised. Under conditions of vasoconstriction (by 5HT/histamine) the junction exponent deviated from its control value but was restored towards 3, both by basal and by acetylcholine-stimulated EDRF activity. In contrast, endothelin-1 caused a dose-dependent reduction in the junction exponent from its optimal value 3. This suggests that the endothelium helps to optimise microvascular function through EDRF but not endothelin-1 release.

Key words: Endothelium; EDRF; endothelin-1; optimality; rabbit ear; microvascular function

Introduction

The physiological adaptation of arterial diameters to acute changes in flow ("flow-dependent dilatation") is thought to be mediated by stimulation of endothelium-derived relaxing factor (EDRF) activity in response to shear stress (14–15). Long-term adaptation to changes in flow rate is also dependent on endothelial cells and may involve chronic modulation of EDRF activity (9, 12). It remains unclear, however, whether the endothelium-derived vasoconstrictor peptide endothelin-1 is involved in arterial responses to changes in flow, although there is evidence that its production is influenced by shear stress and that it exerts a mitogenic effect upon vascular smooth muscle (8, 20). In the present study we have investigated how EDRF and endothelin-1 affect parent (d_0) and daughter (d_1 and d_2) diameters and thus the distribution of flow at arterial bifurcations. The data have been related to "optimality" of branching geometry by analysis of the frequency distributions of the junction exponent x, which is given by the expression $d_0^x = d_1^x + d_2^x$. This parameter can be related to branching angles though optimisation principles based on minimisation of surface area, volume, shear stress (drag) and power losses, and is also an important determinant of the geometrical space-filling properties of vascular networks.

Experimental methods

The x-ray microangiographic technique employed and the topography of the vascular network of the rabbit ear have been described in detail (3–5). Briefly, isolated ear preparations from 2.5 kg New Zealand White rabbits were perfused under conditions of steady flow with oxygenated (95% O_2, 5% CO_2) Holman's buffer at 35° C. Microangiograms were obtained following the introduction of a short pulse of dilute iodinated (~100 mg/ml) radiographic contrast medium into the perfusate after changes in flow rate or addition of drugs when perfusion pressure had restabilized (ca. 10–15 min). In vitro preparations possess low intrinsic tone under resting conditions, so that in some experiments constrictor agonists (0.1 μM 5 HT or the combination of 1 μM 5 HT plus 1 μM histamine) were used to "mimic" the tone present in vivo. Freshly prepared and purified haemoglobin solution (concentration 1 μM) was used to inhibit EDRF activity (2), and the interaction between flow and basal EDRF activity was studied at four flow rates (1, 2, 3.5 and 5 ml/min). Stimulated EDRF release was studied by constructing concentration-response curves to the endothelium-dependent vasodilator acetylcholine after constriction by 1 μM 5HT plus 1 μM histamine. These agonists do not themselves stimulate EDRF release in these preparations (4) and their combination was found necessary to give stable constrictor responses. Endothelin-1 was administered by bolus injection and generally caused sustained (10–60 min) vasoconstriction.

Junction Exponents

Junction exponents x were calculated iteratively from the expression $d_0^x = d_1^x + d_2^x$ at bifurcations between the central ear artery (ca. 700 μm diameter) and its fourth branch generation (ca. 90 μm diameter). Diameters and branching angles were measured with a semi-interactive image analysis system.

Optimality Nomogram

The "optimality" of branching geometry at arterial bifurcations can be studied through mathematical models which minimise the total surface area ($\propto d$), volume ($\propto d^2$), drag/shear stress ($\propto \dot{q}/d^2$) or power losses ($\propto \dot{q}^2/d^4$) involved, assuming in the latter two cases that flow is laminar and blood Newtonian (d = diameter, $\dot{q}$ = flow rate). These models allow calculation of optimal branching angles which can be compared with actual angles (6, 13, 19, 21). Woldenberg and Horsfield used four expressions which relate the optimal angle between the two daughter arteries at a bifurcation to the junction exponent x, and the asymmetry ratio α ($= d_2/d_1$) of the daughter arteries (19). These provide an essentially two-dimensional nomogram for analysis of optimality at arterial bifurcations as plots of the optimal junction exponent/branching angle relationship are insensitive to the exact value of the asymmetry ratio.

Results

Effects of Flow Rate/Basal EDRF Activity

Four different experimental groups were studied: resting ± haemoglobin, 0.1 μm 5HT ± haemoglobin.

a) *Junction Exponents*

The modes of the frequency distributions of the junction exponent x were ca. 3 at each flow rate in resting preparations, both in the absence and the presence of haemoglobin, and in preparations constricted by 0.1 μM 5HT alone (Fig. 1a, b, c). Medians were generally slightly greater than 3 because the distributions were positively skewed. In contrast, after inhibition of EDRF activity in 0.1 μM 5HT-constricted preparations, no well-defined mode could be identified (Fig. 1d), and the median at each flow rate was increased (to 4.2–5.7, $p < 0.05$, unpaired one-tailed Mann-Whitney tests). There was no systematic variation in junction exponents with flow rate in any of the experimental groups ($p < 0.05$, non-parametric Friedman two-way analysis of variance by ranks).

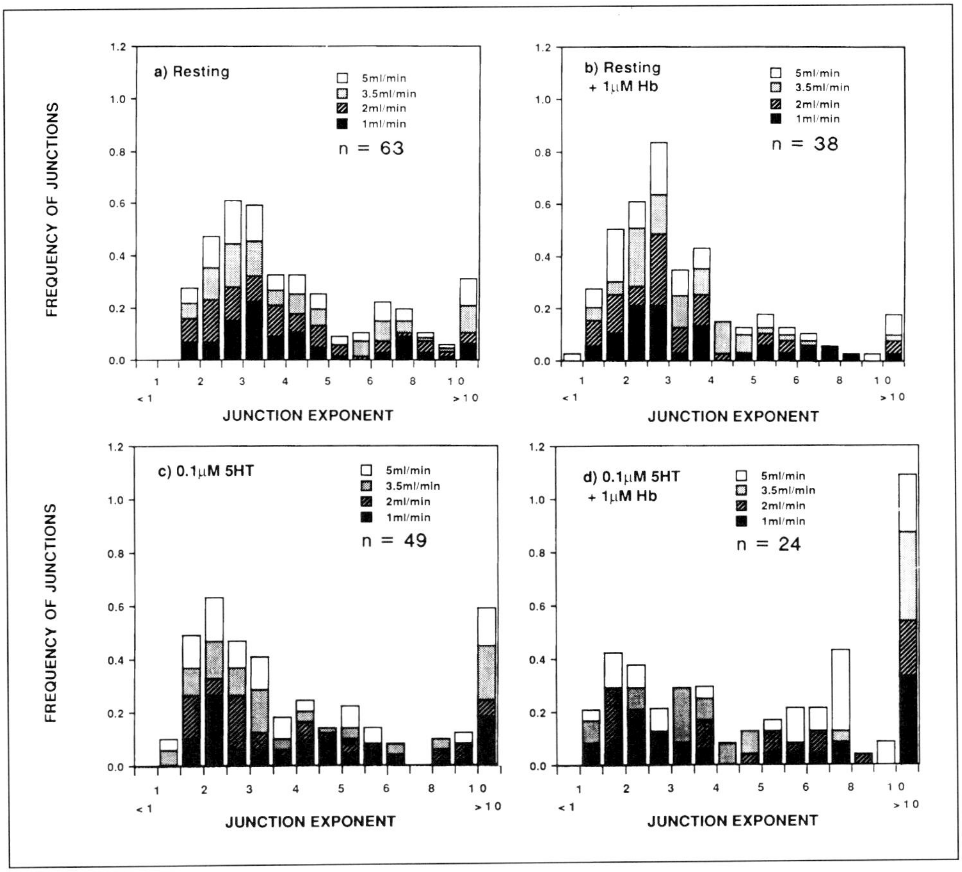

Fig. 1. Frequency distributions of junction exponents at four flow rates stacked in the ordinate direction. Before (**a**) and after (**b**) inhibition of EDRF activity by 1 μM haemoglobin (Hb) in pharmacologically-unconstricted preparations and before (**c**) and after (**d**) inhibition of EDRF activity by haemoglobin in preparations constricted by 0.1 μM 5HT. (n = number of bifurcations studied.)

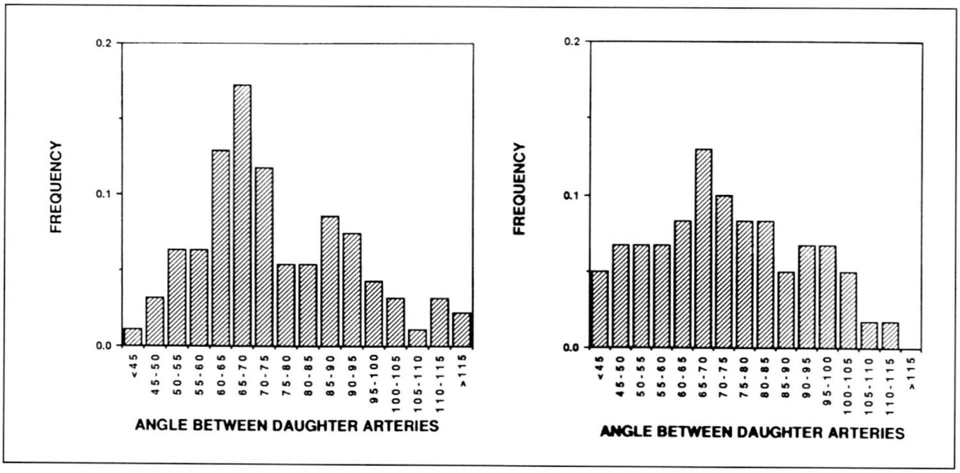

Fig. 2. Frequency distributions of the bifurcation angle between daughter arteries (ψ) for pooled data from the experiments of Fig. 1 (left) and the experiments of Fig. 3 (right). In both cases the median was 72°, and the mode between 65° and 70°

b) *Bifurcation Angles*

Branching angles were not influenced by flow rate or changes in vasomotor tone. A median value for the angle between the two daughter arteries at each bifurcation ψ was calculated for: 1) each of the four experimental groups (70°, 79°, 68°, 75°), and 2) for pooled data (72°) (Fig. 2a, 4). The frequency distribution of the pooled data was positively skewed, with a mode in the range 65–70°.

Median values of x and ψ were plotted on the optimality nomogram for the four minimisation principles. In resting preparations, both in the presence and the absence of haemoglobin, and in preparations constricted by 5HT alone, the experimental data fell close to the intersection of the optimal minimum volume and minimum power loss relationships at all flow rates. In contrast, in 5HT-constricted preparations with haemoglobin (i.e., in the absence of EDRF activity) the experimental data points were displaced above this intersection point (Fig. 4, left).

Effects of Constrictor Tone/Stimulated EDRF Activity

a) *Junction Exponents*

The median x was 2.92 for pooled control data obtained before vasoconstriction by 1 μM 5HT/1 μM histamine or endothelin-1 (Fig. 3). In the presence of 1 μM 5 HT/1 μM histamine the (median) x was decreased to 2.40 but was restored towards the value 3 by acetylcholine in a concentration-dependent manner (Fig. 4, right). Bolus injections of endothelin-1 decreased (median) x in a dose-dependent fashion, the exponent falling to 1.25 (at 60 pmol) (Fig. 4).

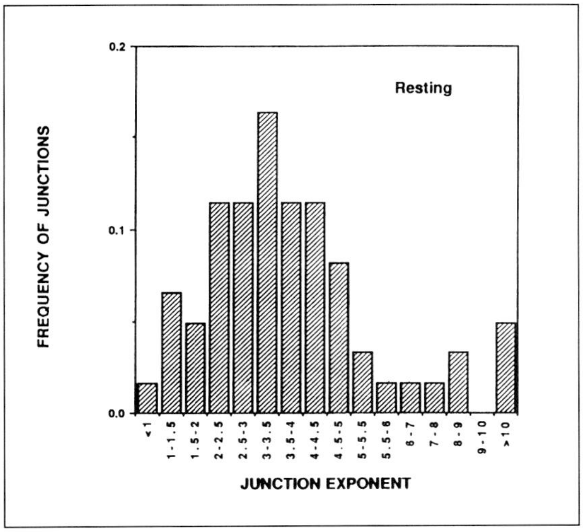

Fig. 3. Frequency distribution of the junction exponent x for the control data obtained before constriction by 5HT plus histamine and by endothelin-1 (n = 66 bifurcations, pooled results). The median was 2.92

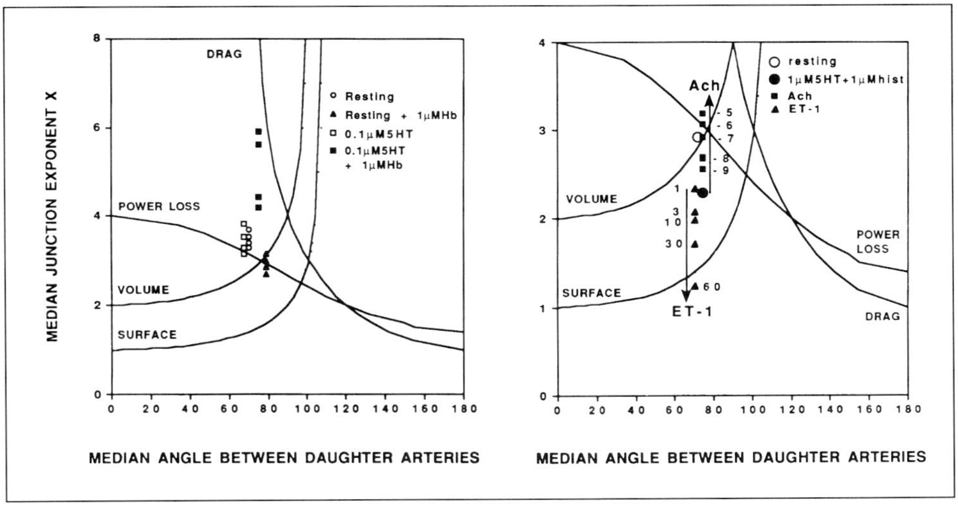

Fig. 4. Plots of the median junction exponent x against corresponding median values of the bifurcation angle between daughter arteries ψ. The continuous curves give the optimal x-ψ relationships for the four minimisation principles indicated. Left: manipulation of flow rate and EDRF activity. The data points lie close to the intersection of the minimum volume and power loss curves at all flow rates, except in 0.1 µM 5HT-constricted preparations after inhibition of EDRF activity by haemoglobin (closed squares). Right: Effect of dilatation by acetylcholine (ACh) at the $\log_{10}$ [molar] concentrations shown (squares) following constriction by the combination of 1 µM 5HT plus 1 µM histamine (closed circle) and of constriction by endothelin-1 (ET-1, pmol) (triangles). The position of the median x before constriction is again close to the intersection of the minimum volume and power loss curves (open circle, pooled data for both sets of experiments). Constriction by either 5HT plus histamine or by endothelin-1 reduced the median x, whereas acetylcholine restored its position towards the "optimal" point

b) *Bifurcation Angles*

The frequency distribution of ψ for pooled data from the 5HT/histamine and endothelin-1 experiments was again positively skewed with a median of 72° and a mode in the range 65–70° (Fig. 2 b).

When median values of x and ψ were plotted on the optimality nomogram, constriction by both endothelin-1 or by 5HT/histamine displaced the data points below the intersection of the minimum volume and power loss curves. Conversely, in 5HT/histamine constricted preparations, acetylcholine restored the data points back towards the "optimal" point ($x=3$) in a concentration-dependent fashion.

Discussion

We have examined the influence of EDRF and endothelin-1 on the "optimality" of the branching geometry of the rabbit ear by plotting junction exponents x, and bifurcation angles ψ on a nomogram of optimal x-ψ relationships for four models which minimise respectively surface, volume, drag and power losses. The minimum volume and minimum power loss relationships always intersect where $x=3$ and when ψ is 75–80° (the exact value being dependent on the asymmetry ratio α) (6, 19). The experiments were performed under conditions of steady laminar flow. The importance of pulsatility is, however, likely to be small as physiological "integration" of the myogenic response damps out pulsatile changes in the diameter of rabbit ear resistance vessels (17).

Murray suggested that arterial diameters (d) and flow rates (q) are matched in such a way as to minimise the sum of viscous power losses and the energetic cost of a high blood volume and showed that the optimal diameter-flow relationship would then be cubic for steady Newtonian flow (i.e., $\dot{q} \propto d^3$) (13). The continuity equation for flow at a bifurcation, $q_0 = q_1 + q_2$, is then transformed to $d_0{}^3 = d_1{}^3 + d_2{}^3$ so that Murray's hypothesis predicts that the optimal junction exponent should be 3.

An alternative explanation for a junction exponent close to 3 has been given by Mandelbrot (10). If the geometry of vascular branching is self-similar (i.e., each vascular division repeats the previous one on a smaller scale) and diameters are small compared to the volume occupied, $x=3$ would generate a vascular network in which the most distal vessels would exactly fill the space available to them. If $x/3$, successive generations either run out of space in which to grow or occupy only part of the space available. Selfsimilarity implies that vascular growth is determined by the ratio of branch width/branch length and the junction exponent x. This would be the simplest rule which could govern angiogenesis and would obviate the necessity to encode deterministic minimisation principles based on physical parameters genetically. Interestingly, a recursively applied self-similar growth and branching rule derived from experimental data with a junction exponent close to 3 generates anatomically accurate models of the renal vasculature (1).

In the present study junction exponents remained close to 3 in both resting and 0.1 μM 5HT-constricted preparations at different flow rates except, in the latter case, when EDRF activity was inhibited by haemoglobin. Moreover, in preparations constricted by the combination of 1 μM 5HT/1 μM histamine, which decreased the junction exponent, the EDRF-dependent vasodilator acetylcholine restored x to a value close to 3. Branching geometry was thus found to remain "optimal" when the level of EDRF activity was sufficiently high to depress exogeneously increased vasomotor tone. Consistent with the idea that vasoconstriction adversely affects the optimality of branching geometry, endothelin-1 caused a dose-dependent decrease in the junction exponent.

Other workers have produced evidence in support of Murray's hypothesis in small conduit and resistance arteries of the rat both in vivo (11) and by analysis of arterial casts (22). In cat skeletal muscle frequency distributions of the junction exponent were similar in shape to those of the present study with modes in the range 2.5 to 4, although their medians were in the range 4–5 (16). In large human pulmonary arteries, where inertial considerations dominate over viscous power losses and the assumptions underlying the derivation of Murray's law are likely to be invalid, junction exponents have been reported to be in the range 1–2 (18).

Physiological significance

Minimisation of power losses at bifurcations would contribute to the "efficiency" of the circulation by reducing cardiac work. The hypothesis that the junction exponent should be close to 3 on the grounds that the geometry of branching would then be "ideally" space-filling and thus provide maximum surface area for the exchange of oxygen and metabolites (or heat in the case of the rabbit ear) has obvious relevance (10). The significance of a minimum volume optimality principle may be related to the fact that large and rapid changes in flow rate are sometimes required in the circulation. During exercise, for example, skeletal muscle resistance falls by over 90% and flow increases by up to 20-fold; it is clearly preferable to increase flow by reducing resistance, than to increase pressure to levels which could impair cardiac function (7). This would be facilitated by a "minimum volume" circulation, where small changes in artery diameters would have a large effect on flow relative to pressure. Arguments that "minimum volume" would facilitate the rapid dissemination of humoral stimuli and reduce the "energetic cost" of blood are unconvincing since the venous system contains such a large proportion of the total blood volume.

Previous workers have noted that branching angles and junction exponents exhibit considerable scatter (16, 22, 23). This was also the case in the present study. The optima of the minimisation principles studied have, however, been shown to be "shallow" in the sense that the total "cost" of a bifurcation is always within a few % of the predicted minimum (23). This also applies to junction exponents: power losses increase by only ca. 5% above those for $x = 3$ over the range 1.5 to 100 (16). Whether the "rules" which govern angiogenesis are physical optimisation principles and/or fractal space-filling considerations, EDRF activity nevertheless appears to be necessary for their accurate operation at different flow rates in the presence of constrictor tone. Impairment of EDRF activity in disease states may therefore be seen as reducing the "efficiency" of vascular perfusion.

Acknowledgements. The work was funded by the British Heart Foundation. The authors thank Miss R St Leger for secretarial assistance and Professor A H Henderson for helpful comments during preparation of the manuscript.

References

1. Bittner HR, Wlczek P, Sernetz M (1989) Characterization of fractal biological objects by image analysis. Acta Stereol 8:31–40
2. Edwards DH, Griffith TM, Ryley HC, Henderson AH (1986) Haptoglobin-haemoglobin complex in human plasma inhibits endothelium-dependent relaxation: evidence that endothelium-derived relaxing factor acts as a local autacoid. Cardiovasc Res 20:549–556
3. Griffith TM, Edwards DH, Davies RLl, Harrison TJ, Evans KT (1987) EDRF coordinates the behaviour of vascular resistance vessels. Nature 329:442–445

4. Griffith TM, Edwards DH, Davies RLl, Harrison TJ, Evans KT (1988) Endothelium-derived relaxing factor (EDRF) and resistance vessels in an intact vascular bed: a microangiographic study of the rabbit isolated ear. Br J Pharmacol 93:654–662
5. Griffith TM, Edwards DH, Davies RLl, Henderson AH (1989) The role of EDRF in flow distribution: a microangiographic study of the rabbit isolated ear. Microvascular Res 37:162–177
6. Griffith TM, Edwards DH (1990) Basal EDRF activity helps to keep the geometrical configuration of arterial bifurcations close to the Murray optimum. J Theor Biol 146:545–573
7. Harris P (1983) Evolution and the cardiac patient: Origins of the blood pressure. Cardiovascular Res 17:373–378
8. Hirata Y, Takagi Y, Fukuda Y, Marumo F (1989) Endothelin is a potent mitogen for rat vascular smooth muscle cells. Atherosclerosis 78:225–228
9. Langille L, O'Donnell F (1986) Reductions in arterial diameter produced by chronic decreases in blood flow are endothelium-dependent. Science 231:405–407
10. Mandelbrot BB (1982) The fractal geometry of nature. Freeman, N.Y. pp 158
11. Mayrovitz HN, Roy J (1982) Microvascular blood flow: evidence indicating a cubic dependence on arteriolar diameter. Am J Physiol 245:H1031–H1038
12. Miller VM, Vanhoutte PM (1988) Enhanced release of endothelium-derived factor(s) by chronic increases in blood flow. Am J Physiol 255:H446–H451
13. Murray CD (1926) The physiological principle of minimum work applied to the angle of branching of arteries. J Gen Physiol 9:835–841
14. Pohl U, Busse R, Kuon E, Bassenge E (1986) Pulsatile perfusion stimulates the release of endothelial autacoids. J Appl Cardiol 1:215–235
15. Rubanyi GM, Romero JC, Vanhoutte PM (1986) Flow-induced release of endothelium-derived relaxing factor. Am J Physiol 250:H1145–H1149
16. Sherman TF, Popel AS, Koller A, Johnson PC (1989) The cost of departure from optimal radii in microvascular networks. J Theor Biol 136:245–265
17. Speden RN, Warren DM (1986) Myogenic adaptation of rabbit ear arteries to pulsatile internal pressure. J Physiol (Lond) 391:313–323
18. Woldenberg MJ, Horsfield K (1983) Finding the optimal lengths for three branches as a junction. J Theor Biol 104:301–318
19. Woldenberg MJ, Horsfield K (1986) Relation of branching angles to optimality for four cost principles. J Theor Biol 122:187–204
20. Yosizumi M, Kurihara H, Sugiyama T, Takaku F, Yanagisawa M, Masaki T, Yazaki Y (1989) Haemodynamic shear stress stimulates endothelin production by cultured endothelial cells. Biochem Biophys Res Comm 161:859–864
21. Zamir M (1976) Optimality principles in arterial branching. J Theor Biol 62:227–251
22. Zamir M, Wrigley SM, Langille BL (1983) Arterial bifurcations in the cardiovascular system of a rat. J Gen Physiol 81:325–335
23. Zamir M, Bigelow DC (1984) Cost of departure from optimality in arterial branching. J Theor Biol 109:401–409

Author's address:
T. M. Griffith, M. D.
Department of Cardiology and Radiology
University of Wales College of Medicine
Health Park
GB-Cardiff
CF4 4XN

Impaired tissue perfusion after inhibition of endothelium-derived nitric oxide

U. Pohl [1] and D. Lamontagne [2]

[1] Institute of Physiology, Med. University of Lübeck, and
[2] Institute of Applied Physiology, University of Freiburg, FRG

Summary: The effects of a blockade of the action or synthesis of endothelium-derived nitric oxide (EDRF) on vascular resistance and reactivity, platelet cGMP and tissue oxygenation were studied. Experiments were performed in isolated perfused rabbit hearts as well as in rabbit hindlimbs in vivo. In isolated hearts, perfusion with hemoglobin (6 μM) or N^G-nitro-L-arginine (30 μM) significantly increased vascular resistance. The cGMP level in platelets passing through the coronary bed was found to be more than 50% lower than with intact EDRF production. EDRF inhibition also resulted in a reduced peak reactive hyperemia, an enhanced reactive vasoconstriction after a rapid increase in perfusion pressure (myogenic response), and in abolition of flow-dependent dilation of coronary resistance vessels. In rabbit hindlimbs, local blockade of EDRF-mediated dilations by gossypol resulted also in an increased vascular resistance and abolition of the increase in platelet cGMP induced by intraarterial infusion of acetylcholine. In addition, the oxygen uptake of the hindlimb (−46%) and the skeletal muscle pO_2 were significantly reduced. It is concluded that continuously released EDRF has a functional role in maintaining adequate tissue perfusion and oxygen supply. Furthermore, the adaption of the vascular bed to rapid changes in flow and pressure is impaired after inhibition of EDRF.

Key words: EDRF; Langendorff heart; vascular resistance; basal release; myogenic response; flow-dependent dilation; pO_2; tissue oxygen supply

Introduction

Numerous investigations have shown that endothelium-derived nitric oxide (EDRF) is a potent vasodilator (3, 6, 16). Since many physiologic and pharmacologic compounds simultaneously stimulate release of EDRF and at the same time elicit direct constrictor effects on vascular smooth muscle (3,6), it is evident that an impaired production of EDRF must have considerable pathophysiologic consequences. Several studies in animals and man suggest that a lack of EDRF might be an important *pathophysiologic* factor in coronary heart disease (13, 14, 27, 31, 32). The *physiologic* role of EDRF in the control of local blood flow and oxygen supply still remains to be determined. However, in cultured endothelial cells and isolated vessels there is evidence for a continuous basal release of EDRF , which might be maintained in part by the pulsatile blood flow (8, 17, 18, 26) and by the stimulatory effects of a reduced pO_2 (21) in small arterioles. Furthermore, studies in several microvascular preparations and intact organs demonstrate that EDRF-mediated dilations do occur in resistance vessels (8, 12, 19, 25, 28). It has also been shown that non-metabolizable analogues of L-arginine, the precursor of nitric oxide, induce an increase in blood pressure which can be explained as inhibition of a basal EDRF-release (24,30). These findings suggest that EDRF is an important factor in the local control of blood flow. Here we report that scavenging of EDRF or inhibition of its synthesis results in an impaired tissue oxygen supply in vitro and in vivo and a reduced adaptation of blood flow to the rapidly changing demands of the tissue.

Methods

Experiments were performed in isolated rabbit hearts (Langendorff preparation) and in autoperfused rabbit hindlimbs.

Isolated rabbit heart

The hearts of mongrel rabbits (1.0–1.5 kg) were excised immediately after administration of a lethal dose of sodium pentobarbital. Flow-controlled perfusion was performed by means of a roller pump using a modified Krebs-Henseleit buffer as described earlier (29). Test solutions and platelet boluses were administered through a Y-connector in the aortic perfusion line. To assess the effects of the coronary endothelium on platelet cGMP, which was determined by a commercially available radioimmunoassay, the coronary effluent was collected following the injection of platelets.

The effect of sudden changes of coronary perfusion pressure on coronary tone (myogenic response was studied under pressure controlled conditions). To this end, the hearts were perfused through a reservoir whose hydrostatic level above the heart could be varied between 50 cm H_2O and 200 cm H_2O.

Injections were performed under control (unstimulated) conditions and 2 min after beginning continuous administration of acetylcholine (1 μM).

Autoperfused rabbit hindlimb in vivo

The femoral arteries of anesthetized rabbits were exposed for electromagnetic flow measurement and insertion of catheters. A multiwire Clark-type surface electrode (Eschweiler, Kiel, FRG) was positioned at the surface of the peroneus muscle distal to the artery for measurement of skeletal muscle surface pO_2 distribution. Samples of femoral arterial and venous blood were taken for determination of pO_2, pCO_2, and hemoglobin concentration to calculate the oxygen uptake of the hindlimb. Femoral blood flow reactivity, tissue oxygen uptake and local muscle pO_2 were studied before and after inhibition of EDRF by gossypol as described earlier (19). In additional experiments increases in platelet cGMP to EDRF stimulation with acetylcholine were compared before and after treatment with gossypol. Platelets were isolated within 25 min after sampling by a washing procedure similar to that described for in vitro experiments in the presence of the phosphodiesterase inhibitor zaprinast.

Drugs

N^G-nitro-L-arginine, obtained from Serva (Heidelberg, FRG) was dissolved by vigorous stirring in warmed (50° C) Tyrode's solution. Bovine hemoglobin (purchased from Sigma) was prepared as described previously (20). All other drugs were obtained from Sigma (Deisenhofen, FRG) and freshly dissolved in Tyrode's solution.

Statistics

Data are presented as means ±SEM. Comparisons were performed by means of paired or unpaired *t*-tests. Differences were considered significant at a *p*-value <0.05.

Results

Isolated heart

Perfusion of isolated perfused rabbit hearts with the EDRF-inhibitors hemoglobin (6 μM) or N^G-nitro-L-arginine (30 μM) did not only selectively block the dilator response to acetylcholine, but also resulted in a significant increase in peripheral resistance. Figure 1 shows a more than 50% reduction of resting coronary flow after treatment with N^G-nitro-L-arginine during pressure-controlled perfusion. Likewise, during flow-controlled perfusion (perfusion rate: 28 ± 2 ml/min), hemoglobin induced a significant increase in perfusion pressure from 51 ± 7 mm Hg to 87 ± 10 mm Hg ($p < 0.01$, n = 11).

Inhibition of EDRF by hemoglobin also resulted in a complete inhibition of the platelet cGMP increase upon stimulation of the coronary endothelium by acetylcholine; also, the basal cGMP level of platelets after passage through the heart was significantly lower (Fig. 2). Similar results were obtained after inhibition of EDRF synthesis with N^G-nitro-L-arginine (control: 0.5 ± 0.1 pmol/mg protein; N^G-nitro-L-arginine: 0.18 ± 0.08 pmol/mg protein; n = 7).

A sudden increase in pump flow (mean: 2.4 fold) under control conditions resulted in a rapid initial increase in perfusion pressure (from 63 to 132 mm Hg; n = 9), followed by a significant secondary decrease to 121 mm Hg within 3 min ($p < 0.05$). After inhibition of EDRF-synthesis by N^G-nitro-L-arginine, the same increase in flow induced a pressure increase from 82 to 153 mm Hg. No significant reduction of perfusion pressure could be

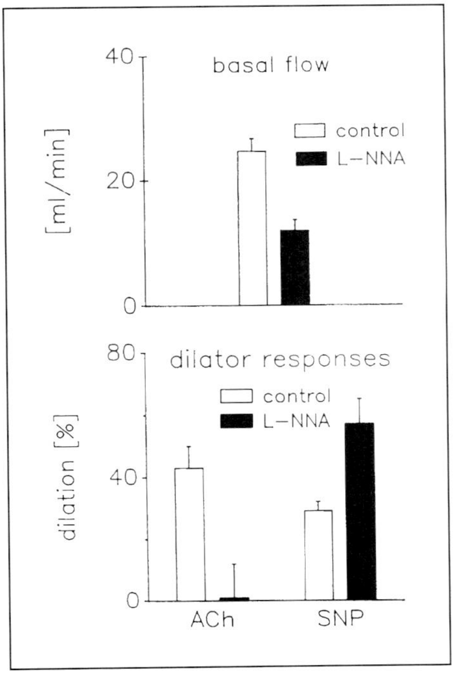

Fig. 1. Effect of the inhibitor of EDRF synthesis N^G-nitro-L-arginine (L-NNA 30 μM) on resting coronary flow and the dilator response to acetylcholine (ACh 1μM) and sodium nitroprusside (SNP, 1 μM); (n = 7)

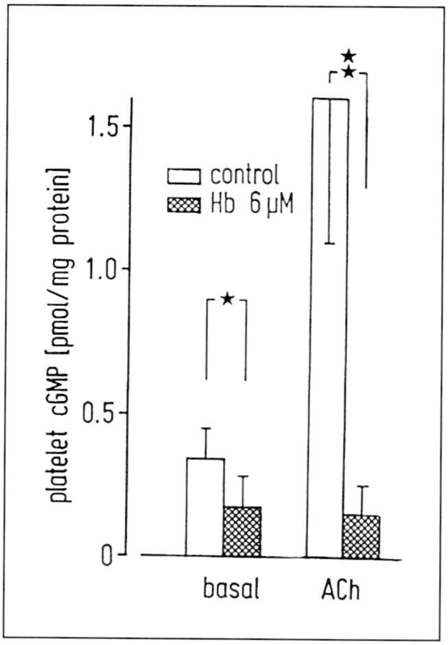

Fig. 2. Platelet cGMP content (pmol/mg platelet protein) after passage through the unstimulated heart (basal), and during EDRF stimulation with acetylcholine (ACh; 1 µM). In the presence of the EDRF-inhibitor hemoglobin (Hb), basal cGMP as well as the ACh-induced increase are significantly suppressed; (n = 11) $*p<0.05$, $**p<0.01$.

observed within 3 min (150 ± 15 mm Hg). In some cases even a further increase of perfusion pressure was observed.

To test whether this further increase in perfusion pressure could be due to an enhanced myogenic response, a pressure-controlled perfusion was performed. A sudden increase in the perfusion pressure from 50 to 120 mm Hg induced an initial increase in flow by 108 ± 13%, corresponding to a decrease in vascular resistance by 22 ± 4%. This was followed within 20 s by a renewed increase in vascular resistance by 12 ± 4%. After N^G-nitro-L-arginine, this increase in vascular resistance was significantly higher (55 ± 15%; $p<0.02$; Fig. 3).

To further test the coronary reactivity and conductivity to rapid changes in tissue demand, the peak reactive hyperemia (pressure-controlled perfusion; 55 mm Hg) was measured after 30 s of flow stop. The peak flow after treatment with N^G-nitro-L-arginine (32 ± 2 ml/min) was significantly lower ($p<0.05$) than during control (48 ± 1) or after treatment with the inactive D-enantiomer N^G-nitro-D-arginine 52 ± 3; n = 5).

In vivo studies

In the autoperfused (resting flow: 6.9 ± 7 ml/min) hindlimb of rabbits, acetylcholine (calculated blood concentration 8 µM) and adenosine (100 µM) infused into a femoral arterial side branch induced similar flow increases by two- to four-fold. Treatment of the hindlimb vasculature by the EDRF-inhibitor gossypol resulted in a significant increase of peripheral resistance of the femoral vascular bed (from 24 ± 3 to 77 ± 18 mmHg·min·min^{-1}), and – similar to that in earlier experiments (19) – in a selective inhibition of the flow response to acetylcholine. In contrast, the flow increase induced by adenosine was not significantly reduced. Likewise, the acetylcholine-induced

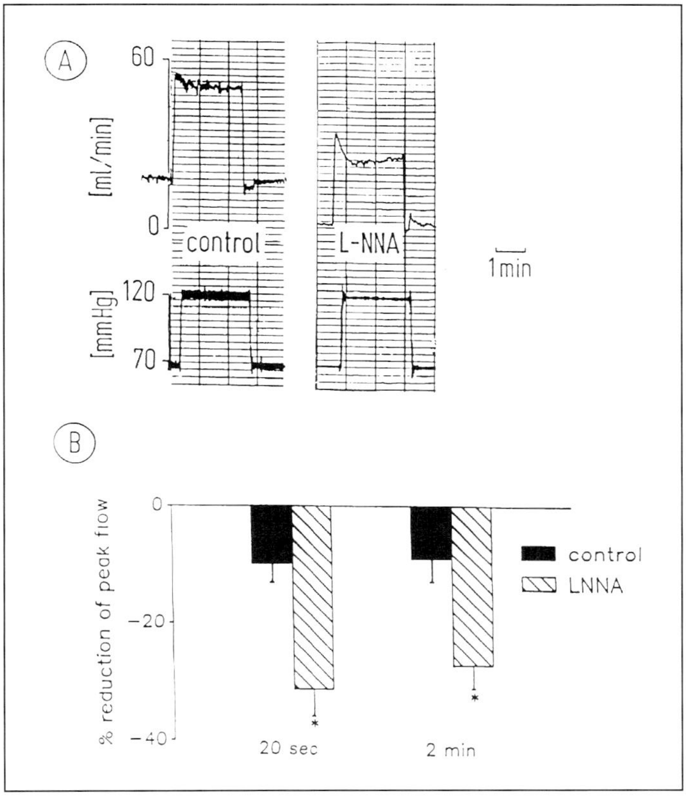

Fig. 3. Coronary flow response to rapid increases in (hydrostatically controlled) perfusion pressure. **A**: With step increase in perfusion pressure (bottom) a rapid increase in flow is observed, followed by a secondary flow reduction that indicates myogenic vasoconstriction of the vascular bed. Original tracings of one experiment before (control) and after treatment with N^G-nitro-L-arginine (L-NNA). **B**: Secondary flow reduction in percent of the peak flow 20 s and 2 min after initiation of pressure increase; (n = 6) $*p < 0.05$.

increase in platelet cGMP by 42 ± 11% was completely inhibited after treatment with gossypol, provided that acetylcholine was perfused only locally into the hindlimb circulation.

Measurements of the tissue pO_2 distribution in the skeletal muscle showed a left shift of the distribution after treatment with gossypol which was reversible upon infusion with exogenous adenosine (Fig. 4). Sham treatment of the vasculature did not significantly alter the oxygen pressure fields (not shown). The calculated oxygen uptake of the hindlimb amounted to 4.35 ± 0.98 ml·100 g^{-1}·min^{-1} and was not significantly altered during infusion of adenosine or acetylcholine. Inhibition of EDRF release by gossypol, however, resulted in a 46 ± 7% ($p < 0.01$) reduction of the oxygen uptake which was completely reversed upon infusion of adenosine.

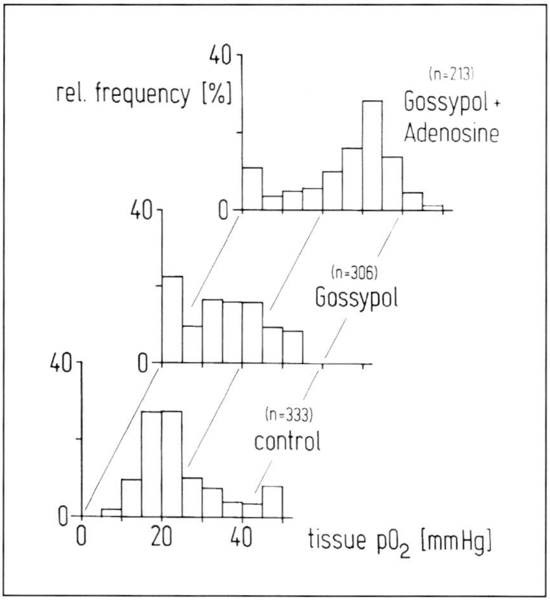

Fig. 4. pO_2 distribution at the surface of the peroneus muscle of four rabbits before (bottom, "control") and after local treatment with the EDRF-inhibitor gossypol (middle panel). The left shift of the histogram was completely reversed in three out of four experiments during adenosine infusion.

Discussion

The experiments in isolated hearts and in the rabbit hindlimb in vivo demonstrate that EDRF is present in resistance arteries and acts as a potent modulator of local blood flow, tissue oxygen supply and platelet cGMP content.

The findings give evidence that there is a considerable continuous basal release of EDRF in the isolated perfused Langendorff heart. First, there was a significantly lower cGMP level in platelets passing through the coronary vascular bed, when the EDRF was scavenged by hemoglobin or its synthesis was blocked by N_G-nitro-L-arginine. It was shown earlier that EDRF is a potent stimulator of the soluble guanylate cyclase located in platelets and that the platelet cGMP can be taken as an indicator of EDRF release (2, 4, 9, 20). Second, both treatments also significantly increased the perfusion resistance already under resting conditions, similar to that shown with other EDRF inhibitors in isolated organs and in man (1, 30). This indicates that basally released EDRF is functionally important for the maintenance of an adequate balance of dilator and constrictor local influences on vascular smooth muscle and that its removal results in enhanced vasoconstriction. In accordance with this, the inhibitor of EDRF synthesis L-monomethyl-arginine induces a significant increase in blood pressure in vivo (7). Local treatment of the hindlimb with gossypol, which selectively inhibits endothelium-dependent vascular responses (19), also increased the peripheral vascular resistance and blocked the EDRF-dependent increase in platelet cGMP. Under these conditions, a reduced oxygen uptake and a left shift of the tissue pO_2 distribution was observed. This is consistent with a significant reduction of the nutritive perfusion of the skeletal muscle. It is apparently due to the lack of endogenously produced EDRF since infusion of an exogenous endothelium-independent dilator largely restored control values. A reduced oxygen uptake associated with an increased lactate release was also observed recently in isolated hearts after treatment with N^G-nitro-L-arginine (23). Therefore, EDRF is obviously a significant factor in the local adaption of blood flow to tissue oxygen demands.

The present study further demonstrates that inhibition of EDRF-synthesis does not only affect basal vascular resistance, but also affects mechanisms which are important in the control of flow adaption to changing tissue demands. In large conduit arteries in vivo and in vitro, it has been demonstrated that increase in flow induce endothelium-dependent dilations (5, 10, 11, 18) that are mediated by enhanced release of EDRF in response to increases in shear stress (15). This flow-dependent dilation improves the conductivity of feeding arteries and therefore reduces pressure losses along arterial sections of the vascular tree during hyperemia (8). The secondary decrease in perfusion pressure observed after a rapid increase in pump flow and its inhibition by N^G-nitro-L-arginine is consistent with the occurrence of EDRF-mediated, flow-dependent dilation in resistance arteries of the coronary bed. Furthermore, the time course of the dilation is consistent with flow-dependent dilation as observed in the canine femoral arteries in vivo (18). Inhibition of EDRF synthesis was also associated with an enhanced vasoconstriction after rapid increases in perfusion pressure, most likely reflecting the myogenic response of the perfused vessels. This increase in myogenic constriction might be, in part, due to the lack of the shear-induced release of EDRF which can normally be expected during myogenic constriction in the intact vascular bed. Recently, it was shown in small mesenteric arteries that the flow-dependent dilation effectively counteracts myogenic responses (22) which occur during simultaneous increases in pressure and flow so that net dilations occurred in the presence of EDRF, and net constrictions occurred in its absence.

Therefore, the reduced peak hyperemic flow after a flow stop, as seen in the isolated heart, indicates a significant reduction of the coronary conductivity which may be based on both reduced flow dependent dilation and enhanced myogenic activity.

In summary, these experiments suggest that EDRF contributes significantly to the control of resting basal tone and to the adaptation of vascular diameter and reactivity to rapid changes in tissue oxygen demand. It appears to be a decisive factor for tissue blood supply and nutrition in the intact organ and in vivo.

Acknowledgements. This work was supported by the Deutsche Forschungsgemeinschaft (DFG Po 307/1–2). D. L. is a fellow of the Heart and Stroke Foundation of Canada. The skillful technical assistance of I. Winter, C. Kircher, and H. Münzel is gratefully acknowledged.

References

1. Amezcua JL, Palmer RMJ, Desouza BM, Moncada S (1989) Nitric oxide synthesized form L-arginine regulates vascular tone in the coronary circulation of the rabbit. Br J Pharmacol 97:1119–1124
2. Azuma H, Ishikawa M, Sekizaki S (1986) Endothelium dependent inhibition of platelet aggregation. Br J Pharmacol 88:411–415
3. Busse R, Trogisch G, Bassenge E (1985) The role of endothelium in the control of vascular tone. Basic Res Cardiol 80:475–490
4. Busse R, Lückhoff A, Bassenge E (1978) Endothelium-derived relaxant factor inhibits platelet activation. Naunyn-Schmiedebergs Arch Pharmacol 336:566–571
5. Drexler H, Zeiher AM, Wollschläger H, Meinertz T, Just H, Bonzel T (1989) Flow-dependent coronary artery dilatation in humans. Circulation 80:466–474
6. Furchgott RF (1983) Role of endothelium in responses of vascular smooth muscle. Circ Res 53:557–573

7. Gardiner SM, Sompton AM, Bennett T, Palmer RMJ, Moncada S (1990) Control of regional blood flow by endothelium-derived nitric oxide. Hypertension 15:486–492
8. Griffith TM, Edwards D, Davies RLI, Harrison TJ, Evans KT (1987) EDRF coordinates the behaviour of vascular resistance vessels. Nature 329:442–445
9. Hogan JC, Lewis MJ, Henderson AH (1988) In vivo EDRF activity influences platelet function. Br J Pharmacol 94:1020–1022
10. Holtz J, Förstermann U, Pohl U, Giesler M, Bassenge E (1984) Flow-dependent, endothelium-mediated dilation of epicardial coronary arteries in conscious dogs: effects of cyclooxygenase inhibition. J Cardiovasc Pharmacol 6:1161–1169
11. Hull SS, Kaiser L, Jaffe MD, Sparks HV (1986) Endothelium-dependent flow induced dilation of canine femoral and saphenous arteries. Blood Vessels 23:183–198
12. Koller A, Messina EJ, Wolin MS, Kaley G (1989) Effects of endothelial impairment on arteriolar dilator responses in vivo. Am J Physiol 257:H1485–H1489
13. Ludmer PL, Selwyn AP, Shook TL, Wayne RR, Mudge GH, Alexander RW, Ganz P (1986) Paradoxical vasoconstriction induced by acetylcholine in atherosclerotic coronary arteries. N Engl J Med 315:1046–1051
14. Maseri A, Kaski JC (1989) Pathogenetic mechanisms of coronary artery spasm. J Am Coll Cardiol 14:610–612
15. Melkumyants AM, Balashov SA, Veselova ES, Khayutin VM (1987) Continuous control of the lumen of feline conduit arteries by blood flow rate.Cardiovasc Res 21:863–870
16. Palmer RMJ, Ashton DS, Moncada S (1988) Vascular endothelial cells synthesize nitric oxide from L-arginine. Nature 333:664–666
17. Pohl U, Busse R, Kuon E, Bassenge E (1986) Pulsatile perfusion stimulates the release of endothelial autacoids. J Appl Cardiol 1:215–235
18. Pohl U, Holtz J, Busse R, Bassenge E (1986) Crucial role of endothelium in the vasodilator response to increased flow in vivo. Hypertension 8:37–44
19. Pohl U, Dézsi L, Simon B, Busse R (1987) Selective inhibition of endothelium-dependent dilation in resistance-sized vessels in vivo. Am J Physiol 253:H234–H239
20. Pohl U, Busse R (1989) EDRF increases cyclic GMP in platelets during passage through the coronary vascular bed. Circ Res 65:1798–1803
21. Pohl U, Busse R (1989) Hypoxia stimulates the release of endothelium-derived relaxant factor (EDRF). Am J Physiol 256:H1595–H1600
22. Pohl U, Herlan K, Huang A, Bassenge E (1990) EDRF-mediated, shear-induced dilation opposes myogenic vasoconstriction. Am J Physiol (in press)
23. Pohl U, Lamontagne D, Bassenge E, Busse R (1990) EDRF augments coronary conductivity through attenuation of myogenic autoregulation. Pflüger Arch 415 (Suppl 1):1262
24. Rees DD, Palmer RMJ, Moncada S (1989) Role of endothelium-derived nitric oxide in the regulation of blood pressure. Proc Natl Acad Sci USA 86:3375–3378
25. Rosenblum WI (1986) Endothelial dependent relaxation demonstrated in vivo in cerebral arterioles. Stroke 17:494–497
26. Rubanyi GM, Romero JC, Vanhoutte PM (1986) Flow-induced release of endothelium-derived relaxing factor. Am J Physiol 250:H1145–H1149
27. Shimokawa H, Flavahan NA, Sheperd JT, Vanhoutte PM (1989) Endothelium-dependent inhibition of ergonovine-induced contraction is impaired in porcine coronary arteries with regenerated endothelium. Circulation 80:643–650
28. Stewart DJ, Holtz J, Pohl U, Bassenge E (1987) Balance between endothelium-mediated dilator and direct constrictor actions of serotonin on resistance vessels in the isolated rabbit heart. Eur J Pharmacol 143:131–134
29. Stewart DJ, Pohl U, Bassenge E (1988) Free radicals inhibit endothelium-dependent dilation in the coronary resistance bed. Am J Physiol 255:H765–H769
30. Vallance P, Collier J, Moncada S (1989) Effects of endothelium-derived nitric oxide on peripheral arteriolar tone in man. Lancet 2:997–1000
31. Yamamoto Y, Tomoike H, Egashira K, Kobayashi T, Kawasaki T, Nakamura M (1987) Pathogenesis of coronary artery spasm in miniature swine with regional intimal thickening after balloon denudation. Circ Res 60:113–121

32. Zeiher AM, Drexler H, Wollschläger H, Saurbier B, Just H (1989) Coronary vasomotion in response to sympathetic stimulation in humans – importance of the functional integrity of the endothelium. J Am Coll Cardiol 14:1181–1190

Author's address:
Dr. Ulrich Pohl
Institute of Physiology
Med. University of Lübeck
Ratzeburger Allee
W-2400 Lübeck, FRG

Endothelial function in pathological conditions

Endothelial dysfunction in myocardial ischemia and reperfusion: role of oxygen-derived free radicals

A. M. Lefer [1] and D. J. Lefer [2]

[1] Department of Physiology, Jefferson Medical College, Thomas Jefferson University, Philadelphia, Pennsylvania, and
[2] Department of Physiology and Pharmacology, Bowman Gray School of Medicine, Wake Forest University, Winston-Salem, North Carolina, USA

Summary: Myocardial ischemia followed by reperfusion results in endothelial dysfunction in cats. This dysfunction is characterized by a loss of endothelium-derived relaxing factor (EDRF) release in response to endothelium-dependent dilators. This loss of endothelium-dependent relaxation (EDR) occurs significantly at 2.5 min post-reperfusion and the dysfunction progresses until it is complete at 20 min post-reperfusion. This reduced EDR is prevented by superoxide dismutase, but not by hydroxyl radical scavengers. In contrast, neutrophil accumulation in the heart, as measured by cardiac myeloperoxidase (MPO) activity, does not reach significant levels until 3 h post-reperfusion, and significant myocardial necrosis does not occur until 4.5 h post-reperfusion. No significant changes in EDR, MPO or cardiac necrosis occurred during the 90 min of ischemia. Thus, endothelial dysfunction is an early and specific marker of reperfusion injury preceding neutrophil involvement and cardiac necrosis. Superoxide radicals appear to play a key role in the decreased EDR observed early after reperfusion.

Key words: Endothelium-derived relaxing factor (EDRF); superoxide radicals; acetylcholine; myeloperoxidase activity; neutrophils; cardiac necrosis

Myocardial ischemia and subsequent reperfusion result in a significant degree of myocardial cell damage related to the severity and duration of the ischemic period. A variety of factors contributes to the myocardial injury, including the hypoxia produced by the initial ischemia, and several factors which occur after reperfusion including neutrophil accumulation in the ischemic area and their subsequent release of cytokines, proteolytic enzymes, and oxygen derived free radicals (1–3). However, recent evidence has focused attention on endothelial dysfunction as an important contributory factor to early post-reperfusion injury. Impairment of release of endothelium-derived relaxing factor (EDRF) has been shown to occur to a significant degree in post-reperfusion myocardial ischemia (4–6). This reduction in EDRF is of considerable significance since EDRF not only is a potent coronary vasodilator, but is a potent inhibitor of platelet aggregation (7) and of neutrophil adherence to the endothelium (8). Additionally, EDRF opposes the actions of a number of adhesive proteins, either expressed on the surface of endothelial cells (ELAM-1 and ICAM-1) or on the surface of adhering neutrophils (CD-11/CD-18) (9). This profile of action of EDRF as well as its location at the blood vasculature interface enables it to function as a key regulatory substance during disease states including myocardial ischemia. Therefore, information on the dynamics of EDRF release, factors which protect EDRF, and the actions of EDRF in post-reperfusion events, are of significance in our understanding of the pathophysiology of myocardial ischemia and reperfusion.

Recently, in a cat model of myocardial ischemia and reperfusion, we assessed the time-course of endothelial dysfunction by determining EDRF release in isolated coronary

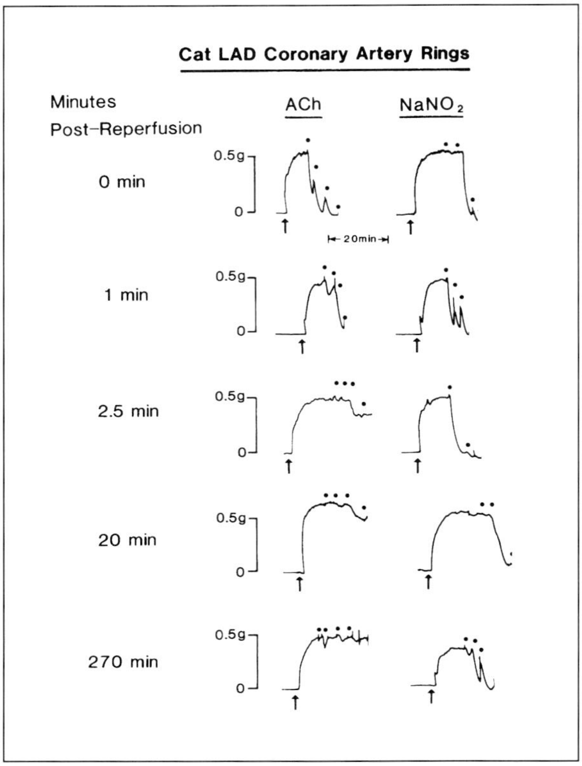

Fig. 1. Representative recordings obtained from left anterior descending (LAD) coronary artery rings of cats subjected to myocardial ischemia and reperfusion of 0, 1, 2.5, 20, and 270 min. At the arrow U-46619 (300 nM) was added to precontract the rings. At the dots (0.01, 0.1, 1, or 10 nM acetylcholine [ACh] or 1, 10, and 10 μM acidified sodium nitrite [$NaNO_2$]) was added. A clear defect to ACh-induced vasorelaxation occurred at 2.5 mm and beyond. No impairment of vasorelaxation occurred to $NaNO_2$, a releaser of NO, at any time.

artery rings. These results were obtained in anesthetized cats subjected to a midline sternotomy. The left anterior descending (LAD) coronary artery was occluded approximately 10 to 12 mm from its origin for 90 min followed by periods of reperfusion of 0 (i.e., no reperfusion), 1, 2.5, 20, and 270 min. At the end of these reperfusion times, the occlusion was reestablished and hearts were stained with Evans blue to delineate the area-at-risk (AAR) by negative staining, and then 2-mm-thick sections of heart were incubated at 37° C for 15 min in 0.1% nitroblue tetrazolium to delineate the necrotic tissue (10). Additional samples were taken for assay of myeloperoxidase (MPO) activity as a marker for neutrophil accumulation (11). At the time of determining area of necrosis and myeloperoxidase activity, the LAD and the left circumflex (LCX) coronary arteries were cut into 3–4 mm wide rings and suspended in tissue baths for study of endothelium-dependent (i.e., acetylcholine [ACh] and A-23187) and endothelium-independent (i.e., acidified $NaNO_2$) vasodilators. This allowed comparison of the vascular responses of the occluded and non-occluded coronary arteries.

Figure 1 illustrates representative responses of LAD coronary artery rings to ACh and $NaNO_2$ at different times following ischemia and reperfusion. At the time of reperfusion (i.e., 0 min), it is clear that a complete vasorelaxation occurred to both ACh and $NaNO_2$, indicating a normal endothelium production of EDRF. Similar results were obtained 1 min post-reperfusion. However, by 2.5 min post-reperfusion, a significant loss of vasorelaxation occurred to ACh, but not to $NaNO_2$. A similar loss of endothelium-dependent relaxation (EDR) occurred with ADP. This signifies a defect in EDRF production or release, which continued through 20 min post-reperfusion. At 270 min, virtually a total loss of EDR had occurred. This dramatic loss of ACh occurring at 2.5 min post-reperfusion also occurred in response to the calcium ionophore A-23187, at 20 min. Thus, this early impairment of EDR cannot be attributed to down regulation of muscarinic receptors on the coronary endothelium. Moreover, it indicates that the observed endothelial dysfunction applies to receptor as well as non-receptor-mediated endothelium-dependent vasodilators. No defect of any kind was observed in the non-occluded LCX coronary arteries at any time.

One possible explanation for this decrease in EDRF release could be severe morphological disruption or denudation of the endothelium following reperfusion. Figure 2 shows representative scanning electron micrographs obtained from critical point dried, gold coated LAD coronary arteries. These photomicrographs show a normal endothelium at the time of reperfusion as well as 270 min after reperfusion. Similar results were observed at the other post-reperfusion times. Therefore, the defect in EDRF production is not due to a sloughing or curling of the endothelium.

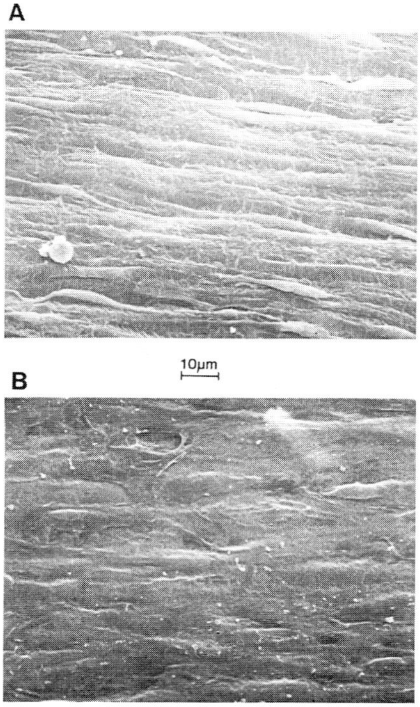

Fig. 2. Representative scanning electron micrographs of cat LAD coronary arteries removed at 0 and 270 min post-reperfusion. A normal endothelial appearance is evident with no curling or sloughing of endothelial cells.

Table 1. Responses of LAD coronary artery rings 20 min post-reperfusion

Group	ACh (10 nM)	A-23187 (100 μM)	$NaNO_2$ (100 μM)
MI + R (vehicle)	17 ± 5*	28 ± 3*	98 ± 5
MI + R (MPG)	28 ± 5*	79 ± 10	104 ± 6
MI + R (h-SOD)	83 ± 4	78 ± 6	106 ± 5

All values are means % relaxation of 6–8 coronary rings pretreated with 300 nM U-46619.
*$p < 0.01$ from vehicle.
LAD = left anterior descending;
MI + R = myocardial ischemia and reperfusion;
h-SOD = human superoxide dismutase;
MPG = N-2 mercapto proprionyl glycine;
ACh = acetylcholine.

In an effort to determine the source of the rapid post-reperfusion endothelial injury, cats were subjected to 90 min of ischemia and 20 min of reperfusion. However, 10 min before reperfusion (i.e., at 80 min of ischemia), either recombinant human superoxide dismutase (h-SOD) 5 mg/kg/h or N-2 mercapto proprionyl glycine (8 mg/kg)/h) was infused for 30 min. Twenty min following reperfusion, at a time when a marked impairment of EDR occurs, coronary artery rings were prepared and responses to ACh, A-23187, and $NaNO_2$ were assessed. Table 1 summarizes the responses in LAD coronary artery rings. In cats receiving only the vehicle (i.e., 0.9% NaCl), both endothelium-dependent dilators (i.e., ACh and A-23187) showed a marked reduction in vasorelaxant responses ($p < 0.01$ from control). Responses to $NaNO_2$ were essentially normal. However, MPG appeared to restore the A-23187 response to normal, although it failed to protect the response to ACh. This may indicate that hydroxyl radicals may play some role in producing the injury to endothelial cells, since MPG is a hydroxyl radical scavenger (12). Even more impressive was the endothelial protective effects of h-SOD, a superoxide ion scavenger (13). h-SOD preserved the vasorelaxant response to both ACh and A-23187. These data are consistent with a mediator role of oxygen derived free radicals in the endothelial dysfunction occurring soon after reperfusion, and also confirm the coronary protective effect of h-SOD in ischemia (14).

In order to relate the endothelial dysfunction to neutrophil accumulation and to myocardial cell injury, we also measured cardiac MPO activity as a marker for neutrophils, and the percent of cardiac necrotic tissue indexed to area-at-risk (i.e., NEC/AAR) at different times following reperfusion. Figure 3 illustrates these temporal relationships. First, it is evident that endothelial dysfunction occurs much earlier than either neutrophil accumulation or cardiac injury. Secondly, neutrophil accumulation does not appear to be an immediate post-reperfusion event, and thus is not responsible for the endothelial dysfunction observed at 2.5 to 20 min post-reperfusion. However, endothelial dysfunction may set the stage for later neutrophil adherence and accumulation in the ischemic region. Thirdly, neutrophil accumulation closely parallels myocardial injury, and the neutrophils may be an important contributory factor in inducing cardiac myocyte injury. Finally, significant cardiac injury does not occur until 3 to 4.5 hours post-reperfusion, a time much later than that required for endothelial dysfunction. Treatment delayed beyond 20–30 min following reperfusion is generally ineffective, thus indicating that there is only a moderately short window of opportunity for therapeutic intervention in preserving myocardial integrity in cats.

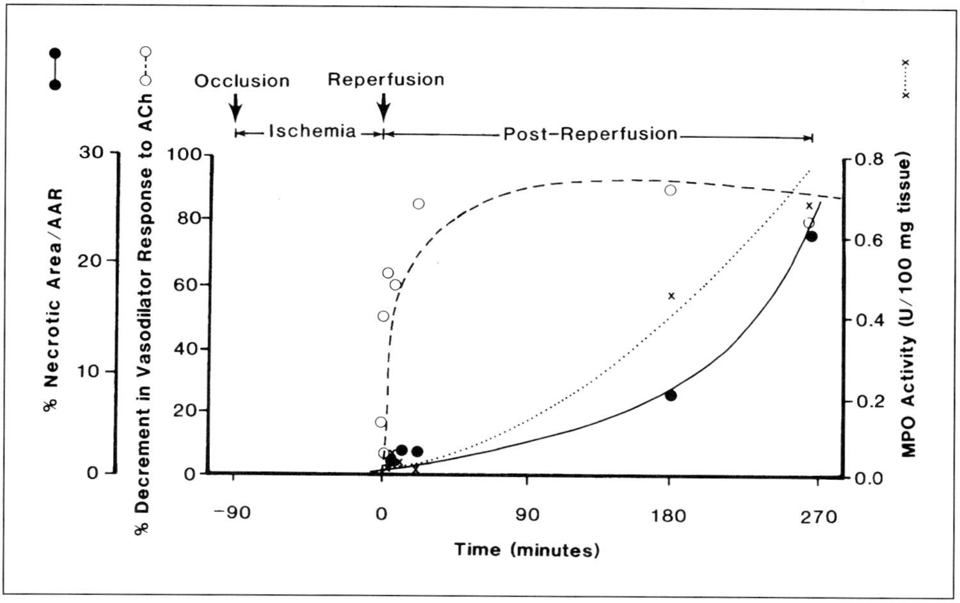

Fig. 3. Time-course of endothelial dysfunction (o---o), cardiac myeloperoxidase (MPO) activity in the ischemic region (x...x) and cardiac necrosis as a percent of area-at-risk (NEC/AAR) (●---●) over time. Endothelial dysfunction is an early event (i.e., 2.5 to 20 min post-reperfusion) preceding both MPO accumulation and cardiac necrosis which occur 3 to 4.5 h post-reperfusion.

Since h-SOD preserved endothelial integrity at 20 min, we decided to ascertain whether h-SOD given over the period of 10 min prior to reperfusion and extending over the first 20 min of the post-reperfusion period, could preserve myocardial integrity at 4.5 h post-reperfusion. Table 2 summarizes the major results of these experiments. Clearly, h-SOD markedly attenuated plasma CK activity at 4.5 h post-reperfusion. Additionally, h-SOD preserved the integrity of the coronary vascular endothelium to endothelium-dependent vasodilators (e.g., acetylcholine; ACh) at 4.5 h post-reperfusion. Moreover, h-SOD dramatically reduced the degree of necrosis normalized to area-at-risk ($p < 0.001$) and the cardiac myeloperoxidase activity ($p < 0.01$) in the area-at-risk. These data clearly show that h-SOD given over the critical period (i.e., the first 20 min of reperfusion) can exert a significant cardioprotective effect measured at 4.5 h post-reperfusion. These findings strongly implicate superoxide radicals as important mediators in the pathogenesis of reperfusion injury following myocardial ischemia, and are in close agreement with the work of Stewart et al. (15) who obtained similar results in perfused rabbit hearts.

A schematic diagram of the postulated concepts involved in the pathogenesis of myocardial ischemia followed by reperfusion is shown in Fig. 4. The central role of the endothelium is indicated. Under normal conditions the endothelium produces EDRF, indicated here as nitric oxide (NO), the most likely chemical form of EDRF. NO prevents neutrophils and platelets from being activated in the vicinity of the endothelial cell surface, and clearly prevents adherence of these blood cells to the endothelium. Thus, NO can increase cyclic GMP in vascular smooth muscle cells and coronary vasorelaxa-

Table 2. Protective effects of h-SOD in myocardial ischemia reperfusion in anesthetized cats

Variable	MI + R + Vehicle	MI + R + h-SOD*	Significance
Plasma creatine kinase activity (IU/mg protein × 10^{-3})	45.5 ± 5.5	15.0 ± 1.4	$p<0.01$
Vasorelaxation to ACh (Percent relaxation)	24 ± 8	76 ± 4	$p<0.01$
Cardiac Myeloperoxidase Activity (U/100 mg tissue)	1.09 ± 0.28	0.26 ± 0.16	$p<0.01$
Cardiac Necrotic Area (% Area-at-Risk)	20.4 ± 3.0	1.8 ± 1.0	$p<0.001$

All values are means taken at 4.5 h post-reperfusion ± SEM for 5 cats in each group.
* h-SOD was given intravenously at 5 mg/kg/h over a 30-min period beginning 10 min prior to reperfusion

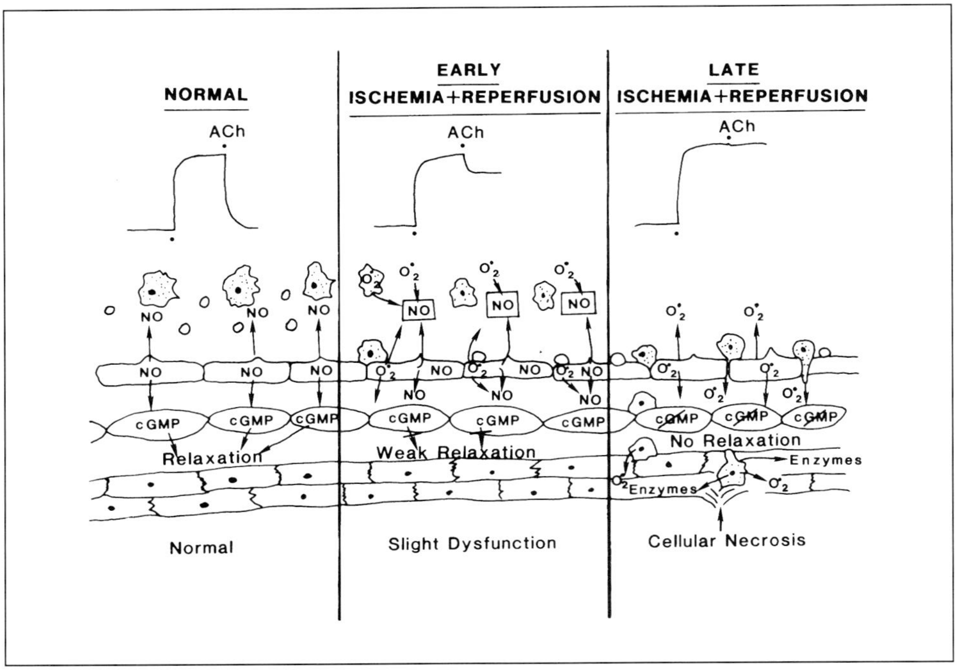

Fig. 4. Schematic diagram of coronary microvasculature prior to ischemia (i.e., normal), early ischemia + reperfusion (i.e., 2.5 to 20 min post-reperfusion), and late ischemia + reperfusion (i.e., 3–4.5 h post-reperfusion). Nitric oxide (NO) is shown as EDRF. Neutrophils and platelets are in the lumen. Endothelial vascular smooth muscle (containing cyclic GMP) and myocardial cells are shown.

tion occurs. In this environment, myocardial cells are normal in structure and function. However, early after myocardial ischemia and reperfusion, endothelial dysfunction occurs, less NO is produced and neutrophils and platelets can become activated. Some of these cells will adhere to the endothelium and release oxygen derived free radicals. These free radicals can also originate from endothelial cells themselves (16). The free radicals, particularly superoxide (O_2) can also inactivate NO (17), and impair endothelial derived vasorelaxation, as well as remove the protective effect of NO in platelets and neutrophils. This results in a significant degree of endothelial dysfunction, but only a slight degree of myocardial injury. Later (i.e., 3–4 hours post-reperfusion), further endothelial dysfunction occurs (i.e., EDR is totally impaired) and neutrophils probably diapedese through the endothelium to the myocardium where they continue to release free radicals, hydrolytic enzymes, and cytokines, all of which accelerate myocardial cell injury and result in cardiac necrosis.

Thus, endothelial cell dysfunction resulting in impaired EDRF production is a pivotal event early in reperfusion injury and significantly contributes to the myocardial cell necrosis and cardiac injury occurring several hours later.

References

1. Mullane KM (1988) Myocardial ischemia-reperfusion injury. Role of neutrophils and neutrophil derived mediators. In: Marone G (ed) Human inflammatory disease: clinical immunology, vol. 1. Burlington, Ontario, Canada, B. C. Decker; pp. 143–198
2. Romson JL, Hook BG, Kunkel SL, Abrams GD, Schork MA, Lucchesi BR (1983) Reduction of the extent of ischemic myocardial injury by neutrophil depletion in the dog. Circulation 67:1016–1023
3. Engler RL, Dahlgren MD, Morris D, Peterson MA, Schmid-Schoenbein G (1986) Role of leukocytes in the response to acute myocardial ischemia and reflow in dogs. Am J Physiol 251:H307–H313
4. Ku DD (1982) Coronary vascular reactivity after acute myocardial ischemia. Science 218:576–578
5. Van Benthuysen KM, McMurtry IF, Horowitz LD (1987) Reperfusion after acute coronary occlusion in dogs impairs endothelium-dependent relaxation to acetylcholine and augments contractile reactivity in vitro. J Clin Invest 79:265–274
6. Mehta JL, Nichols WW, Donnelly WH, Lawson DL, Saldeen TGP (1989) Acetylcholine and bradykinin after occlusion-reperfusion. Circ Res 64:43–54
7. Furlong B, Henderson AH, Lewis MJ et al. (1987) Endothelium-derived relaxing factor inhibits in vitro platelet aggregation. Br J Pharmacol 90:687–692
8. McCall T, Whittle BJR, Boughton-Smith NK, Moncada S (1988) Inhibition of FMLP-induced aggregation of rabbit neutrophils by nitric oxide. Br J Pharmacol 95–517P
9. Tonnensen MG (1989) Neutrophil-endothelial cell interactions: mechanisms of neutrophil adherence to vascular endothelium. J Invest Dermatol 93:53S–58S
10. Johnson G III, Furlan LE, Aoki N, Lefer AM (1990) Endothelium and myocardial protecting actions of Taprostene, a stable prostacyclin analog, following acute myocardial ischemia and reperfusion in cats. Circ Res 66:1362–1370
11. Mullane KM, Kraermer R, Smith B (1985) Myeloperoxidase activity as a quantitative assessment of neutrophil infiltration into ischemic myocardium. J Pharmacol Meth 14:157–167
12. Bolli R, Jeroudi MO, Patel BS, Aruoma OI, Halliwell B, Kai EK, McCay PB (1989) Marked reduction of free radical generation and contractile dysfunction by antioxidant therapy begun at the time of reperfusion. Evidence that myocardium "stunning" is a manifestation of reperfusion injury. Circ Res 65:607–622
13. McCord JM, Fridovich I (1969) Superoxide dismutase: an enzymatic function for erythrocuprein (hemocuprein). J Biol Chem 244:6049–6055

14. Aoki N, Bitterman H, Brezinski ME, Lefer AM (1988) Cardioprotective action of human superoxide dismutase in two reperfusion models of myocardial ischemia in the rat. Br J Pharmacol 95:735–740
15. Stewart DJ, Pohl U, Bassenge E (1988) Free radicals inhibit endothelium-dependent dilation in the coronary resistance bed. Am J Physiol 255:H765–H769
16. Zweier JL, Flaherty JT, Weisfeldt ML (1987) Observation of free radical generation in the postischemic heart. Proc Natl Acad Sci USA 84:1404–1407
17. Rubanyi GM, Vanhoutte PM (1986) Oxygen-derived free radicals, endothelium, and responsiveness of vascular smooth muscle. Am J Physiol 250:H815–H821

Author's adress:

Dr. Allan M. Lefer
Department of Physiology
Jefferson Medical College
1020 Locust Street
Philadelphia, PA 19107, USA

Interactions between nitric oxide and prostacyclin in myocardial ischemia and endothelial cell cultures

K. Schrör, I. Woditsch, H. Strobach and H. Schröder

Summary: This study investigates biochemical and functional interactions between NO and PGI_2 that generate pathways in two different in vitro assays: porcine aortic endothelial cells (PAEC) and reperfused ischemic Langendorff hearts of rabbits. Using cGMP as an index of NO generation and 6-oxo-$PGF_{1\alpha}$ as an index for PGI_2 production in endothelial cells, it is demonstrated that the two metabolic pathways for NO and prostacyclin formation act independent of each other. Moreover, NO appears to have an autocrine function in endothelial cells which does not exist with PGI_2, probably because of a lack of PGI_2 receptors. Endothelial damage in the course of myocardial ischemia is associated with a marked increase in mediator release whose inhibition has consequences for both myocardial and coronary function: inhibition of NO formation also inhibits PGI_2 release and the recovery of coronary vessel tone with only minor if any effect on myocardial contractility. In contrast, inhibition of PGI_2-generation results in marked deterioration of myocardial recovery with only minor changes in coronary perfusion. It is concluded from these data that PGI_2 in endothelial injury is important for preservation of myocardial function while NO might mainly be involved in control of local vessel tone.

Key words: Endothelial cells; myocardial ischemia; prostacyclin; cGMP; cAMP; nitric oxide (NO)

Introduction

Prostacyclin (PGI_2) and nitric oxide (NO) are two major mediators of local control in vessel tone (2, 7, 21). Both are potent vasodilators that are released in response to appropriate stimulation. In the cardiovascular system, the vascular endothelium is the major site of biosynthesis, i.e., the generation from liberated arachidonic acid or hydroxylation of arginine. Both compounds have a short half-life that focuses the biological activity to the site of formation. However, there are significant differences in cellular signal transmission. Thus, cyclic AMP is considered the intracellular messenger system, in most cases, for PGI_2, and cyclic GMP, generated by the soluble guanylate cyclase, for NO (6, 12, 20, 22, 29).

Because of the apparent similarities in intercellular signal transmission between these two mediators on vessel tone and platelet function, the question arises of whether or not interactions exist between the two at the level of mediator generation and/or action. It has been shown recently that endothelial cells inhibit platelet aggregation by two separate, but synergistic mechanisms involving PGI_2-induced cAMP stimulation and NO-induced cGMP stimulation (1). Whereas the role of PGI_2 and NO in paracrine signaling between endothelial and other vascular cells is widely accepted (2, 21), only preliminary information is available about a possible autocrine function of PGI_2 and NO in the endothelial generator cell (28). This problem is particularly relevant in local endothelial injury, for example, in the course of myocardial ischemia.

This study investigates biochemical and functional interactions of PGI_2 and NO in two well-defined in vitro assay systems: isolated porcine aortic endothelial cells (PAEC) and reperfused ischemic Langendorff-hearts of the rabbit.

Materials and methods

Endothelial cells from pig aorta

Porcine aortic endothelial cells (PAEC) were isolated and cultured according to Gryglewski et al. (9). After reaching confluence, cells were trypsinized and subcultured in 35-mm culture dishes. Washed cells were exposed for 10 min to the L-arginine antagonist N^G-monomethyl-L-arginine (L-NMMA) (25) or arginine enantiomers at 37° C in a balanced salt solution (24) containing 0.5 mM isobutyl-methylxanthine. A23187, iloprost, or forskolin were added and the incubation continued for another 10 min. The supernatant was used for determination of 6-oxo-$PGF_{1\alpha}$, an index metabolite for PGI_2, by radioimmunoassay (34). Cyclic nucleotide levels were also measured by radioimmunoassay after terminating the reaction by addition of ethanol and subsequent evaporation as described previously (5, 27, 35).

Langendorff-hearts of rabbits

Langendorff-hearts were prepared from New Zealand White rabbits (body weight 1600–2200 g), following previously described procedures (31–33). The hearts were perfused at a constant rate of 22 ml/min with Krebs-Henseleit-buffer, equilibrated with 95% oxygen +5% CO_2 at 37° C using a membrane oxygenator (Eschweiler, Kiel, FRG). Left-ventricular actively developed pressure (LVSP), left ventricular enddiastolic pressure (LVEDP) (balloon technique), and coronary perfusion pressure (CPP) were monitored continuously by using Statham transducers. In some experiments, the buffer solution contained indomethacin (3 μM) to prevent endogenous prostaglandin formation, or L-NMMA (30 μM) or N^G-nitro-L-arginine (100 μM) (23) to inhibit nitric oxide formation. Hearts were made globally ischemic by reducing the perfusion rate to 1.25 ml/min for 2 h. Particular care was taken to maintain the temperature of the heart at 37° C at this time. Thereafter, the hearts were reperfused for 30 min. 6-oxo-$PGF_{1\alpha}$ was determined in aliquots of the coronary effluent as described above. NO-formation was determined by the oxyhemoglobin technique (4, 11, 15–17) with some modifications as previously described (32). For this purpose, purified oxyhemoglobin was always present in the perfusion fluid at a constant concentration of 3 μM. The difference in extinction at 402 and 411 nm was continuously monitored by a dual-wave-length spectrophotometer (Aminco DW-2000, Colora Lorch, FRG). NO-release was quantified after assessing the molar extinction coefficient (ε). ε was found to be 32 mmoles-1 min-1, i.e., similar to values, reported in the literature (11).

Statistics

The data are mean ± SEM of n determinations. Statistical analysis was performed by the two-tailed *t*-test or the *u*-test (changes in coronary perfusion pressure) as appropriate. p levels of <0.05 were considered to be significant.

Results

Endothelial cells

A23187 (0.3–3 µM) stimulated endothelial cGMP levels concentration-dependently with a maximal 55-fold stimulation at 3 µM. Therefore, this concentration was used for the further experiments. Coincubation with L-NMMA (1–100 µM) produced a concentration-dependent inhibition of cGMP accumulation, an index for nitric oxide generation. L-arginine (2 mM), but not D-arginine (2 mM), completely restored in cGMP response to A23187. Neither of these interventions are associated with any change in 6-oxo-$PGF_{1\alpha}$ accumulation (Table 1).

Table 1. Effects of L-NMMA on A23187 (3 µM)-induced cyclic GMP and 6-oxo-$PGF_{1\alpha}$ accumulation in cultured porcine aortic endothelial cells

Additions	Cyclic GMP (pmol/10^6 cells)	6-oxo-$PGF_{1\alpha}$ (pmol/10^6 cells)
None (control)	153.2 ± 9.3	46.0 ± 1.2
1 µM L-NMMA	54.1 ± 3.6*	42.1 ± 3.1
10 µM L-NMMA	19.9 ± 2.0*	46.9 ± 4.3
100 µM L-NMMA	16.1 ± 0.5*	50.0 ± 7.0
100 µM L-NMMA + 2 mM L-NMMA	156.7 ± 12.2	48.4 ± 2.0
100 µM L-NMMA + 2 mM L-NMMA	11.4 ± 1.5*	43.3 ± 4.0

* $p < 0.05$; treatment vs control

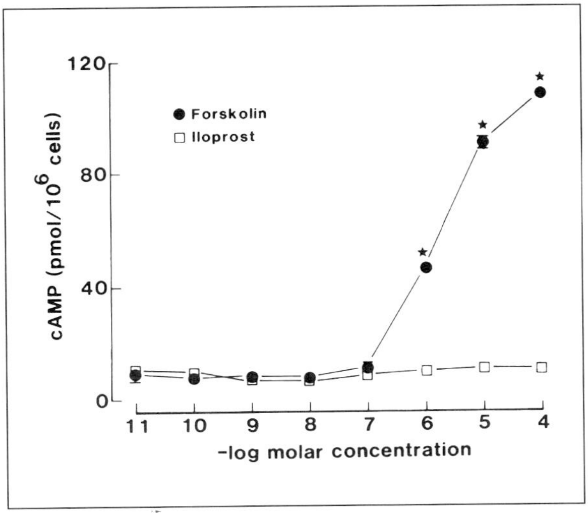

Fig. 1. Stimulation of cAMP formation in porcine aortic endothelial cells by forskolin, but not by iloprost. The data are mean ± SEM of n = 6 experiments

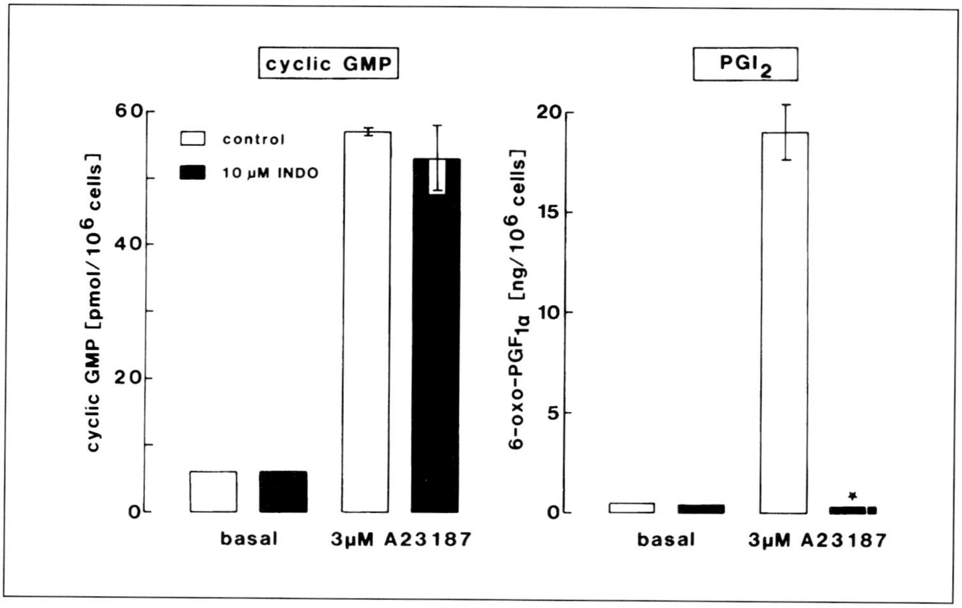

Fig. 2. Failure of indomethacin to modify A23187-induced cyclic GMP accumulation in isolated porcine aortic endothelial cells despite an almost complete inhibition of stimulated prostacyclin formation (for further explanation, see text). The data are mean ± SEM of n = 6 experiments

A23187 increased the endothelial PGI_2 formation in a concentration-dependent manner, amounting to 31-fold stimulation at 3 μM. This increase in PGI_2 formation was not accompanied by any stimulation of cAMP formation. Similarly, the stable PGI_2 mimetic iloprost in concentrations up to 0.1 mM did not modify endothelial cAMP synthesis. In contrast, forskolin (1–100 μM) increased endothelial cAMP levels concentration-dependently with a 12-fold stimulation at 100 μM. These data are shown in Fig. 1. There was also no effect of inhibition of PGI_2 generation on cGMP accumulation. As shown in Fig. 2, treatment of the endothelial cells with indomethacin did not alter cGMP formation.

Rabbit hearts

There was a small but constant release of PGI_2 into the coronary effluent prior to ischemia, but a sharp and marked rise of PGI_2 release during early reperfusion. As expected, no significant PGI_2 release was seen in indomethacin treated hearts (not shown). However, both antagonists of NO formation also induced significant reductions in PGI_2 overflow. These data are shown in Fig. 3. Figure 4 summarizes the changes in NO release. In contrast to PGI_2, the overflow of NO rose continuously throughout the reperfusion period. As expected, treatment with L-NMMA or nitro-arginine reduced NO formation. However, treatment with indomethacin had apparently the same effect, also resulting in a considerably reduced NO release.

The functional consequences of reduced NO and PGI_2 generation, respectively, were impressive and completely different. As summarized in Tables 2 and 3, blockade of

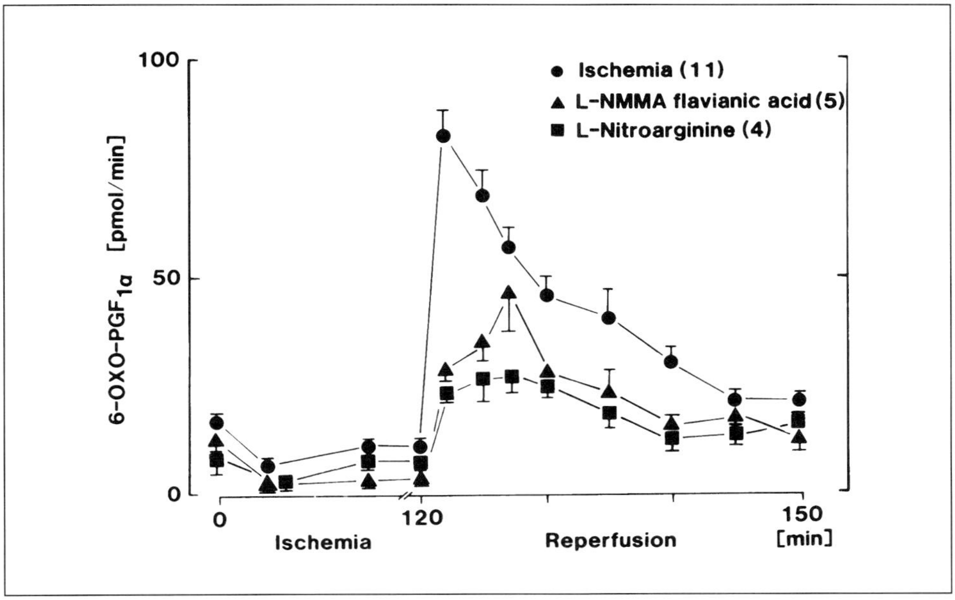

Fig. 3. 6-oxo-PGF$_{1\alpha}$ release into the coronary effluent of Langendorff-perfused rabbit hearts during ischemia and reperfusion and its modification by L-nitroarginine and L-NMMA. The data are mean ± SEM of (n) experiments

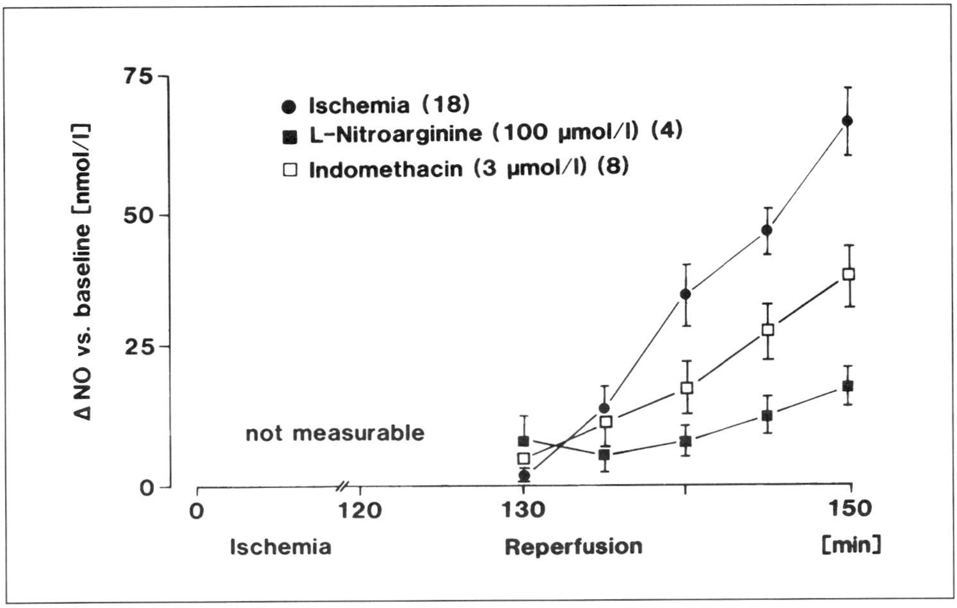

Fig. 4. NO release into the coronary effluent of Langendorff-perfused rabbit hearts during reperfusion and its modification by L-nitroarginine and indomethacin. The data are mean ± SEM of (n) experiments

Table 2. Coronary perfusion pressure [mmHg] of isolated rabbit hearts at the end of ischemia and reperfusion

	Additional treatment		
	None (control) (11)	Indomethacin (3 μmol/l) (8)	L-NMMA (30 μmol/l) (5)
Before ischemia	39 ± 4	32 ± 3	41 ± 5
Ischemia	0	0	0
Reperfusion	75 ± 4	44 ± 5*	102 ± 9*

* $p < 0.05$ (Indomethacin and L-NMMA vs control)

Table 3. End-diastolic left-ventricular pressure [mmHg] of isolated rabbit hearts at the end of ischemia and reperfusion

	Additional treatment		
	None (control) (11)	Indomethacin (3 μmol/l) (8)	L-NMMA (30 μmol/l) (5)
Before ischemia	0	0	0
Ischemia	46 ± 8	62 ± 3	41 ± 13
Reperfusion	32 ± 7	58 ± 7*	35 ± 12

* $p < 0.05$ (Indomethacin vs control and L-NMMA)

endogenous NO formation by L-NMMA or nitro-arginine did not modify left ventricular enddiastolic pressure in comparison to controls. However, there was an about 2-fold increase in coronary perfusion pressure ($p<0.05$). In indomethacin-treated hearts, the rise in coronary perfusion pressure after reperfusion was significantly attenuated, while the deterioration of myocardial function was markedly enhanced, associated with a considerable increase in left ventricular enddiastolic pressure and a marked fall in left ventricular actively developed pressure (not shown).

Discussion

These data demonstrate that endothelial cGMP stimulation by the calcium ionophore A23187 is strictly L-arginine-dependent and can thus be attributed to autocrine activation of the L-arginine/NO pathway. This is in good agreement with previous findings that demonstrated the presence of soluble guanylate cyclase in endothelial cells (18, 19). It is conceivable that NO-induced cGMP stimulation in endothelial cells serves as a negative feedback mechanism or switch-off signal for NO formation. This is supported by a recent study showing that 8-bromo-cGMP inhibits endothelium-dependent relaxation (3). In contrast to NO, PGI_2 in our study failed to activate its respective second messenger system in endothelial cells, although the receptor-independent stimulator of adenylate cylase, forskolin, was active. Thus, the observed inability of PGI_2 or its stable analogue iloprost to activate endothelial adenylate cyclase is probably due to a lack of PGI_2 receptors in the plasma membrane or in uncoupling of PGI_2 binding sites and stimulatory G-proteins. In LLC-PK_1 kidney epithelial cells (30) kept under the same culture conditions, a marked PGI_2-induced cAMP-stimulation was observed (data not shown). This precludes that the culture conditions used promote a down-regulation or artificial loss of PGI_2 binding sites. Our findings are in contrast to previous investigations reporting endothelial cAMP stimulation by PGI_2 (13, 26). However, these authors were unable to demonstrate a PGI_2-dependent activation of adenylate cyclase in endothelial membrane preparations which has to be postulated for a receptor-dependent activation of the adenylate cyclase/cAMP system. Although little is known about the distribution of PGI_2 receptors in the vasculature and possible species-dependent variations, recent findings suggest the absence of PGI_2 receptors in vascular endothelial membranes (10). These observations are in line with the lack of PGI_2-induced cAMP stimulation in endothelial cells reported here. In contrast to cytotoxic NO formation by macrophages (36), PGI_2 generation by endothelial cells may not require a negative feedback mechanism via cAMP stimulation in the endothelial generator cell.

In contrast to this more physiological situation where PGI_2 and NO pathways were independently regulated, clear connections between the two messenger systems were found in endothelial injury as exemplified with myocardial ischemia. Thus, inhibition of prostacylin formation not only resulted in profound deterioration of recovery of myocardial function (31, 33), but also in a significantly reduced NO formation. We previously reported that administration of PGI_2 (31) or its mimetic iloprost (33) to these preparations at non-vasoactive concentrations significantly improves recovery of myocardial function. This suggests that PGI_2 generation by the injured endothelial cells may not be sufficient to afford myocardial protection. Alternatively, endothelial PGI_2 formation may become rapidly inactivated because of inhibition of prostacyclin synthase. In any case, these data, together with the cell culture data, would suggest that reduced NO formation after indomethacin may be another expression of endothelial dysfunction.

Interestingly, inhibition of NO formation did result in marked elevations of coronary vascular resistance, but with no apparent effects on myocardial contractile function. This might be due to the particular experimental conditions, i.e., the maintenance of constant flow despite the considerable increase in coronary vascular resistance. It could, however, also suggest that NO formation is less important for cardiac myocyte function. In contrast to the vascular endothelium, there is no evidence that the NO/cGMP system plays a role for cardiac myocyte function (8). On the other hand, inhibition of soluble guanylate cyclase activation by L-NMMA should have major effects on coronary smooth muscle. This exactly was found and underlines the significance of NO formation for local control of vessel tone (7, 14).

In summary, our data demonstrate two independent pathways for NO and prostacyclin formation in endothelial cells, both being coupled to two different cellular mediator systems: the adenylate cyclase and soluble guanylate cyclase, respectively. Endothelial damage is associated with a marked increase in mediator release whose inhibition has consequences for myocardial and coronary function: inhibition of NO formation also inhibits PGI_2 release and the recovery of coronary vessel tone with only minor if any effects on myocardial contractility. In contrast, inhibition of PGI_2 generation results in marked deterioration of myocardial recovery with only minor changes in coronary perfusion. It is concluded from these data that PGI_2 is important for preservation of myocardial function while NO might mainly be involved in control of local vessel tone.

Acknowledgements. The authors thank Christine Machunsky for technical assistance. This study was supported by the Deutsche Forschungsgemeinschaft (Schr 194/7-2).

References

1. Alheid U, Reichwehr I, Förstermann U (1989) Human endothelial cells inhibit platelet aggregation by separately stimulating platelet cyclic AMP and cyclic GMP. Eur J Pharmacol 164:103–110
2. Botting R, Vane JR (1989) The receipt and dispatch of chemical messengers by endothelial cells. Prog Clin Biol Res 301:1–11
3. Evans HG, Smith JA, Lewis MJ (1988) Release of endothelium-derived relaxing factor is inhibited by 8-bromo-cyclic guanosine monophosphate. J Cardiovasc Pharmacol 12:672–677
4. Feelisch M, Noack EA (1987) Correlation between nitric oxide formation during degradation of organic nitrates and activation of guanylate cyclase. Eur J Pharmacol 139:19–30
5. Friedl A, Harmening C, Schuricht B, Hamprecht B (1985) Rat atrial natriuretic peptide elevates the level of cyclic GMP in astroglia-rich brain cell cultures. Eur J Pharmacol 111:141–142
6. Gorman R, Bunting S, Miller O (1977) Modulation of human platelet adenylate cyclase by prostacyclin (PGX). Prostaglandins 13:377–388
7. Griffith TM, Edwards DH, Davies RLl, Harrison TJ, Evans KT (1988) Endothelium-derived relaxing factor (EDRF) and resistance vessels in an intact vascular bed: a microangio-graphic study of the rabbit isolated ear. Br J Pharmacol 93:654–662
8. Groschner K, Holzmann S, Kukovetz W (1986) Lack of second messenger function of cyclic GMP in acetylcholine induced negative inotropism. J Cardiovasc Pharmacol 8:1154–1157
9. Gryglewski RJ, Moncada S, Palmer RMJ (1986) Bioassay of prostacyclin and endothelium-derived relaxing factor (EDRF) from porcine aortic endothelial cells. Br J Pharmacol 87:685–694
10. Halushka PV, Mais DE, Mayeux PR, Morinelli TA (1989) Thromboxane, prostaglandin and leukotriene receptors. Ann Rev Pharmacol Toxicol 29:213–239
11. Haussmann HJ, Werringloer J (1985) Oxidative denitrosation and activation of N-nitrosodimethylamine. Biochem Pharmacol 34:411–412
12. Holzmann S (1982) Endothelium-induced relaxation by acetylcholine associated with larger rises in cyclic GMP in coronary arterial strips. J Cyclic Nucleotide Protein Phosphor Res 8:409–419
13. Hopkins NK, Gorman RR (1981) Regulation of endothelial cells cyclic nucleotide metabolism by prostacyclin. J Clin Invest 67:540–546
14. Inoue T, Tomoike H, Hisano K, Nakamura M (1988) Endothelium determines flow-dependent dilation of the epicardial coronary artery in dogs. J Am Coll Cardiol 11:187–191
15. Kelm M, Feelisch M, Spahr R, Piper HM, Noack E, Schrader J (1988) Quantitative and kinetic characterization of nitric oxide and EDRF released from cultured endothelial cells. Biochem Biophys Res Commun 154:236–244
16. Kelm M, Schrader J (1988) Nitric oxide release from the isolated guinea pig heart. Eur J Pharmacol 155:317–321
17. Kelm M, Schrader J (1990) Control of coronary vascular tone by nitric oxide. Circ Res 66:1561–1575
18. Kukovetz WR, Holzmann S, Schmidt K (1988) Freisetzung von EDRF durch Kaliumionen, Bradykinin and Kalzium-Ionophor (A23187) aus Endothelzellen. CorVas 4:163–168
19. Martin W, White DG, Henderson AH (1988) Endothelium-derived relaxing factor and atriopeptin II elevate cyclic GMP levels in pig aortic endothelial cells. Br J Pharmacol 93:229–239
20. Moncada S, Palmer RMJ, Higgs EA (1987) Prostacyclin and endothelium-derived relaxing factor: biological interactions and significance. In: Verstraete M, Vermylen J, Lijnen R, Arnout J (eds) Thrombosis and haemostasis. Leuven University Press, Leuven, pp 587–618
21. Moncada S, Radomski MW, Palmer RMJ (1988) Endothelium-derived relaxing factor. Identification as nitric oxide and role in the control of vascular tone and platelet function. Biochem Pharmacol 37:2495–2501

22. Mülsch A, Böhme E, Busse R (1987) Stimulation of soluble guanylate cyclase by endothelium-derived relaxing factor from cultured endothelial cells. Eur J Pharmacol 135:247–250
23. Mülsch A, Busse R (1990) N^G-nitro-L-arginine (N^5-[imino-(nitroamino)methyl]-L-ornithine) impairs endothelium-dependent dilations by inhibiting cytosolic nitric oxide synthesis from L-arginine. Naunyn-Schmiedeberg's Arch Pharmacol 341:143–147
24. Ogura A, Ozaki K, Kudo Y, Amano T (1986) Cytosolic calcium elevation and cGMP production induced by serotonin in a clonal cell of glial origin. J Neurosci 6:2489–2494
25. Palmer RMJ, Rees DD, Ashton DS, Moncada S (1988) L-Arginine is the physiological precursor for the formation of nitric oxide in endothelium-dependent relaxation. Biochem Biophys Res Commun 153:1251–1256
26. Schafer AI, Gimbrone MA Jr, Handin RI (1980) Endothelial cell adenylate cyclase: activation by catecholamines and prostaglandin I_2. Biochem Biophys Res Commun 96:1640–1647
27. Schröder H, Leitman DC, Bennett BM, Waldman SA, Murad F (1988) Glyceryl trinitrate-induced desensitization of guanylate cyclase in cultured rat lung fibroblasts. J Pharmacol Exp Ther 245:413–418
28. Schröder H, Machunsky C, Strobach H, Schrör K (1990) Nitric oxide but not prostacyclin has an autocrine function in porcine aortic endothelial cells. Adv Prostaglandin Thromboxane Leukotriene Res 21:671–674
29. Schröder H, Ney P, Woditsch I, Schrör K (1990) Cyclic GMP mediates SIN-1-induced inhibition of human polymorphonuclear leukocytes. Eur J Pharmacol 182:211–218
30. Schröder H, Schrör K (1989) Cyclic GMP stimulation by vasopressin in LLc-PK1 kidney epithelial cells is L-arginine-dependent. Naunyn-Schmiedeberg's Arch Pharmacol 340:475–477
31. Schrör K, Darius H, Addicks K, Köster R, Smith EF III (1982) PGI_2 prevents ischaemia-induced alterations in cardiac catecholamines without influencing nerve-stimulation induced catecholamine release in non-ischaemic conditions. J Cardiovasc Pharmacol 4:741–748
32. Schrör K, Förster S, Woditsch I, Schröder H (1989) Generation of NO from molsidomine (SIN-1) in vitro and its relationship to changes in coronary vessel tone. J Cardiovasc Pharmacol 14:(suppl 1)S29–S34
33. Schrör K, Funke K (1985) Prostaglandins and myocardial noradrenaline overflow after sympathetic nerve stimulation during ischemia and reperfusion. J Cardiovasc Pharmacol 7:(suppl 5)S50–S54
34. Schrör K, Seidel H (1988) Blood vessel-wall arachidonate acid metabolism and its pharmacological modification in a new in vitro assay system. Naunyn-Schmiedeberg's Arch Pharmacol 337:177–182
35. Steiner AL, Parker CW, Kipnis DM (1972) Radioimmunoassay for cyclic nucleotides. J Biol Chem 247:1106–1113
36. Stuehr DJ, Nathan CF (1989) Nitric oxide – a macrophage product responsible for cytostasis and respiratory inhibition in tumor target cells. J Exp Med 169:1543–1555

Author's address:

K. Schrör
Institut für Pharmakologie
Heinrich-Heine-Universität Düsseldorf
Moorenstraße 5
W-4000 Düsseldorf 1, FRG

Effects of native and oxidized low-density lipoproteins on endothelium-dependent and endothelium-independent vasomotion

J. Galle and E. Bassenge

Department of Applied Physiology, University of Freiburg, FRG

Summary: Native and oxidized low-density lipoproteins (LDL) were investigated for their direct influence on EDRF-formation, EDRF-activity, and vascular smooth muscle tone. Native (n) LDL, isolated from fresh human plasma, was oxidized by Cu^{2+}-incubation. EDRF released from cultured endothelial cells was inactivated by both n-LDL and ox-LDL (1 mg/ml) as detected in a bioassay system. n-LDL reduced the EDRF-mediated vasodilations of the detector segments by $38.5 \pm 5.3\%$, and ox-LDL by $55.5 \pm 4.6\%$. The effects of lipoproteins on EDRF-formation were studied on cultured endothelial cells, preincubated with either n-LDL or ox-LDL (1 mg/ml, 1 h) and stimulated for EDRF-release with bradykinin after washout of the lipoproteins. EDRF was assessed by measuring its stimulatory effect on the activity of a purified soluble guanylate cyclase. Preincubation with both n-LDL and ox-LDL did not reduce the bradykinin-induced EDRF-formation. Accordingly, acetylcholine-induced, EDRF-mediated dilations of intact rabbit femoral artery segments were not impaired by luminal exposure to n-LDL or ox-LDL (1 h, 1mg/ml).

Effects of n-LDL and ox-LDL on vascular smooth muscle tone were investigated in isolated perfused rabbit femoral arteries. Perfusion of endothelium-intact and -denuded segments with ox-LDL (80–500 μg protein/ml) caused no or only weak vascoconstrictions in the absence of contractile agonists. However, in the presence of ox-LDL, vasoconstrictions to threshold concentrations of norepinephrine (NE), serotonin (5-HT), phenylephrine (PE) or potassium were significantly enhanced. Native LDL (80–1000 μg/ml) had no effect on vascular tone, neither in presence nor in absence of contractile agonists. Preincubation with verapamil, diltiazem, and nitrendipine inhibited vasoconstrictions evoked by ox-LDL. The contractile responses to ox-LDL were significantly greater in endothelium-denuded segments than in endothelium-intact segments.

In conclusion, neither n-LDL nor ox-LDL acutely impair the formation of EDRF, but do inactivate EDRF after its release from endothelial cells. n-LDL has no direct influence on vascular smooth muscle tone, but ox-LDL greatly enhances vasoconstrictions to various contractile agonists by direct interaction with vascular smooth muscle. Thus, in regions of lipoprotein-accumulation in the arterial wall, both n-LDL and ox-LDL may favor inappropriate vasoconstrictions.

Key words: Hypercholesterolemia; atherosclerosis; vasospasm; endothelium-derived relaxant factor (EDRF); vascular smooth muscle; lipid peroxidation

Introduction

The crucial role of low-density lipoproteins (LDL) for the development of atherosclerosis is well established, and recent evidence suggests that oxidation of LDL is a key event in this process (38). Since endothelium-dependent vasodilations are impaired in atherosclerosis (3, 22, 32, 43), and an arterial hyperresponsiveness to different vasoconstrictors in hypercholesterolemic animals (3, 18, 20, 36, 41, 45) has been shown, interest has focused on a possible link between lipoproteins and changes in vascular tone (1, 25, 40, 42). However, conflicting results have been reported with regard to the attenuation of endothelium-dependent vasodilations by short-term exposure to n-LDL and ox-LDL in vitro, and it also remains controversial, whether lipoproteins directly affect arterial smooth muscle tone.

It was the aim of the present study to clarify whether different methodological approaches account for these conflicting results. Therefore, we studied separately the effects of n-LDL and ox-LDL on the formation of EDRF in cultured endothelial cells, on its inactivation after the release from endothelial cells, on endothelium-dependent vasodilations of arterial rings and segments, and on vascular smooth muscle tone. Special care has been taken to avoid lipoprotein oxidation during preparation of n-LDL to clearly differentiate between n-LDL and ox-LDL, since the biological activity of LDL critically depends on its state of oxidation (19).

Material and methods

Preparation and oxidation of native LDL

Plasma was separated from freshly drawn human blood, and LDL (density 1.019–1.063 g/ml) was isolated by sequential ultracentrifugation at 200000 g (17) in the presence of ethylene-diamine-tetraacetic acid (EDTA, 0.2 mM), butylated-hydroxy-toluene (BHT, 20 μM), chloramphenicol (10 mg/dl) and phenyl-methyl-sulphonyl-fluoride (PMSF, 1 mM) to avoid autoxidation, proteolytic digestion, and bacterial growth (10). Thereafter, LDL was concentrated and purified by gel filtration in presence of EDTA 0.2 mM and BHT 20 μM. Stock solutions of LDL (8–12 mg protein/ml, dissolved in Tyrode's solution) were sterilized by filtration (millex, Millipore, pore size 0.22 μM) and kept in the dark at 4° C for no longer than 3 weeks. LDL prepared by this method is referred to as native-LDL (n-LDL). Protein content was measured as described by Bradford (4).

For oxidation, n-LDL was separated from EDTA and BHT by gel filtration, and incubated with $CuSO_4$ (5 μM) for 24 h at 23° C in phosphate-buffered saline. The degree of oxidation in comparison to n-LDL was quantified by three different methods: i) the absorption at $\lambda = 234$ nm increased, indicating an increase in diene formation of fatty acids (12), ii) the relative mobility on agarose gel increased to up to 1.60 times that of n-LDL, indicating an enhanced negative charge of ox-LDL (39), and iii) sodium-dodecyl-sulfate polyacrylamid gel electrophoresis (SDS-PAGE) demonstrated fractionation of apoprotein B 100 (20). Finally, ox-LDL was separated from $CuSO_4$ by gel filtration and concentrated as n-LDL.

Electrophoresis

Sodium-dodecyl-sulfate polyacrylamid gel electrophoresis (SDS-PAGE) was performed according to the Laemmli' method using 3–20% gradient gels (26). Visualization of the protein bands was achieved by Coomassie blue (26). n-LDL migrated as a single, apo-B 100-protein band. ox-LDL was completely depleted of apo-B 100-protein, and fractionated into multiple protein bands of minor molecular weight. Agarose gel electrophoresis was performed to measure relative mobility of ox-LDL compared to n-LDL as index for lipoprotein oxidation (39). Electrophoresis kits (lipidophor) were purchased from Immuno (Heidelberg, FRG).

Drugs

Phenylephrine, indomethacin, serotonin, bradykinin, thimerosal, and verapamil were purchased from Sigma (Munich, FRG). Indomethacin was dissolved in ethanol-0.1 M $NaHCO_3$ (1:3) vol/vol and diluted with Tyrode's solution. Norepinephrine (Arterenol, Hoechst, Frankfurt, FRG), diltiazem hydrochloride (Dilzem, Goedecke, Berlin, FRG), and acetylcholine hydrochloride (Sigma, Munich, FRG) were also dissolved in Tyrode's solution. For stock solutions of potassium-rich Tyrode's solution, sodium was replaced isotonically by potassium to gain a potassium concentration of 140 mM. Nitrendipine (Bayer, Leverkusen, FRG) was dissolved in absolute ethanol, and further diluted with Tyrode's solution.

Endothelial cell culture

For bioassay experiments with femoral segments, bovine aortic endothelial cells were isolated and cultured as described elsewhere in detail (28). Briefly, the endothelium was scraped off freshly obtained aortae and grown on standard culture dishes. For bioassay experiments with endothelium-denuded artery segments, cells were subcultured on microcarrier beads (Biosilon, Nunc-Intermed, Wiesbaden, FRG), and packed into a column. The endothelial cell column was perfused with oxigenated Tyrode's solution (PO_2 about 140 mmHg) at a rate of 30 ml/h, and stimulated for continuous EDRF-release with thimerosal (5 μM) (14). The outflow tubing of the cell column was connected with the inflow cannula of a preconstricted artery segment which served as detector for EDRF (Fig. 1). The dilator compound released from the cell columns were characterized as EDRF, as in earlier experiments (28).

To investigate whether lipoproteins inactivate released EDRF, the lipoproteins could be applicated distally to the endothelial cell columns by a T-connection (Fig. 1). The perfusion rate through this sideway was 1/10 of the perfusion rate through the endothelial cell columns, and the lipoproteins (stock solution concentration: 10 mg/ml) were administered through this sideway in change with Tyrode's solution to give a final concentration of 1 mg/ml.

While testing the inhibitory action of lipoproteins, a second detector segment not perfused with the lipoproteins served as control for continuous and stable EDRF-release. Therefore, the effluent of the endothelial cell columns could be perfused, alternatively through the segments.

Inactivation of EDRF by the lipoproteins is expressed as percent of the vasodilations in absence of lipoproteins.

Guanylate cyclase assay

EDRF-release from cultured endothelial cells was detected by a guanylate cyclase assay as described elsewhere in detail (29, 30). Endothelial cells grown on plates were exposed to n-LDL, ox-LDL, or lipoprotein-deficient serum as control (1 mg/ml, 1 h, respectively). The cells were then washed and stimulated with bradykinin (30 nM). The supernatant covering the cells was transferred into a test tube containing purified soluble guanylate cyclase from bovine lung. The activity of guanylate cyclase was determined by measuring the formation of $[^{32}P]$cGMP from $[\alpha-^{32}P]$GTP.

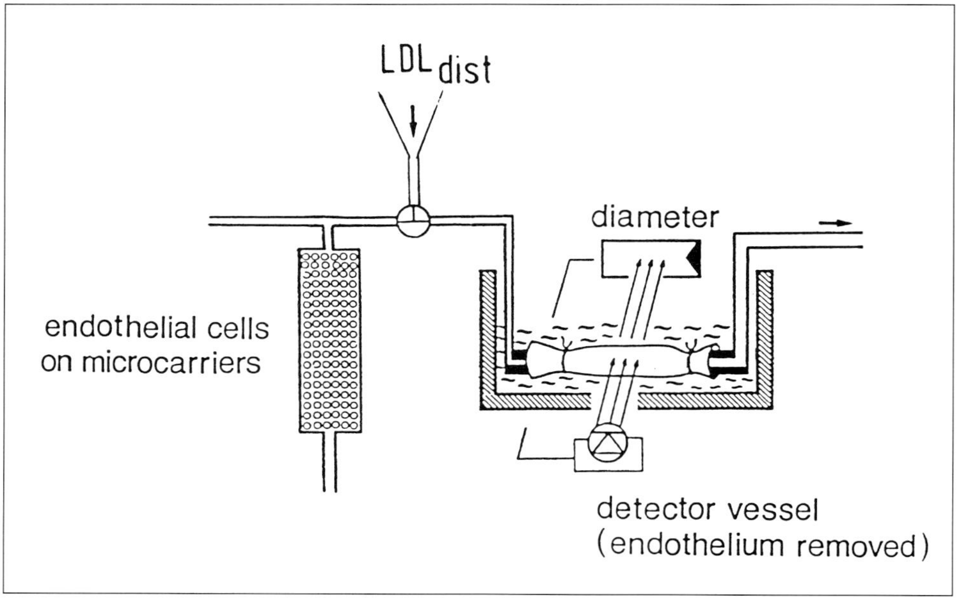

Fig. 1. Experimental setup used for bioassay of EDRF released from cultured endothelial cells after stimulation with thimerosal (5 μM). A preconstricted, endothelium-denuded detector vessel was perfused either by the EDRF-containing effluent of an endothelial cell column or by Tyrode's solution. Lipoproteins could be administered distal to the endothelial cell column. External diameter of the detector segment was recorded by a photoelectrical device

Vessel preparation

Intact segments of the fermoral artery were obtained from rabbits of either sex (2.5–3.5 kg). For part of the experiments, the endothelium was removed mechanically by gently rubbing the segments over a rough steel cannula. Intactness or absence of endothelium was tested as described earlier (5). The segments were fixed between two steel cannulas and placed in an organ bath (37° C) containing oxygenated Tyrode's solution (pH 7.4). The solution was perfused through the organ bath at a rate of 0.66 ml/min. In addition to organ bath perfusion the segments were perfused intraluminally (Tyrode's solution: PO_2 130 mmHg, PCO_2 28 mmHg, pH 7.38, at a rate of 0.5 ml/min).

Outer vascular diameters were recorded continuously by a photoelectric device. The transmural pressure was adjusted hydrostatically to 40 mmHg (isobaric conditions). Resting diameter was 1755 ± 22 μm) (n = 28) under these conditions. Full details of this experimental set-up (Fig. 1) have been published (5).

Endothelium-dependent vasodilations before and after 1 h incubation with n-LDL or ox-LDL (1 mg/ml) were elicited by intraluminal perfusion with cumulative dosages of acetylcholine (0.03–1 μM).

For bioassay experiments, the segments were preconstricted with norepinephrine (0.1 μM) applied to the organ bath, and the effluent of the endothelial cell columns was perfused intraluminally through the endothelium-denuded segments as described above. Since ox-LDL has an enhancing effect on norepinephrine-induced vasoconstrictions

(15), the norepinephrine concentration in the organ bath was lowered in presence of ox-LDL to achieve the same level of preconstriction as under reference conditions without ox-LDL.

Effects of the lipoproteins on smooth muscle tone were tested in each experiment in segments with and without endothelium simultaneously. n-LDL (50–500 µg), ox-LDL (50–500 µg/ml), acetylcholine (Ach, 0.5 µM), indomethacin (10 µM), verapamil (1µM), diltiazem (10 µM) and nitrendipine (1 µM) were administered at the intimal side by adding to the intraluminal perfusate. Norepinephrine (NE, 1–100 nM), phenylephrine (PE, 0.01–1 µM), serotonin (5-HT, 0.01–1 µM), and potassium (K^+, 20–40 mM) were added to the organ bath (if not otherwise indicated). For experiments with (sub)threshold concentrations of the contractile agonists, concentrations were choosen which evoked no or minimal vasoconstrictions. Concentration-response relations of NE and PE with and without ox-LDL were performed by adding the compounds to the intraluminal perfusate.

In an additional series of experiments, we compared the influence of n-LDL on endothelium-dependent vasorelaxations in arterial ring preparations with those in arterial segments. Pairs of rings and segments were prepared from the same rabbit aorta. The aortic rings (4 mm in diameter, 3-mm wide) were mounted in a force transducer (Biegestab K 30, H. Sachs, Hugstetten, FRG) under 1.5 g resting tension, and superfused with oxygenated Tyrode's solution (95% O_2 – 5% CO_2, pH 7.4, 37° C, 40 ml/h). After 30 min equilibration time, the rings were precontracted with norepinephrine (0.1 µM), and endothelium-dependent relaxations were elicited by 1 µM acetylcholine before and after 30-min superfusion with n-LDL (1 mg/ml) or Tyrode's solution without n-LDL (control). Relaxations are expressed as percent of precontraction. In each experiment, aortic rings and segments obtained from the same animal were investigated simultaneously.

Statistics

All data are presented as means ± SEM. Paired Student's *t*-test was used to evaluate statistical significance of differences. For multiple comparison of data, Bonferroni' correction was performed. $p \leqq 0.05$ was considered to be statistically significant. $* = p < 0.05$.

Results

Formation of EDRF in cultured endothelial cells after incubation with n-LDL and ox-LDL

Figure 2 shows the release of EDRF from cultured endothelial cells after stimulation with bradykinin (30 nM). Prior to stimulation, endothelial cells were incubated with either n-LDL, ox-LDL, or lipoprotein-deficient serum as control (1 mg/ml, 1 h, respectively). Following bradykinin-stimulation of the endothelial cells, the guanylate cyclase (GC) activity in the assay increased more than three fold in all groups. The increase in GC-activity did not differ between the groups.

Inactivation by n-LDL and ox-LDL of EDRF released from cultured endothelial cells

Figure 3a illustrates the EDRF-inactivating effect of n-LDL (1 mg/ml) on a detector segment preconstricted with norepinephrine. The EDRF-mediated vasodilation of the

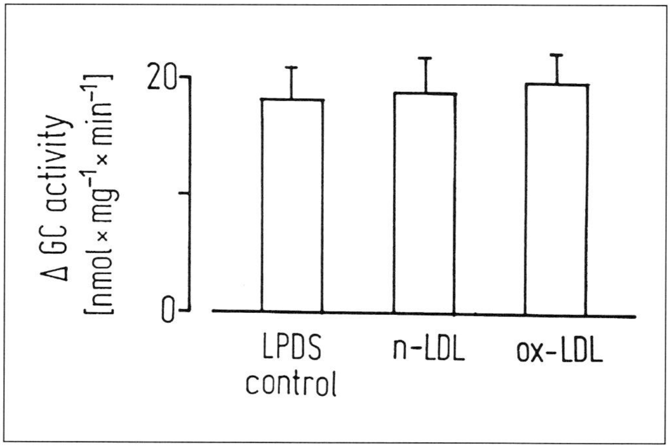

Fig. 2. Effects of incubation with n-LDL and ox-LDL (1 h, 1 mg/ml) on bradykinin (BK) – induced EDRF-release from cultured endothelial cells. EDRF-release was measured as stimulation of the activity of guanylate cyclase (GC). Stimulation of the cells with bradykinin (30 nM) caused a significant increase of basal GC-activity in the control group (LPDS, lipoprotein-deficient serum), which did not differ from the increase in the lipoprotein-incubated groups (middle and right columns). n = 8

detector segment was markedly reduced when n-LDL was added to the effluent of an endothelial cell column. The same holds true for administration of ox-LDL. Figure 3 b illustrates the time-course of the EDRF-inactivation by n-LDL during continuous EDRF-perfusion of a detector segment. Addition of n-LDL to the effluent caused immediate suppression of the vasodilation, which was also immediately reversible when the n-LDL perfusion was stopped.

Data of the EDRF-inactivation by n-LDL and ox-LDL are summarized in Fig. 4: addition of n-LDL reduced the vasodilations of the detector segments by 38.5 ± 5.3%, and addition of ox-LDL by 55.5 ± 4.6% (n = 12).

Endothelium-mediated dilatation in perfused femoral segments preincubated with n-LDL and ox-LDL

Dose-response relations of preconstricted rabbit femoral arteries to acetylcholine before and after 1-h incubation with n-LDL or ox-LDL (1 mg/ml) are shown in Figs. 5 a and 5 b. Throughout the whole concentration range, dilations to acetylcholine did not differ significantly between lipoprotein-incubated segments and control segments. Thus, n-LDL and ox-LDL did not impair acetylcholine-induced endothelium-dependent vasodilations in perfused segments.

Comparison of the influence of n-LDL on endothelium-dependent relaxations in aortic rings and aortic segments

As in femoral segments, vasodilations of aortic segments to acetylcholine (1 μM) were not impaired after 1-h incubation with 1 mg/ml n-LDL: 81 ± 5% dilation before vs

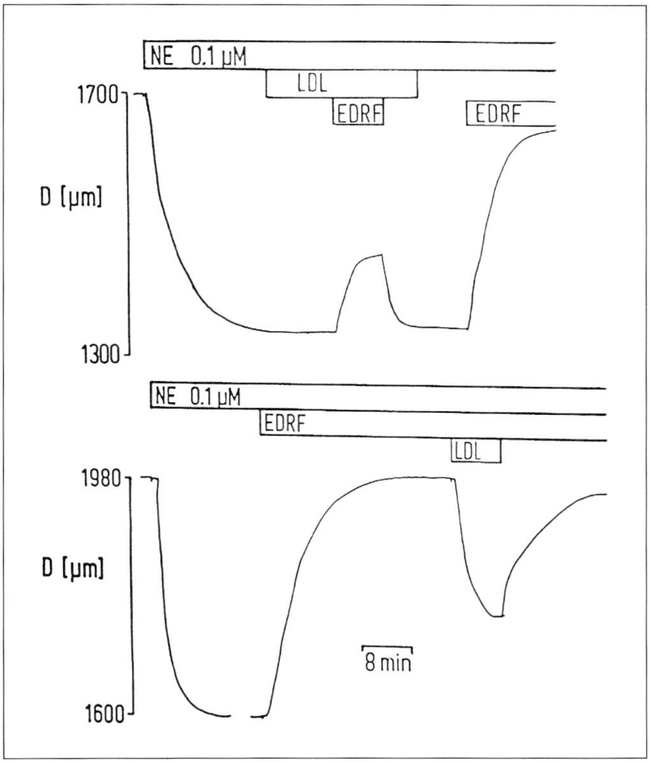

Fig. 3. Diameter (D) recordings of an endothelium-denuded rabbit femoral-artery segment, perfused with either Tyrode's solution or the EDRF-containing effluent from an endothelial cell column stimulated with thimerosal (5 µM). The detector segment was preconstricted with norepinephrine 0.1 µM, and vasodilations were elicited by switching the intraluminal perfusate from Tyrode's solution to the EDRF containing effluent from the endothelial cell column. **a** (upper part): In presence of n-LDL (1 mg/ml) added to the effluent distally to the endothelial cell column, the EDRF-mediated vasodilation was markedly reduced. **b** (lower part): Adding n-LDL to the EDRF-containing effluent caused immediate suppression of the vasodilation, which was also immediately reversible

79 ± 5% dilation after incubation with n-LDL (n = 4). In contrast, relaxations of aortic rings to acetylcholine (1 µM) were markedly reduced after 30-min superfusion with n-LDL: 81 ± 8% relaxation vs 36 ± 15% relaxation (n = 4). Relaxations of control rings without incubation with lipoproteins did not change within this time interval.

Effects of n-LDL and ox-LDL upon unstimulated segments

Intraluminal perfusion of unstimulated segments (no contractile agonists present in the organ bath) with n-LDL in concentrations between 50 and 500 µg protein/ml did not elicit any vasoconstriction. Ox-LDL caused no or only weak vasoconstrictions (17 ± 4 µm, max. 2% of resting diameter, n = 26) at concentrations below 150 µg pro-

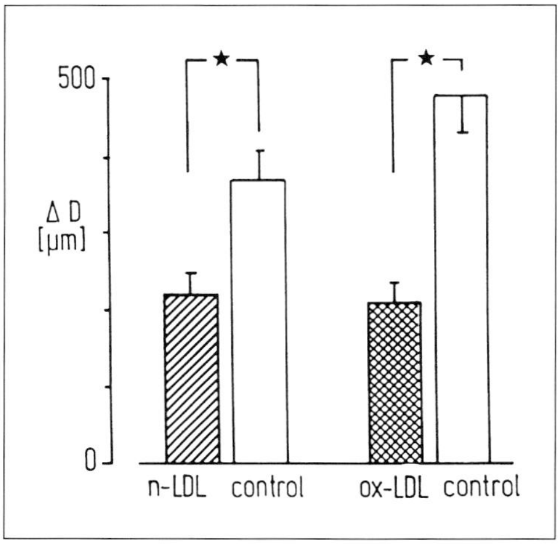

Fig. 4. Effects of 1 mg/ml n-LDL and ox-LDL on EDRF released from endothelial cell columns on its transfer to endothelium-denuded detector vessels. Addition of n-LDL is effluent from endothelial cell columns reduced the vasodilations of the detector segments by 38.5±5.3% (left pair of columns), and addition of ox-LDL by 55.5±4.6% (right pair of columns). n=12. * = p<0.05

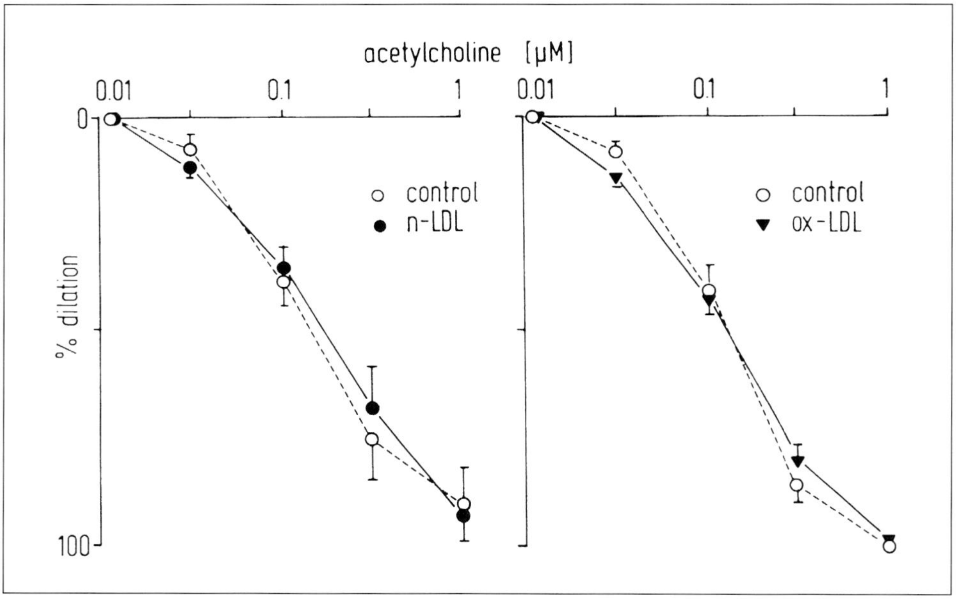

Fig. 5a, b. Vasodilations evoked by acetylcholine in intact rabbit-femoral artery segments prior to and after 1 h incubation with 1 mg/ml n-LDL or ox-LDL. Acetylcholine was perfused intraluminally through the segments in cumulative dosages (0.03, 0.1, 0.3, 1 μM). Vasodilations are expressed as % of preconstriction (induced by norepinephrine 0.1 μM). **a** (left): vasodilations before (control, -○-) and after incubation with n-LDL (-●-). n=7. **b** (right): vasodilations before (control, -○-) and after incubation with ox-LDL (-▼-). n=9. The vasodilations did not differ significantly tein/ml. When ox-LDL was administered at higher concentrations, moderate vasoconstrictions (139 ± 11 μm, max. 8% of resting diameter, n = 16) were observed.

Effects of n-LDL and ox-LDL upon stimulated segments

As shown by the diameter recording in Fig. 6, ox-LDL caused markedly augmented contractile responses in the presence of the contractile agonist phenylephrine, which was administered at threshold concentrations.

Figure 7 demonstrates that this potentiating effect of ox-LDL takes place also with other contractile agonists: contractile responses to norepinephrine (NE), phenylephrine (PE), serotonin (5-HT), and potassium (K^+), all administered at threshold concentrations, were significantly augmented in the presence of ox-LDL (80 μg/ml). Native LDL did not enhance the contractile responses to these agonists. For each agonist, the enhancement was significantly greater in endothelium-denuded than in endothelium-intact segments. In the case of NE and PE, cumulative concentration-response relations were obtained with and without ox-LDL. As shown in Fig. 8, ox-LDL increased the potency of NE and PE in endothelium-intact and endothelium-denuded segments. Again, the enhancement of the contractile response was significantly greater in endothelium-denuded than in endothelium-intact segments.

In additional experiments, ox-LDL derived by prior incubation with activated macrophages also enhanced contractile responses to norepinephrine (data not shown).

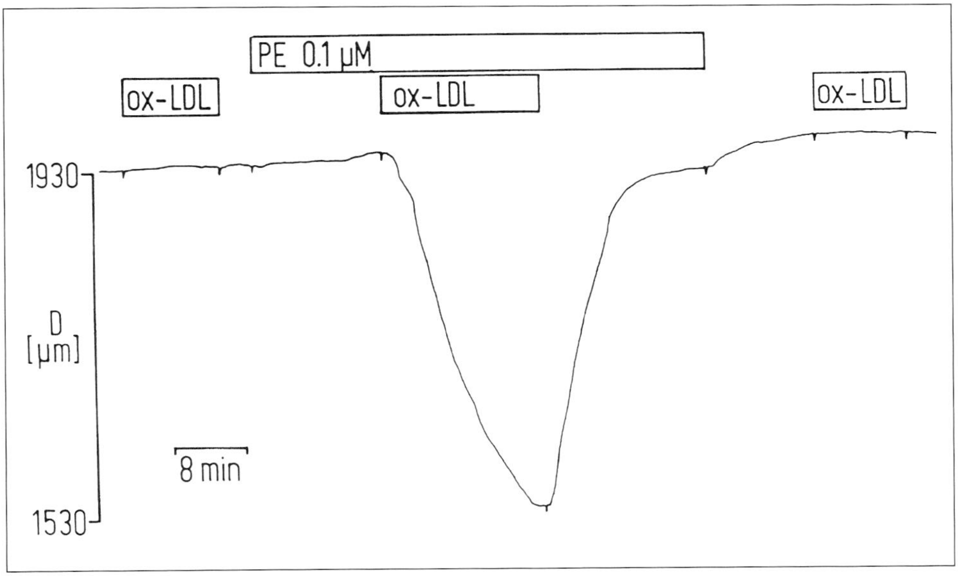

Fig. 6. Diameter (D) recording of a rabbit femoral-artery segment intraluminally perfused with ox-LDL (80 μg/ml), either in absence or in presence of phenylephrine (PE) in subthreshold concentration (0.1 μM). ox-LDL caused no vasoconstriction on its own, but substantial vasoconstriction in presence of phenylephrine. Bars indicate the presence of ox-LDL or phenylephrine

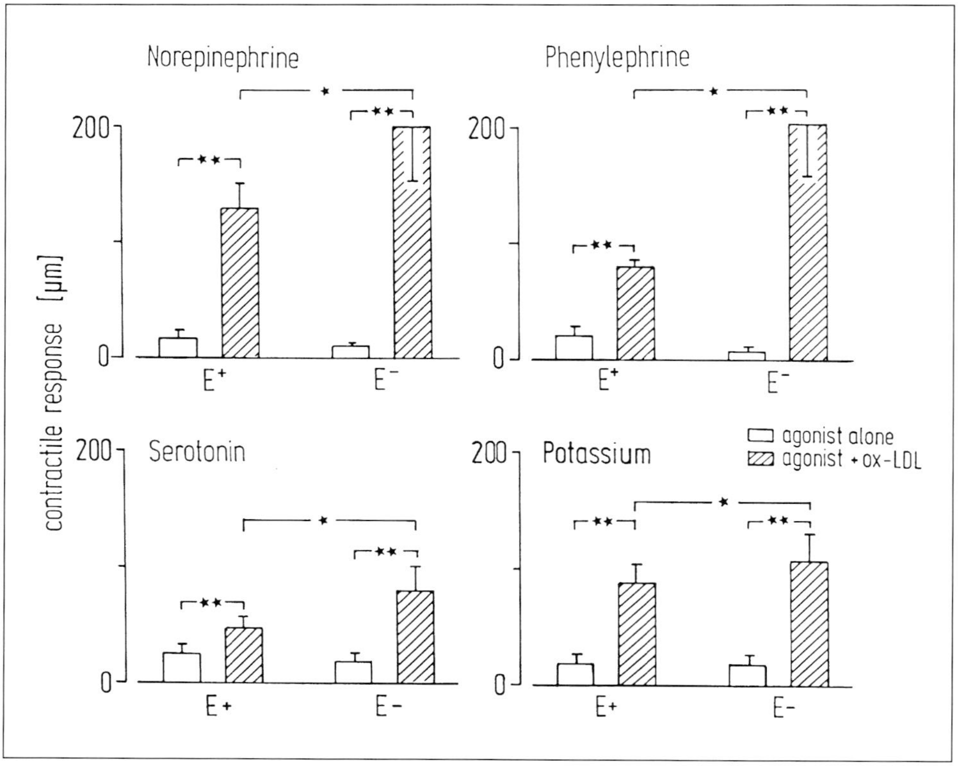

Fig. 7. Perfusion with ox-LDL enhances contractile responses to various agonists. Agonists were administered to the organ bath at threshold concentrations which evoked only marginal vasoconstrictions in segments with (E^+) and without endothelium (E^-): NE = norepinephrine [1–3 nM, 17 ± 8 μm (E^+), 12 ± 5 μm (E^-)], PE = phenylephrine [10–30 nM, 7 ± 5 μm (E^+), 21 ± 9 μm (E^-)], 5-HT = serotonin 10–50 nM, 26 ± 7 μm (E^+), 20 ± 7 μm (E^-)], and K^+ = potassium [20–30 mM, 20 ± 8 μm (E^+), 19 ± 8 μm (E^-)]. Ox-LDL (80 μg/ml) was perfused intraluminally and caused only minimal vasoconstrictions [9 ± 2 μm (E^+), 17 ± 4 μm (E^-)] in absence of agonists. Contractile responses (μm) are expressed as means ± SEM. Each panel shows the enhancement of contractile responses to one agonist by ox-LDL in endothelium-intact and endothelium-denuded segments. * = $p < 0.05$, ** = $p < 0.01$. n = 7 for each group

Effects of Ca^{2+}-antagonists and indomethacin upon ox-LDL evoked vasoconstrictions

To investigate whether the ox-LDL evoked vasoconstrictions are linked to a transmembraneous Ca^{2+}-influx, we pre-incubated segments with three structurally different types of Ca^{2+}-channel blockers: diltiazem, verapamil, and nitrendipine. As shown in Fig. 9, the ox-LDL-induced vasoconstrictions were nearly equally suppressed by diltiazem, verapamil, and nitrendipine in the presence of norepinephrine. These inhibitory effects were more pronounced in endothelium-denuded than in endothelium-intact segments (Fig. 9 and Table 1). However, the Ca^{2+} antagonist-induced suppression was different for the specific agonists used (Table 1).

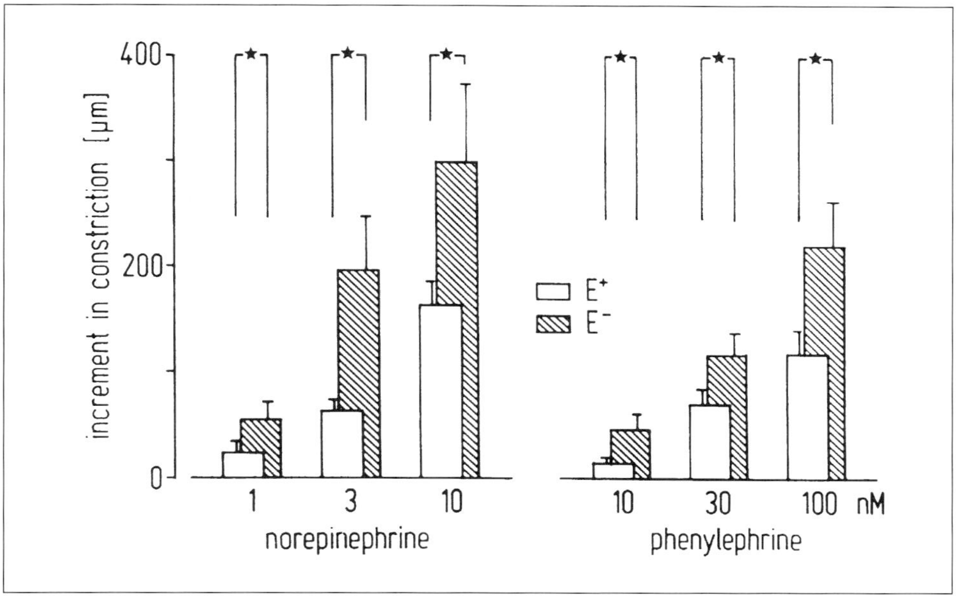

Fig. 8. Increase in potency of norepinephrine (NE) and phenylephrine (PE) by ox-LDL in rabbit femoral arteries. NE (0.3–10 nM) and PE (0.3–30 nM) were administered in cumulative doses to the intraluminal perfusion, with and without ox-LDL (80 µg/ml). Open columns represent increments of contractile responses (means ± SEM) to NE (left) and PE (right) when ox-LDL was additionally administered to the intraluminal perfusion of endothelium-intact (E^+) segments; hatched columns represent increments of contractile responses by ox-LDL in endothelium-denuded (E^-) segments. In segments without endothelium the increments of contractile responses were significantly greater than in segments with endothelium. Ox-LDL alone caused no vasoconstriction. * = $p < 0.05$

Table 1. Suppression of ox-LDL evoked vasoconstrictions in the presence of various contractile agonists by diltiazem. Percent suppression of contractile responses by diltiazem[a].

	ox-LDL[a] + NE[b]	n	ox-LDL[a] + PE[b]	n	ox-LDL[a] + 5-HT[b]	n	ox-LDL[a] + K^{+b}	n
E^+	48 ± 16	6	81 ± 9	6	67 ± 14	5	100 ± 0	6
E^-	87 ± 3[c]	6	95 ± 3[c]	6	93 ± 3[c]	6	85 ± 12	6

[a] ox-LDL = oxidized low-density-lipoprotein (80 µg/ml) and diltiazem (10 µM) were administered intraluminally
[b] NE = norepinephrine (1–3 nM), PE = phenylephrine (10–30 nM), 5-HT = serotonin (10–50 nM), and K^+ = potassium (20–40 mM) were administered extraluminally
Effects of diltiazem are expressed as means ± SEM of % suppression of contractile responses. Endothelium-intact = E^+, endothelium-denuded = E^-
[c] suppression in E^--segments was significantly greater than in E^+-segments ($p < 0.05$)

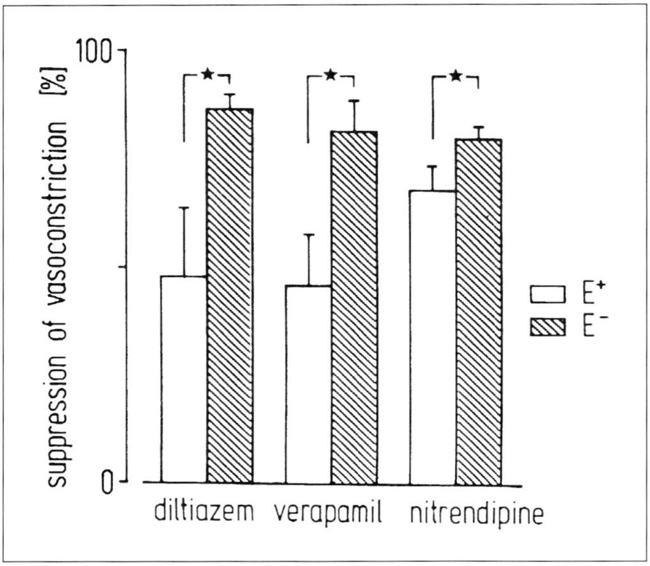

Fig. 9. Suppression of ox-LDL (80 μg/ml) evoked contractile responses by the Ca^{2+}-antagonists verapamil (1 μM), diltiazem (10 μM), and nitrendipine (1 μm) in presence of norepinephrine (n = 6). Suppression is expressed in percent of the contractile response. The suppression by diltiazem, verapamil, and nitrendipine was more effective in endothelium-denuded segments (E^-, hatched columns) than in endothelium-intact segments (E^+, open columns). * = $p < 0.05$

Similar results as obtained in the presence of norepinephrine were also found in the absence of contractile agonists. The vasoconstriction induced by ox-LDL alone was reduced by verapamil by 52 ± 4% (diltiazem: 65 ± 6%) in endothelium-intact segments, and by 71 ± 5% (diltiazem: 77 ± 5%) in endothelium-denuded segments (n = 6).

When the segments were perfused with the cyclooxygenase inhibitor indomethacin (10 μM), no change in the potentiation of contractile responses to ox-LDL was detected (data not shown).

Discussion

The data presented in this study show that both n-LDL and ox-LDL inactivate EDRF after its release from endothelial cells, and that not native LDL, but its oxidized derivatives enhance contractile responses of the isolated rabbit femoral artery to various contractile agonists. However, the formation of EDRF – which is most likely identical with NO (34) – both in cultured endothelial cells and in isolated arterial segments remained unaffected after 1-h incubation with n-LDL and ox-LDL.

There is strong evidence indicating that both native and oxidized LDL are present in the arterial wall in hypercholesterolemia (9, 23, 33, 46). Thus, it is conceivable that the inactivation of EDRF by n-LDL and ox-LDL contributes to the impairment of endothelial function in hypercholesterolemia, as it has been observed in numerous studies (3, 8, 22, 32, 41, 43). Also, the markedly reduced responsiveness of atherosclerotic arteries to EDRF/NO-superfusion (44) can be explained by this direct inactivating effect of n-LDL and ox-LDL accumulating in fatty streaks and atherosclerotic plaques. Furthermore, the increase responsiveness to vasoconstricting agents observed in arteriosclerotic human (3) and animal arteries (3, 18, 20, 22, 36, 41) and their increased disposition for vasospasms might be explained by the potentiating effect of ox-LDL on vascular smooth muscle contractions.

However, our observation that neither a short exposure (1 h) to n-LDL nor to ox-LDL attenuates the formation of EDRF, is in contrast to conclusions drawn by others. In studies performed with arterial-strip preparations, Andrews et al. (1) and Tomita et al. (40) found impairment of endothelium-dependent vasodilations already after less than 30-min incubation with "native" LDL. Henry and associates observed impairment of endothelial function with ox-LDL (2-h incubation) (24), and Vedernikov et al. (42) found (dependent on the route of LDL-application and on the origin of the lipoproteins) both endothelium-dependent vasorelaxations induced by LDL and impairment of acetylcholine-induced vasodilations (after 30-min LDL-incubation).

Different techniques applied for investigation of effects of the lipoproteins on vasomotion could explain the various findings. In our experimental approach with intact segments, endothelium-mediated vasodilations induced by acetylcholine were not impaired after incubation with n-LDL or ox-LDL. However, incubation of arterial ring preparations with n-LDL inhibited such relaxations. One can speculate that arterial ring or strip preparations are more easily permeated by lipoproteins than intact segments. This rapid permeation would render the direct EDRF-inactivating effect of n-LDL and ox-LDL, and thus explain why endothelium-dependent vasodilations were attenuated after relatively short incubation with lipoproteins in ring and strip preparations (1, 24, 40, 42), but not in intact segments.

Furthermore, the comparison of studies undertaken with n-LDL or ox-LDL is associated with major difficulties. Absence of adequate measures against lipid peroxidation favors the development of oxidatively modified LDL. Hence, without detection of the oxidative state of the LDL preparation (40, 42), the observed effects cannot be attributed unequivocally to "native" LDL. More complicating, "oxidized LDL" is not clearly defined. During the lipid peroxidation process, a variety of – partly instable – biologically active substances is formed (11). ox-LDL can be cytotoxic to endothelial cells (19, 21, 31), but its composition can differ depending on the plasma origin and the oxidative conditions (13). With respect to this problem, we used lipoproteins prepared following a standardized protocol throughout a whole series of experiments in all the systems studied. A biological test for our standardization was that oxidized LDL had the capacity to potentiate vasoconstrictions as reported in a previous study (15).

The fact that EDRF-formation was not attenuated by 1-h incubation with the potentially cytotoxic ox-LDL can be explained by the rather short incubation time, which must be clearly differentiated from chronic effects. Thus, we may have missed cytotoxic effects of ox-LDL occurring after more protracted exposure. The molecular mechanism responsible for inactivation of EDRF/NO by LDL is unknown. A possible desensitization of the vascular smooth muscle to EDRF by the lipoproteins seems unlikely. When n-LDL was added in the bioassay experiments during continuous EDRF-perfusion of the detector segment, vasodilations were suppressed immediately. Also, the suppression was immediately reversible by lipoprotein washout. This suggests rather a direct inactivation of EDRF by the lipoproteins than an effect on the target organ smooth muscle.

The highly hydrophobic core of the LDL particle may act as a sink for EDRF/NO, which is about eight-fold more soluble in hydrophobic than in hydrophilic media (27). The NO radical could be consumed by reaction with hydrocarbonic radicals inside the LDL particle. However, the exact mechanism of NO inactivation by LDL remains to be clarified.

The mechanism of the ox-LDL-induced enhancement of contractile responses remains also to be determined. The enhancing effect was observed in endothelium-intact segments and, even more pronounced, in endothelium-denuded segments, providing evidence that the site of action is rather at the smooth muscle itself than at the endothelium. Further evidence that the endothelium was not involved in the enhancing mechanism is based on an undisturbed production of EDRF even after 2-h incubation of the segments with ox-LDL in concentrations which already markedly augmented agonist-induced vasoconstrictions. This certainly does not rule out that ox-LDL can be cytotoxic, but if so, it would predominantly act on the smooth muscle cells.

The fact that the enhancing effect of ox-LDL was more pronounced in endothelium-denuded segments might be due to the loss of basal release of EDRF (16). This enhancement of contractile responses following endothelium removal has already been described in earlier studies (2, 16, 7, 6).

The suppression of the contractile responses by the Ca^{2+}-antagonists diltiazem, verapamil, and nitrendipine was also more effective in endothelium-denuded segments. Similar findings were made with different nitrovasodilators, which also were more effective in endothelium-denuded than in endothelium-intact arterial segments (35, 37).

The suppressor effect of the Ca^{2+}-antagonists on vasoconstrictions elicited by ox-LDL both in the presence and in the absence of contractile agonists suggests that ox-LDL induces predominantly an increased transmembraneous Ca^{2+}-influx. However, an additional release of Ca^{2+} from intracellular stores cannot be excluded.

The possibility that ox-LDL sensitizes the contractile apparatus to Ca^{2+} is less likely. The enhancing effect started after a few minutes, and washout reversed the effect also within 10 min. It is not conceivable that ox-LDL enters and leaves the smooth muscle cells within this short period of time.

Since the enhancing effect is observed with various receptor binding agonists, and also with the receptor-independent K^+-depolarization, ox-LDL seems to act distally to the receptor-coupled signal transduction cascade. One can speculate that ox-LDL modulates via stimulation of phosphatidylinositol metabolism the voltage-gated Ca^{2+}-channels, and, thus, the transmembraneous Ca^{2+}-influxes in the plasma membrane. However, further investigations are needed to clarify the molecular mechanism.

In conclusion, our findings demonstrate that both native and oxidized LDL directly inactivate EDRF, and that oxidized LDL enhances agonist-induced vasoconstrictions by direct interaction with vascular smooth muscle. Formation of EDRF was not attenuated after short-term exposure of endothelial cells and intact segments to the lipoproteins. The EDRF-inactivating effect of both lipoproteins and the vasoconstriction-potentiating effect of ox-LDL may be of particular pathophysiological relevance in regions with lipoprotein accumulation in the vessel wall, like fatty streaks and atherosclerotic plaques, and may favor the initiation of inappropriate vasoconstriction.

References

1. Andrews HE, Bruckdorfer KR, Dunn RC, Jacobs M (1987) Low-density lipoproteins inhibit endothelium-dependent relaxation in rabbit aorta. Nature 327:237–239
2. Bassenge E, Busse R (1988) Endothelial modulation of coronary tone. Prog Cardiovasc Dis 30:349–380
3. Bossaller C, Habib GB, Yamamoto H, Williams C, Wells S, Henry PD (1987) Impaired muscarinic endothelium-dependent relaxation and cyclic guanosine 5′-monophosphate formation in atherosclerotic human coronary artery and rabbit aorta. J Clin Invest 79:170–174
4. Bradford M (1975) A rapid and sensitive method for the quantitation of microgram quantities of protein utilizing the principle of protein dye binding. Anal Biochem 72:248–254

5. Busse R, Pohl U, Kellner C, Klemm U (1983) Endothelial cells are involved in the vasodilatory response to hypoxia. Pflügers Arch 397:78–80
6. Chiba S, Tsukada M (1984) Potentiation of KCl-induced vasoconstriction by saponin treatment in isolated canine mesenteric arteries. Japan J Pharmacol 36:535–537
7. Cohen RA, Zitnay KM, Weisbrod RM, Tesfamariam B (1988) Influence of the endothelium on tone and the response of isolated pig coronary artery to norepinephrine. J Pharmac Exp Ther 244:550–555
8. Cox DA, Vita JA, Treasure CB, Fish RD, Alexander RW, Ganz P, Selwyn AP (1989) Atherosclerosis impairs flow-mediated dilation of coronary arteries in humans. Circulation 80:458–465
9. Daugherty A, Zweifel BS, Sobel BE, Schonfeld G (1988) Isolation of low density lipoprotein from atherosclerotic vascular tissue of Watanabe heritable hyperlipidemic rabbits. Arteriosclerosis 8:768–777
10. Edelstein C, Scanu AM (1986) Precautionary measures for collecting blood destinated for lipoprotein isolation. In: Segrest JP, Albers JJ (eds) Methods in enzymology. Academic Press Inc, pp 151–155
11. Esterbauer H, Jürgens G, Quehenberger O, Koller E (1987) Autoxidation of human low density lipoprotein: loss of polyunsaturated fatty acids and vitamin E and generation of aldehydes. J Lipid Res 28:495–509
12. Esterbauer H, Striegel G, Puhl H, Rotheneder M (1989) Continuous monitoring of in vitro oxidation of human low density lipoprotein. Free Radical Res Comm 6:67–75
13. Esterbauer H, Rotheneder M, Striegel G, Waeg G, Ashy A, Sattler W, Jürgens G (1989) Vitamin E and other lipophilic antioxidants protect LDL against oxidation. Fat Sci Technol 8:316–324
14. Förstermann U, Goppelt-Strübe M, Frölich JC, Busse R (1986) Inhibitors of acyl-coenzyme A: lysolecithin acyltransferase activate the production of endothelium-derived vascular relaxing factor. J Pharmacol Exp Ther 238:352–359
15. Galle J, Bassenge E, Busse R (1990) Oxidized low density lipoproteins potentiate vasoconstrictions to various contractile agonists by direct interaction with vascular smooth muscle. Circ Res 66:1287–1293
16. Griffith TM, Henderson AH, Edwards DH, Lewis MJ (1984) Isolated perfused rabbit coronary artery and aortic strip preparations: the role of endothelium-derived relaxant factor. J Physiol (London) 351:13–24
17. Havel RJ, Eder HA, Bragdon JH (1955) The distribution and chemical composition of ultracentrifugally separated lipoproteins in human serum. J Clin Invest 34:1345–1353
18. Heistad DD, Armstrong ML, Marcus ML, Piegors DJ, Mark AL (1984) Augmented responses to vasoconstrictor stimuli in hypercholesterolemic and atherosclerotic monkeys. Circ Res 54:711–718
19. Hennig B, Chow CK (1988) Lipid peroxidation and endothelial cell injury: implications in atherosclerosis. Free Radical Biol Med 4:99–106
20. Henry PD, Yokoyama M (1980) Supersensitivity of atherosclerotic rabbit aorta to ergonovine. Mediation by a serotonergic mechanism. J Clin Invest 66:306–313
21. Hessler JR, Robertson AL, Chisolm JR, Chisolm GM (1979) LDL induced cytotoxicity and its inhibition by HDL in human vascular smooth muscle and endothelial cells in culture. Atherosclerosis 32:213–229
22. Hof RP, Hof A (1988) Vasoconstrictor and vasodilator effects in normal and atherosclerotic conscious rabbits. Br J Pharmacol 95:1075–1080
23. Hoff HF, Morton RE (1985) Lipoproteins containing apoB extracted from human aortas. Ann NY Acad Sci 454:183–194
24. Kugiyama K, Bucay M, Morrisett JD, Roberts R, Henry PD (1989) Oxidized LDL impairs endothelium-dependent arterial relaxation (abstract). Circulation 80 (Suppl 2):279
25. Kugiyama K, Kerns SA, Morrisett JD, Roberts R, Henry PD (1990) Impairment of endothelium-dependent arterial relaxation by lysolecithin in modified low density lipoproteins. Nature 344:160–162
26. Laemmli UK (1970) Cleavage of structural proteins during the assembly of the head of bacteriophage T4. Nature 227:680–685
27. Link WF (1965) Solubilities of inorganic and metal-organic compounds. American Chemical Society, Washington, DC, Vol. 2, 4th ed., p. 792

28. Lückhoff A, Busse R, Winter I, Bassenge E (1987) Characterization of vascular relaxant factor released from cultured endothelial cells. Hypertension 9:295–303
29. Lückhoff A, Mülsch A, Busse R (1990) cAMP attenuates autacoid release from endothelial cells: relation to internal calcium. Am J Physiol 258:H960–H966
30. Mülsch A, Böhme E, Busse R (1987) Stimulation of soluble guanylate cyclase by endothelium-derived relaxing factor from cultured endothelial cells. Eur J Pharmacol 135:247–250
31. Morel DW, Hessler JR, Chisolm GM (1983) Low density cytotoxicity induced by free radical peroxidation of lipid. J Lipid Res 24:1070–1076
32. Osborne JA, Lento PH, Siegfried MR, Stahl GL, Fusman B, Lefer AM (1989) Cardiovascular effects of acute hypercholesterolemia in rabbits. J Clin Invest 83:465–473
33. Palinski W, Rosenfeld ME, Ylä-Herttuala S, Gurtner GC, Socher SS, Butler SW, Parthasarathy S, Carew TE, Steinberg D, Witzum JL (1989) Low density lipoprotein undergoes oxidative modification in vivo. Proc Natl Acad Sci USA 86:1372–1376
34. Palmer RMJ, Ferrige AG, Moncada S (1987) Nitric oxide release accounts for the biological activity of endothelium-derived relaxing factor. Nature 327:524–526
35. Pohl U, Busse R (1987) Endothelium-derived relaxant factor inhibitits the effect of nitrocompounds in isolated arteries. Am J Physiol 252:H307–H313
36. Rosendorf C, Hoffman JIE, Verrier ED, Rouleau J, Boerboom LE (1981) Cholesterol potentiates the coronary artery response to norepinephrine in anesthetized and conscious dogs. Circ Res 48:320–329
37. Shirasaki Y, Su C (1985) Endothelium removal augments vasodilation by sodium nitroprusside and sodium nitrite. Eur J Pharmacol 114:93–96
38. Steinberg D, Parthasarathy S, Carew TE, Khoo JC, Witztum JL (1989) Beyond cholesterol: modifications of low-density lipoprotein that increase its atherogenicity. N Engl J Med 320:915–924
39. Steinbrecher UP, Witztum JL, Parthasarathy S, Steinberg D (1987) Decrease in reactive amino groups during oxidation or endothelial cell modification of LDL. Correlation with changes in receptor-mediated catabolism. Arteriosclerosis 7:135–143
40. Tomita T, Ezaki M, Miwa M, Nakamura K, Inoue Y (1990) Rapid and reversible inhibition by low density lipoprotein of the endothelium-dependent relaxation to hemostatic substances in porcine coronary arteries. Heat and acid labile factors in low density lipoprotein mediate the inhibition. Circ Res 66:18–27
41. Tomoike H, Egashira K, Yamamoto Y, Nakamura M (1989) Enhanced responsiveness of smooth muscle, impaired endothelium-dependent relaxation and the genesis of coronary spasm. Am J Cardiol 63:33E–39E
42. Vedernikov Y, Lankin V, Tikhaze A, Vikhert A (1988) Lipoproteins as factors in vessel tone and reactivity modulation. Basic Res Cardiol 83:590–596
43. Verbeuren T, Jordaens F, Zonnekeyn L, Van Hove C, Coene M, Herman A (1986) 1. Endothelium-dependent and endothelium-independent contractions and relaxations in isolated arteries of control and hypercholesterolemic rabbits. Circ Res 58:552–564
44. Verbeuren TJ, Jordaens FH, Van Hove CE, Van Hoydonck AE, Herman AG (1990) Release and vascular activity of the endothelium-derived relaxant factor in atherosclerotic rabbit aorta. Eur J Pharma 191:173–184
45. Wines PA, Schmitz JM, Pfister SL, Clubb FJ, Buja LM, Willerson JT, Campbell WB (1989) Augmented vasoconstrictor responses to serotonin precede development of atherosclerosis in aorta of WHHL rabbit. Arteriosclerosis 9:195–202
46. Ylä-Herttuala S, Palinsky W, Rosenfeld ME, Parthasarathy S, Carew TE, Butler S, Witzum JL, Steinberg D (1989) Evidence for the presence of oxidatively modified low density lipoprotein in atherosclerotic lesions of rabbit and man. J Clin Invest 84:1086–1095

Author's address:

Dr. J.-Chr. Galle
Institut für Angewandte
Physiologie und Balneologie
Universität Freiburg
Hermann-Herder-Str. 7
W-7800 Freiburg, FRG

Endothelium-dependent control of vascular tone: effects of age, hypertension and lipids

T. F. Lüscher [1,2], Y. Dohi [2], F. C. Tanner [2], C. Boulanger [2]

[1] Department of Medicine, Division of Cardiology, and
[2] Department of Research, Laboratory of Vascular Research,
University Hospital, Basel, Switzerland

Summary: As a source of several vasoactive factors, the endothelium takes part in the regulation of vascular tone. The most important endothelium-derived vasoactive substances are nitric oxide, prostacyclin, endothelin-1 and contracting factors requiring the activity of cyclooxygenase. The endothelium is an obvious target organ of cardiovascular risk factors. Accordingly, functional alterations do occur with aging, hypertension, and lipids. All three conditions are associated with a decreased basal and stimulated release of endothelium-derived nitric oxide. On the other hand, the release of endothelin-1 appears to increase with age, while the sensitivity to the peptide markedly decreases under the same conditions. In the spontaneously hypertensive rat, acetylcholine and stretch evoke the release of cyclooxygenase-dependent endothelium-derived contracting factor, most likely prostaglandin H_2. The sensitivity and circulating levels of endothelin-1, on the other hand, are reduced in this experimental model of hypertension. In the porcine coronary circulation, oxidized low-density lipoproteins selectively reduce endothelium-dependent relaxations to aggregating platelets, serotonin, and thrombin which are mediated by nitric oxide. The alterations of endothelial function occurring with aging, hypertension, and hyperlipidemia may have important clinical implications for the pathogenesis of cardiovascular disease.

Key words: Endothelium-derived contracting factor; endothelin; low-density lipoproteins; nitric oxide; prostaglandins

Introduction

Age, hypertension, and lipids are major risk factors for the development of cardiovascular disease. The mechanisms of vascular injury, however, are not well-understood. The endothelium, due to its anatomical location, is an obvious target organ of hypertension and lipids. As the endothelium plays an important protective role in the circulation by the release of substances which inhibit platelet function and evoke vasodilatation such as endothelium-derived relaxing factor (EDRF), changes in endothelial function occurring with aging, hypertension, and hyperlipidemia could contribute to the development of myocardial infarction, vasospasm, and stroke.

This manuscript focuses on alterations in endothelium-dependent responses in aging, hypertensive and hyperlipidemic blood vessels, and updates previous reviews of that field (40–43, 45).

Endothelium-derived substances and blood pressure control

Infusion of hemoglobin – an inhibitor of endothelium-derived relaxing factor (EDRF) – increases arterial blood pressure in normal subjects (60). Intravenous infusion of L-N^G-monomethylarginine (L-NMMA), an inhibitor of the formation of nitric oxide from L-arginine (53, 56), augments arterial blood pressure in rats and rabbits (55, 70), Likewise,

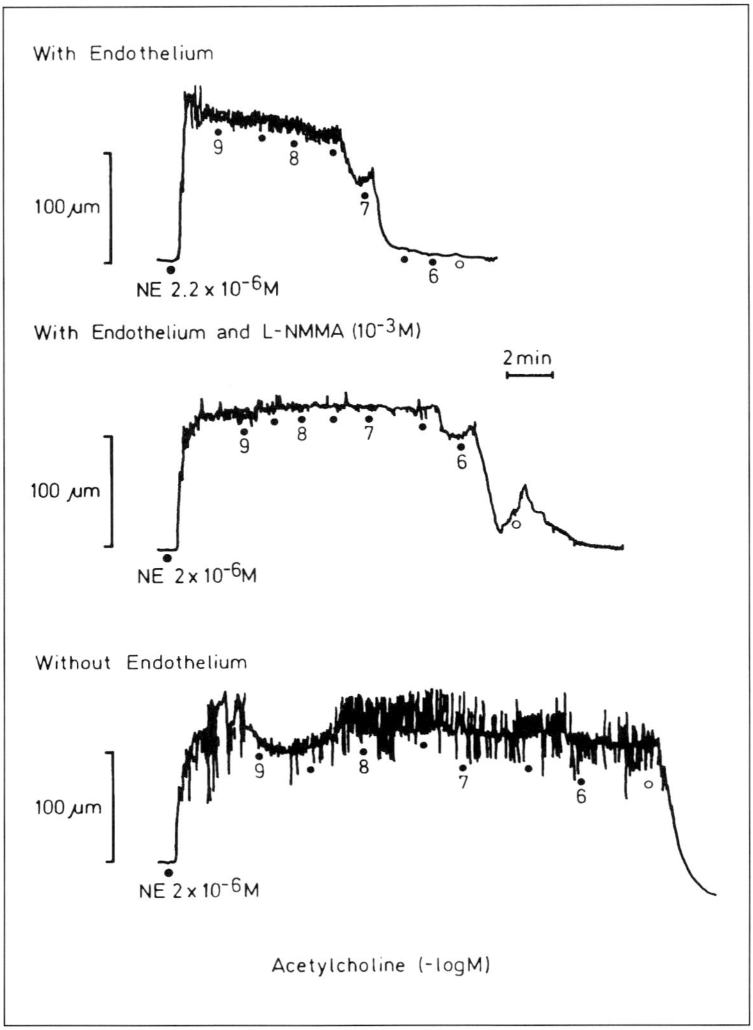

Fig. 1. Endothelium-dependent relaxations to extraluminal acetylcholine in pressurized mesenteric resistance artery obtained from 16–20-week-old WKY rats. In preparations contracted with norepinephrine (NE), acetylcholine evokes potent relaxations in the presence of the endothelium (top panel; vascular diameter: 225 µm), but not in the absence of the endothelium (lower panel; vascular diameter: 201 µm). The inhibitor of nitric oxide formation L-N^G-monomethyl arginine (L-NMMA) inhibits, but does not prevent the relaxations induced by the muscarinic agonist (middle panel). [From 15, by permission.]

intraarterial application of L-NMMA in the human forearm decreases local blood flow (72). Thus, the continuous release of endothelium-derived nitric oxide contributes to the regulation of peripheral vascular resistance. Alterations in the basal release of endothelium-derived vasoactive factors, on the other hand, could contribute to the increase in peripheral vascular resistance characteristic of hypertension.

Systemic application of endothelium-dependent vasodilators such as acetylcholine, adenosine diphosphate (ADP), and substance P markedly decreases blood pressure in the rabbit (18). In the forearm of healthy human subjects, intraarterial administration of acetylcholine evokes a profound increase in forearm blood flow (29). The vasodilator effects of acetylcholine are unaffected by acetylsalicylic acid and phentolamine, indicating that prostacyclin and inhibition of adrenergic neurotransmission do not contribute (29). As infusion of L-NMMA blunts the vasodilator effects of acetylcholine in the human forearm circulation (72), endothelium-derived nitric oxide must at least, in part, mediate the response. Similarly, in perfused and pressurized mesenteric arteries of rats, endothelium-dependent relaxations to acetylcholine are inhibited by L-NMMA, suggesting an important role of nitric oxide in microcirculation [Fig. 1; (15)].

In the rat and rabbit, intravenous infusion of endothelin-1 causes a profound and long-lasting increase in blood pressure (81). In the human forearm circulation, the peptide increases peripheral vascular resistance and decreases local blood flow (7, 30). In the porcine aorta, endothelin is continuously released in an endothelium-dependent manner as it is in endothelial cells in culture (6, 61). The release of the peptide can be further stimulated with thrombin and the calcium ionophore A 23187 (6, 61, 81). The production of endothelin is regulated further by endothelium-derived nitric oxide which is concomitantly formed during stimulation with thrombin (6, 45). Hence, L-NMMA augments the thrombin-induced stimulation of endothelin production to a similar degree as the inhibitor of soluble guanylate cyclase methylene blue (6). On the other hand, superoxide dismutase (which prevents the inactivation of nitric oxide by superoxide radicals) and the stable analogue of cyclic GMP 8-bromo-cyclic GMP inhibits the thrombin-induced formation of the peptide (6). This suggests that endothelium-derived nitric oxide inhibits the thrombin-induced formation of endothelin from intact blood vessels via a cGMP-dependent mechanism.

Aging

In perfused and pressurized mesenteric resistance arteries of Wistar-Kyoto rats (WKY), the presence of the endothelium reduces the sensitivity and the maximal response to norepinephrine. Since this effect can, in large part, be prevented by L-NMMA and the endothelium reduces the contraction induced by phenylephrine to a similar extent as that induced by norepinephrine, basally released nitric oxide must reduce the response of the microcirculation to vasoconstrictor stimuli (15). The basal release of nitric oxide is decreased with advancing age (15).

In large conduit arteries of the rat, endothelium-dependent relaxation to calcium ionophore A23187, histamine and adenosine triphosphate decreases with age (24, 51, 65). However, decreased (24, 65) and increased (23) endothelium-dependent relaxation to muscarinic agonists were reported in the aged rat. In resistance arteries of rats, endothelium-dependent relaxation to acetylcholine decreases with increasing age (16). Since the relaxation induced by nitric oxide donor SIN-1 does not alter with age, the decreased response to the muscarinic agonist must be due to a decreased production and/or release of endothelium-derived nitric oxide after the stimulation with acetylcholine (16).

In perfused and pressurized mesenteric resistance arteries of Fischer 344 rats, the sensitivity, but not the maximal response, to endothelin-1 markedly decreases with age [Fig. 2; (16)]. Since contractions induced by norepinephrine in the same preparations are not affected by aging, the alteration is specific for endothelin-1 (16). The decreased

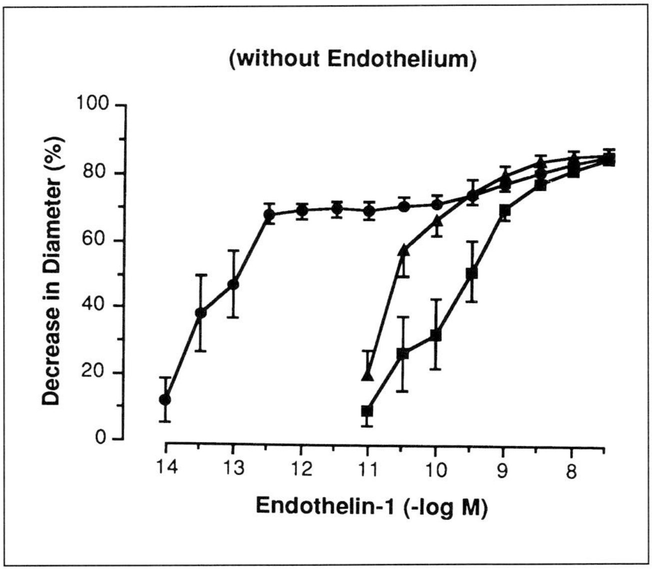

Fig. 2. Vascular effects of endothelin-1 in perfused and pressurized rat mesenteric resistance arteries without endothelium obtained from 4-month (●). 9-month (▲), and 27-month-old (■) Fischer 344 rats. Note the extremely high sensitivity to endothelin-1 in young rats and its big decrease in adult and old rats ($p < 0.05$–0.005). In contrast, the maximal contraction induced by the peptide is identical in all three age groups [From (16), by permission.]

sensitivity to the peptide may be explained by down-regulation of endothelin-1 receptors on the smooth muscle cells. In line with that interpretation, the circulating levels of endothelin increase with advancing age in the human (50). The inhibitory effects of the endothelium against the contraction induced by endothelin-1 are also attenuated in aged rats (16).

Hypertension

Basal release of EDRF

In young, and even more pronounced, in adult spontaneously hypertensive rats (SHR), the inhibitory effect of the endothelium against contraction induced by norepinephrine is reduced, indicating a diminished basal formation of endothelium-derived nitric oxide in hypertensive mesenteric resistance arteries [Fig. 3; (15)]. A contribution of prostacyclin can be excluded as indomethacin does not affect the response.

Removal of the endothelium enhances the response to sodium nitroprusside in mesenteric resistance arteries, most likely due to an inhibitory effect of basally released endothelium-derived relaxing factor [Fig. 4; (24)]. This augmentation of the response to sodium nitroprusside is reduced in stroke-prone SHR as compared to WKY, again suggesting that the basal release of endothelium relaxing factor is impaired in hypertensive resistance arteries (15).

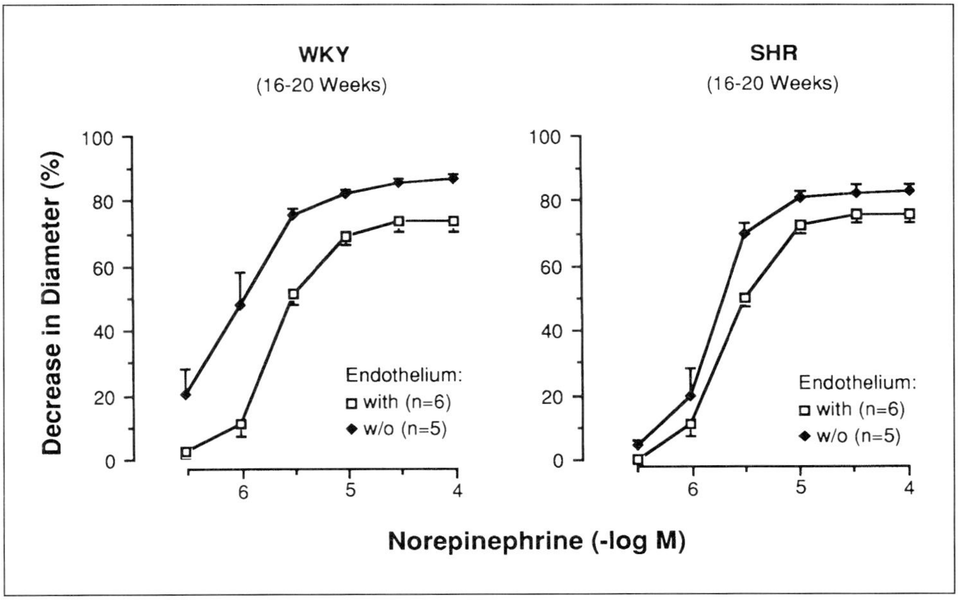

Fig. 3. Contractions induced by extraluminal norepinephrine in pressurized mesenteric resistance arteries with and without endothelium obtained from 16–20-week-old WKY (left) and SHR (right). In both animals, removal of the endothelium significantly augmented the contractions induced by norepinephrine ($p < 0.05$–0.005). The shift caused by removal of the endothelium was smaller in SHR (1.4-fold) than in WKY (2.9-fold). [From (15), by permission.]

Endothelium-dependent relaxations

The endothelium-dependent relaxations to acetylcholine are attenuated in the aorta of rats with spontaneous hypertension [Fig. 5; (27, 28, 35, 41)], renal hypertension, salt-induced hypertension, coarctation, and DOCA-salt induced hypertension (31, 38, 48, 64, 74–76). Similar alterations occur in the carotid artery, but not in the renal artery of adult SHR (24, 39).

In the aorta of the Dahl rat, the reduction of the endothelium-dependent relaxations to acetylcholine is directly related to the level of systolic blood pressure (37). Normalization of blood pressure with antihypertensive drugs (reserpine, hydrochlorothiazide plus hydralazine) restores endothelium-dependent relaxations in hypertensive Dahl rats [Fig. 6; (36, 37)]. Similarly, in rats with aortic coarctation, endothelium-dependent relaxations are maintained in the aortic segment distal to the stenosis (31, 48). This suggests that in these forms of hypertension the impaired endothelium-dependent relaxations are a consequence, rather than a cause of the high blood pressure.

The endothelium-dependent relaxations to thrombin are reduced in Dahl hypertensive, but not in SHR (32, 38, 40). By contrast, those to ADP are impaired in the aorta and in the carotid artery of both hypertensive strains (24, 32, 36, 38). Serotonin and aggregating platelets do not evoke endothelium-dependent relaxations in the aorta or in the carotid artery of the rat (32, 39), but in the aorta of normotensive rats the contractions evoked by aggregating platelets are inhibited in the presence of the endothelium (32). By

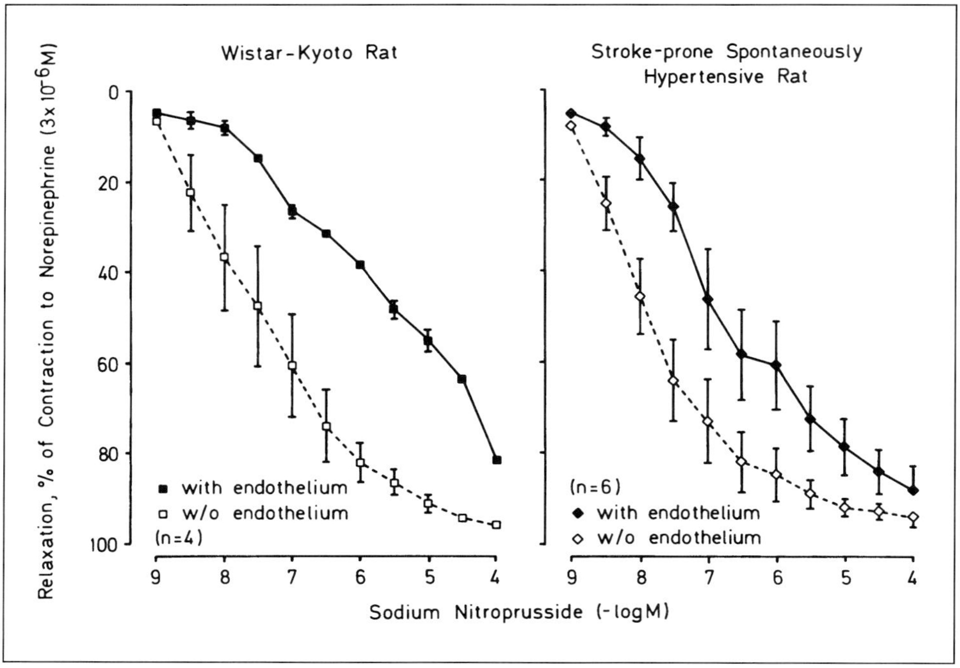

Fig. 4. Effects of sodium nitroprusside in rings of mesenteric resistance arteries with (closed symbols) or without endothelium (open symbols) obtaind from Wistar-Kyoto rats (left panel) or stroke-prone SHR (right panel). The preparations were studied in a myograph system. Note that removal of the endothelium enhances the response to sodium nitroprusside in both strains, but more so in the normotensive rats. Accordingly, relaxations obtained by sodium nitroprusside are reduced in preparations with endothelium obtained from normotensive rats, while the response in preparations without endothelium was comparable in both strains. [From (14), by permission.]

contrast, in SHR the endothelium loses its inhibitory capacity against platelet-induced contractions (32).

In mesenteric resistance arteries of the SHR studied in a myograph system, the endothelium-dependent relaxations to acetylcholine and bradykinin are reduced [Fig. 7; (12–14, 44, 77)]. As in large arteries, the relaxations are reduced predominantly at higher concentrations of the muscarinic agonist. Similarly, in pressurized perfused mesenteric resistance arteries contracted with norepinephrine (15, 69) and in mesenteric microvessels of the SHR studied in vivo (8), the endothelium-dependent relaxations to acetylcholine are reduced. The defect primarily involves the intraluminal activation of the endothelial cell by acetylcholine, suggesting that this part of the endothelial cell most exposed to high blood pressure and shear stress exerted by the circulating blood becomes progressively dysfunctional in hypertension [Fig. 8; (15)]. Both in perfused mesenteric resistance arteries (15) and in those studied in the myograph system (12, 21), endothelium-dependent relaxations become impaired as blood pressure rises.

In the cerebral microcirculation of the anesthetized stroke-prone SHR, the vasodilator responses to acetylcholine (but not those to nitroglycerin) and that to ADP and serotonin are attenuated or converted into contraction (46, 47).

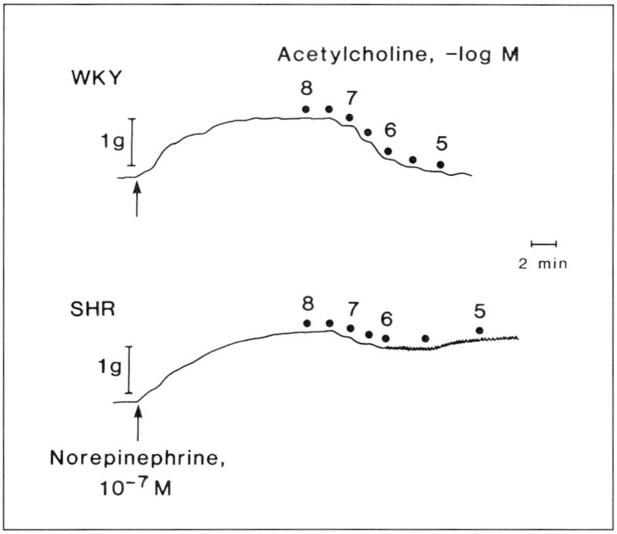

Fig. 5. Endothelium-dependent relaxations to acetylcholine in an aortic ring obtained from a normotensive Wistar-Kyoto rat (WKY, top panel) and a SHR (SHR; lower panel). Note the impaired response in the hypertensive rat. NE = norepinephrine. [From (41), by permission.]

In the hindlimb circulation of the rabbit, hypertension does not induce marked changes in vascular reactivity; the maximal relaxation evoked by acetylcholine, however, is reduced (80). In the perfused hindlimb of rats with psycho-social hypertension, the endothelium-dependent relaxations to acetylcholine are even enhanced (79).

In the forearm of hypertensive patients, the dilatation evoked by intraarterial acetylcholine is attenuated [Fig. 9; (29)]. Since the response to sodium nitroprusside – which as endothelium-derived relaxing factor activates cyclic GMP in vascular smooth muscle – is not significantly reduced, the impaired response to acetylcholine most likely involves an endothelial defect.

Endothelium-dependent contractions

Acetylcholine causes endothelium-dependent contractions in the aorta of the adult SHR, while the responses are weak or absent in normotensive WKY of the same age [Fig. 10; (35)]. In old rats (12 months of age), endothelium-dependent contractions to acetylcholine occur also in normotensive rats and are even more pronounced in spontaneously hypertensive animals (26). Thus, the occurrence of endothelium-dependent contractions to acetylcholine may reflect the premature aging of the hypertensive arterial wall.

The endothelium-dependent contractions to acetylcholine are abolished by inhibitors of phospholipase A_2 or of cyclooxygenase, demonstrating that the metabolism of endogenous arachidonic acid is involved (35). It most likely represents prostaglandin H_2 (25). Indeed, the contractions to exogenous prostaglandin H_2 are prevented by thromboxane receptor antagonists, but unaffected by inhibitors of the synthesis of the prostanoid (25).

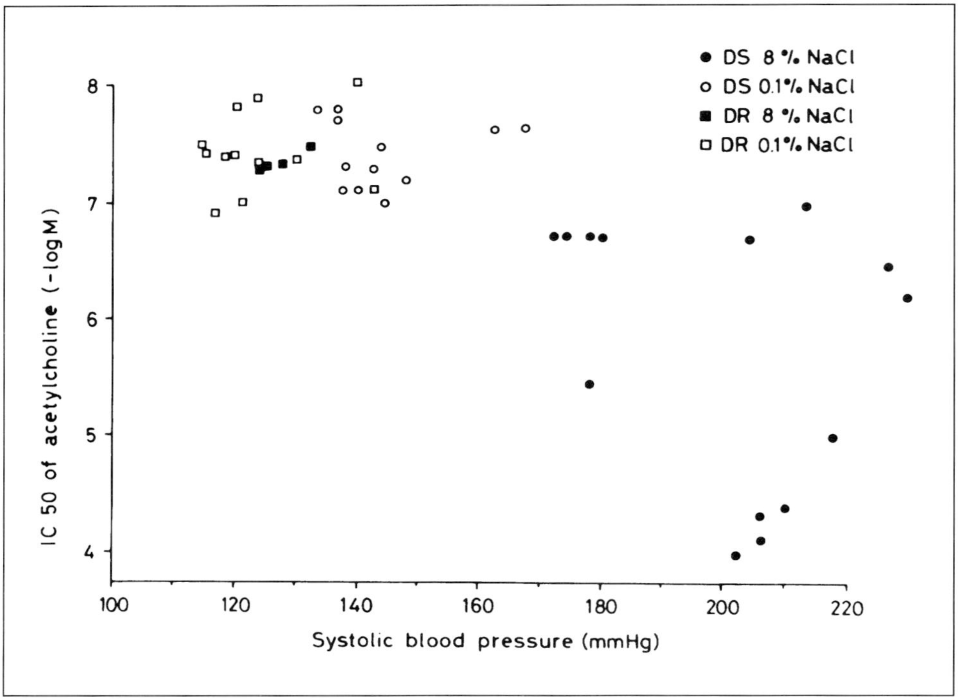

Fig. 6. Endothelium-dependent relaxations to acetylcholine in Dahl salt-sensitive (DS) and Dahl salt-resistant (DR) rats on different diets. Note that the IC_{50}-value of acetylcholine (negative log M), that is, the concentration of the muscarinic agonist required to evoke 50% relaxation of the contraction induced by norepinephrine, is negatively correlated with the level of systolic blood pressure. Closed circle = DS on 8% NaCl; open circle = DS on 0.1% NaCl; closed square = DR on 8% NaCl; open square = DR on 0.1% NaCl [From (37), by permission.]

Isolated aortae obtained from normotensive rats contract when stretched, a response which is larger in arteries from DOCA-hypertensive rats (58). Removal of the endothelium reduces the stretch-induced increase in tension without affecting contractions to norepinephrine (58). These observations indicate that hypertension promotes stretch-induced endothelium-dependent contractions.

Platelet-derived products

The altered endothelial function, together with the greater aggregability of the platelets from hypertensives (1, 3, 11, 20, 22, 52, 73), may favor the occurrence of vasoconstriction and thrombusformation in hypertensive blood vessels. Various abnormalities of platelet function and alterations in the vascular responses to platelet-derived products occur in hypertension (52, 73). In the aorta of the SHR contracted with prostaglandin $F_{2\alpha}$, serotonin causes larger contractions in rings with, than in those without endothelium (32). These differences are particularly apparent in the presence of ketanserin, which blocks 5-HT_2-serotonergic receptors on vascular smooth muscle. Under these condi-

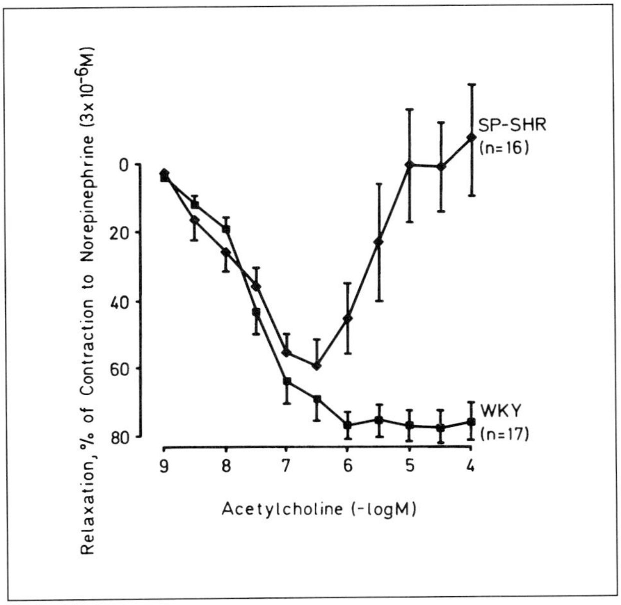

Fig. 7. Endothelium-dependent relaxations to acetylcholine in mesenteric resistance arteries obtained from normotensive Wistar-Kyoto rats (WKY) or stroke-prone SHR (SHR SP). Note the reversal of the relaxations induced by acetylcholine at higher concentrations of the muscarinic agonist in the hypertensive animals. [From (14), by permission.]

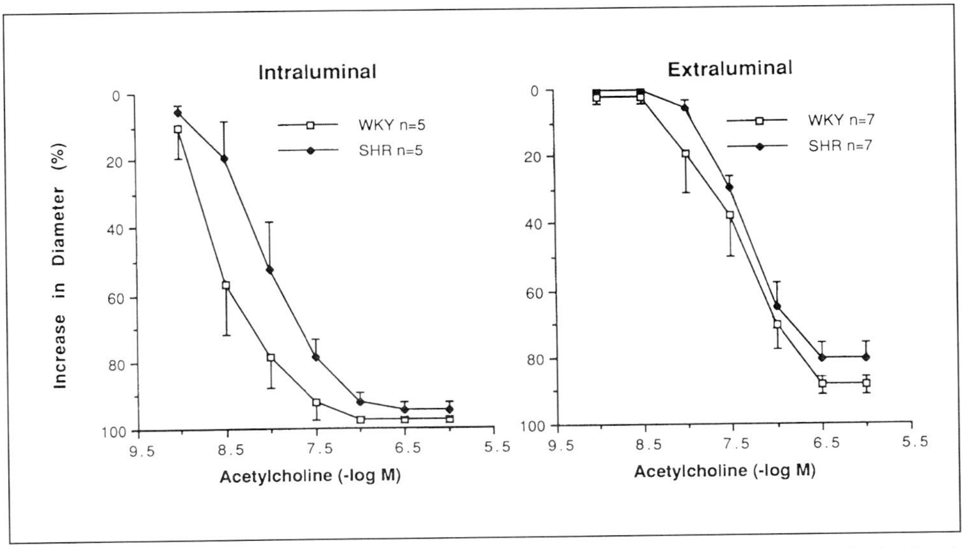

Fig. 8. Endothelium-dependent relaxations to intraluminal (left panel) and extraluminal (right) acetylcholine in perfused and pressurized mesenteric resistance arteries from normotensive Wistar-Kyoto rats (WKY; open symbol) on spontaneously hypertensive rats (SHR; closed symbol). Note the relaxations to intraluminal, but not extraluminal acetylcholine are reduced in SHR as compared to WKY. [Data from (15), by permission.]

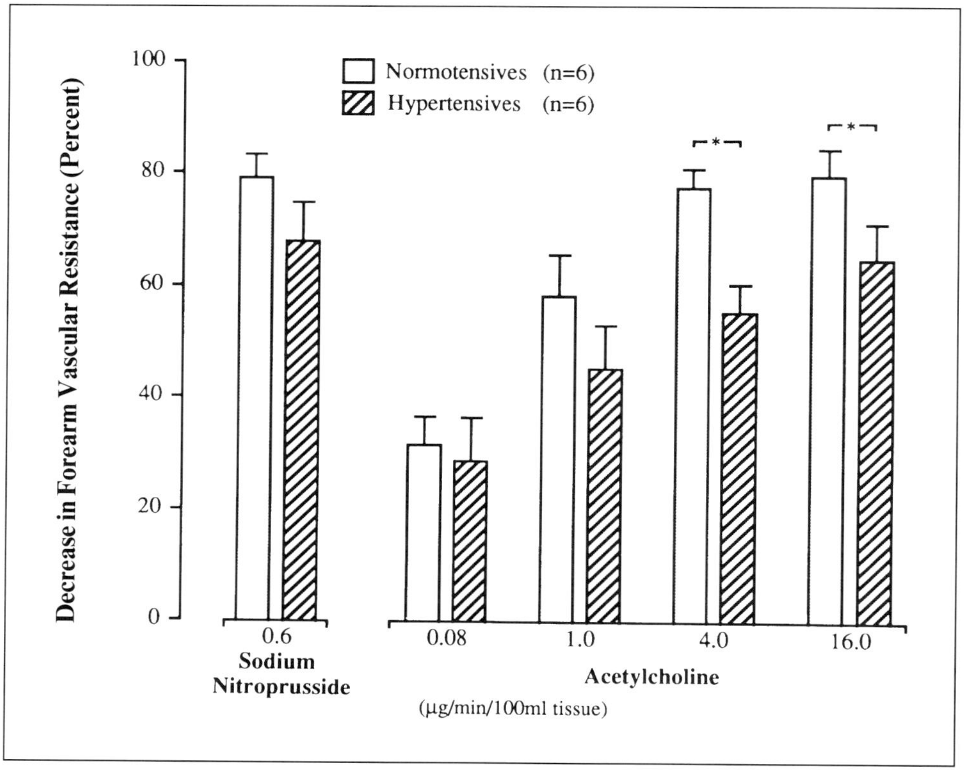

Fig. 9. Effects of intraarterially infused acetylcholine on forearm vascular resistance in normotensive subject (open bars) and patients with essential hypertension (shaded bars). Note the reduced vasodilatation to acetylcholine in the hypertensive patients. * = $p < 0.05$ [From (29), by permission.]

tions, an inhibitory effect of the endothelium against contractions induced by serotonin is apparent in aortas obtained from normotensive rats, while in hypertensive aortas, the monoamine facilitates contractions induced by serotonin (32).

In isolated perfused hearts from WKY, the monoamine induces moderate increases in flow, while marked decreases in flow occur in hearts from SHR (33). The constrictor effect of serotonin in the coronary circulation of hypertensive hearts can be blocked by indomethacin. Similarly, in the cerebral microcirculation of SHR, the dilator effects of adenosine diphosphate and serotonin are lost or converted into contractions, respectively; indomethacin unmasks relaxations in response to the platelet-derived mediators (46, 47). The results of these studies are consistent with the concept that, under these conditions, a cyclooxygenase-dependent endothelium-derived contracting factor ($EDCF_2$) is liberated in response to the platelet products (40).

Endothelin

The plasma levels of endothelin-1 in SHR, but not DOCA-salt hypertensive rats, are lower than those in age-matched normotensive controls (67). There is little or no

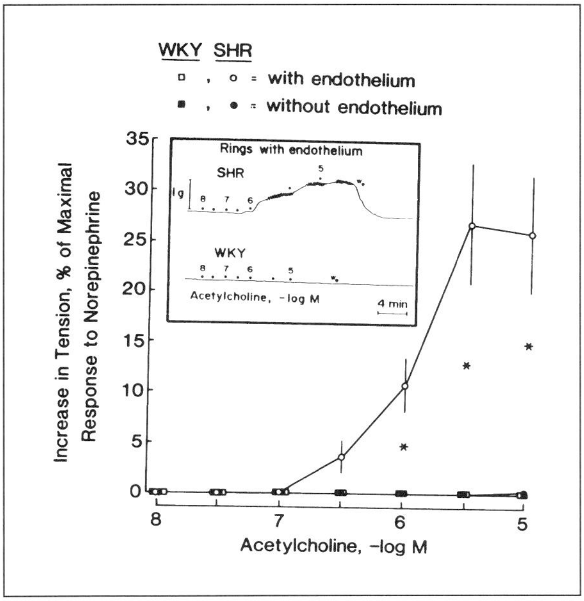

Fig. 10. Quiescent rings with and without endothelium were studied in parallel and exposed to increasing concentrations of acetylcholine (10^{-8}–10^{-5} M). Results are expressed as percent of the maximal response to norepinephrine (10^{-4} M). Asterisk indicates significant difference between rings from SHR with and without endothelium ($p<0.05$; $n=7$). Inset: Original recordings of isometric tension in rings (with endothelium) of aortas from SHR and WKY. [From (35), by permission of the American Heart Association.]

endothelin-3 in rat plasma (59). The circulating levels of endothelin in patients with essential hypertension have been reported to be normal (10, 50) or increased (63). On the other hand, plasma levels of endothelin are increased in patients with renal insufficiency, cardiogenic shock, and in the coronary sinus of patients with coronary artery disease (19, 62, 66).

The first reports on the responsiveness of isolated blood vessels from hypertensive rats to endothelin yielded conflicting results (9, 13, 17, 49, 71). Indeed, while some authors reported a reduced sensitivity to endothelin in the aorta and renal artery and in perfused mesenteric resistance arteries of SHR (17, 45), others reported normal (in mesenteric resistance arteries of stroke-prone SHR studied in the myograph; (13) or augmented responses (49, 71).

Lipids

Elevated circulating levels of plasma lipids are a major cardiovascular risk factor. Plasma lipids, in particular low density lipoproteins (LDL), can profoundly affect endothelial function of isolated blood vessels. In addition, lipids may affect the responsiveness of vascular smooth muscle cells to vasoconstrictor stimuli (see Galle and Bassenge pp 127–142) and vascular smooth muscle cell proliferation.

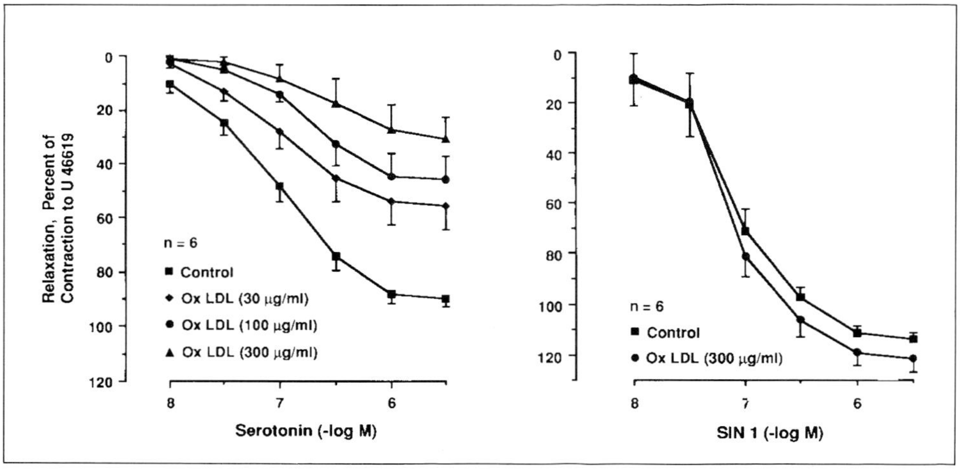

Fig. 11. Effect of oxidized low density lipoproteins (Ox LDL) on endothelium-dependent (left panel) and endothelium-independent (right panel) relaxations of porcine coronary arteries. Endothelium-dependent relaxations to serotonin were performed in the presence of the 5-HT_2-serotonergic antagonist ketanserin (10^{-5} M) to minimize the direct contractile effects of serotonin on vascular smooth muscle. Oxidized LDL inhibited relaxations to the monoamine in a concentration-dependent manner from 30 to 300 µg/ml. In contrast, endothelium-independent relaxations to the nitric oxide donor SIN-1, the active metabolite of molsidomine, were unaffected by the lipoproteins

In the aorta of the rabbit, LDL, and in particular, oxidized LDL which has been isolated from atherosclerotic lesions (82) inhibit endothelium-dependent relaxations to acetylcholine, while high density lipoproteins (HDL) do not appear to have a significant effect (2, 28). Similarly, in the porcine coronary artery, oxidized LDL severely attenuates endothelium-dependent relaxations to serotonin and thrombin [Fig. 11; (68)]. As the response to serotonin can be prevented by L-NMMA, as well as hemoglobin and methylene blue (57), the lipids must either interfere with the production, release or action of endothelium-derived nitric oxide. The latter possibility can be excluded as vessels treated with the lipids can fully relax in response to nitrovasodilators [Fig. 11; (68)]. In contrast, endothelium-dependent relaxations to bradykinin are unaffected by oxidized LDL as well as by L-NMMA, hemoglobin and methylene blue (57, 68). This suggests that the porcine coronary circulation releases two different endothelium-derived relaxing factors (one representing EDRF, and a second factor distinct from it) and oxidized LDL appears to interfere primarily with responses mediated by endothelium-derived nitric oxide. As serotonin is the major mediator of endothelium-dependent relaxations to aggregating platelets in the porcine coronary artery, these effects of oxidized LDL profoundly affect the platelet-vessel wall interaction in this preparation (68).

Studies with porcine aortic endothelial cells in culture provide further evidence that oxidized LDL does interfere with the release of endothelium-derived relaxing factors. Cultured porcine endothelial cells release a relaxing factor upon stimulation with bradykinin which behaves like nitric oxide (5, 53, 82). In cells incubated with oxidized LDL for 1 h, the release of endothelium-derived nitric oxide evoked by bradykinin is blunted in a concentration-dependent manner. In contrast, native LDL only interferes with the release of endothelium-derived relaxing factor at very high concentrations (i.e.,

2 mg/ml). Since oxidized LDL accumulate in early lesions of the atherosclerotic blood vessel wall (82), they may play a key role in the impairment of endothelial function occurring in atherosclerosis. A blunted release of endothelium-derived nitric oxide would decrease the capacity of the endothelium to inhibit platelet adhesion and – aggregation, and would favor the occurrence of vasospasm.

Acknowledgements. The authors wish to thank Bernadette Libsig and Sabine Bohnert for technical assistance. Original research reported in this manuscript was made possible by grants of the Swiss National Research Foundation (grant No. 32-25468.88), Swiss Cardiology Foundation, the Helmut Horten Foundation, and the Schweizerische Rentenanstalt. The first author is recipient of a career development award of the Swiss National Research Foundation (SCORE-grant No. 3231-025150).

References

1. Amstein R, Fetkovska N, Lüscher TF, Kiowski W, Bühler FR (1988) Age and the platelet serotonin vasoconstrictor axis in essential hypertension. J Cardiovasc Pharmacol 11 (Suppl 1): 35–40
2. Andrews HE, Bruckdorfer KR, Dunn RC, Jacobs M (1987) Low-density lipoproteins inhibit endothelium-dependent relaxation in rabbit aorta. Nature 327:237–239
3. Badouin-Legros M, Dard B, Guicheney P (1986) Hyperreactivity of platelets from spontaneously hypertensive rats. Hypertension 8:694–699
4. Boulanger C, Bühler FR, Lüscher TF (1989) Low density lipoproteins impair the release of endothelium-derived relaxing factor from cultured porcine endothelial cells (abstract). Eur Heart J 10:331
5. Boulanger C, Hendrickson H, Lorenz RR, Vanhoutte PM (1989) Release of different relaxing factors by cultured porcine endothelial cells. Circ Res 64:1070–1078
6. Boulanger C, Lüscher TF (1990) Release of endothelin from the porcine aorta: Inhibition by endothelium-derived nitric oxide. J Clin Invest 85:587–590
7. Brian SD, Crossman DC, Buckley TL, Williams TJ (1989) Endothelin-1: demonstration of potent effects on the microcirculation of humans and other species. J Cardiovasc Pharmacol 13 (Suppl 5):147–149
8. Carvalho MHC, Scivoletto R, Fortes ZB, Nigro D, Cordellini S (1987) Reactivity of aorta and mesenteric microvessels to drugs in spontaneously hypertensive rats: role of the endothelium. J Hypertension 5:377–382
9. Criscione L, Nellis P, Riniker B, Thomann H, Burdet R (1989) Reactivity and sensitivity of mesenteric vascular beds and aortic rings of SH and WKY rats to endothelin: effect of calcium entry blockers. Br J Pharmacol 99:31–36
10. Davenport AP, Ashby MJ, Easton P, Ella S, Bedford K, Dickerson C, Nunez DJ, Capper SJ, Brown MJ (1990) A sensitive radioimmunoassay measuring endothelin-like immunoreactivity in human plasma: comparison of levels in patients with essential hypertension and normotensive control subjects. Clin Sci 78:261–264
11. De Clerck F (1986) Blood platelets in human essential hypertension. Agents Actions 18:-563–580
12. De Mey JG, Gray SD (1985) Endothelium-dependent reactivity in resistance vessels. Prog Appl Microcirc 88:181–187
13. Diederich D, Yang Z, Bühler FR, Lüscher TF (1989) Endothelium derived relaxing factor and endothelin in resistance arteries of hypertensive rats (abstract). J Vasc Med Biol 1/3:167
14. Diederich D, Yang Z, Bühler FR, Lüscher TF (1990) Impaired endothelium-dependent relaxations in hypertensive resistance arteries involve the cyclooxygenase pathway. Am J Physiol 258:H445–H451

15. Dohi Y, Thiel MA, Bühler FR, Lüscher TF (1990) Activation of the endothelial L-arginine pathway in pressurized mesenteric resistance arteries: effect of age and hypertension. Hypertension 16:170–179
16. Dohi Y, Lüscher TF (1990) Aging differentially affects direct and indirect actions of endothelin-1 in perfused mesenteric resistance arteries of the rat. Br J Pharmacol 100:889–893
17. Dohi Y, Lüscher TF (1990) Hypertension differentially affects intra- and extraluminal activation of the endothelium (Abstract). Hypertension 6:315
18. Dudel C, Förstermann U (1988) Gossypol attenuates selectively the blood pressure lowering effect of endothelium-dependent vasodilators in the rabbit in vivo. Eur J Pharmacol 145:217–221
19. Emori T, Hirata Y, Aizawa T, Ando K, Shichiri M, Marumo F (1989) Plasma endothelin levels in patients with coronary artery disease undergoing percutaneous coronary angioplasty. Circulation 80 (Suppl II):22327
20. Fetkovska N, Amstein R, Ferracin F, Regenass M, Pletscher A, Bühler FR (1990) 5-hydroxytryptamine kinetics and activation of blood platelets in patients with essential hypertension. Hypertension 15:267–273
21. Gray SD, De Mey JG (1985) Vascular reactivity in neonatal spontaneously hypertensive rats. Progr Appl Microcirc 8:173–180
22. Guicheney P, Legros M, Marcel D, Kamal L, Meyer P (1985) Platelet serotonin content and uptake in spontaneously hypertensive rats. Life Sci 36:679–685
23. Hynes MR, Duckles SP (1987) Effect of increasing age on the endothelium-mediated relaxation of rat blood vessels in vitro. J Pharmacol Exp Ther 241:387–392
24. Hongo K, Nakagomi T, Kassell NF, Sasaki T, Lehmann M, Vollmer DG, Tsukahara T, Ogawa H, Torner J (1988) Effect of aging and hypertension on endothelium-dependent vascular relaxation in rat carotid artery. Stroke 19:892–897
25. Kato T, Iwama Y, Okumura K, Hashimoto H, Itô T, Satake T (1990) Prostaglandin H_2 may be the endothelium-derived contracting factor released by acetylcholine in the aorta of the rat. Hypertension 15:475–481
26. Koga T, Takata Y, Kobayashi K, Takishita S, Yamashita Y, Fujishima M (1989) Age and hypertension promote endothelium-dependent contractions to acetylcholine in the aorta of the rat. Hypertension 14:542–548
27. Konishi M, Su C (1983) Role of endothelium in dilator responses of SHR arteries. Hypertension 5:881–886
28. Kugiyama K, Kerns SA, Morrisett JD, Roberts R, Henry PD (1990) Impairment of endothelium-dependent arterial relaxation by lysolecithin in modified low-density lipoproteins. Nature 344:160–162
29. Linder L, Kiowski W, Bühler FR, Lüscher TF (1990) Indirect evidence of the release of endothelium-derived relaxing factor in human forearm circulation in vivo: blunted response in essential hypertension. Circulation 81:1762–1767
30. Kiowski W, Lüscher TF, Linder L, Bühler FR (1991) Endothelin-1-induced vasoconstriction in humans: reversal by calcium channel blockade but not by nitrovasodilators or endothelium-derived relaxing factor. Circulation 83:469–475
31. Lockette WE, Otsuha Y, Carretero OA (1986) Endothelium-dependent relaxation in hypertension. Hypertension 8 (Suppl II):61–66
32. Lüscher TF, Vanhoutte PM (1986) Endothelium-dependent responses to aggregating platelets and serotonin in spontaneously hypertensive rats. Hypertension 8 (Suppl II):55–60
33. Lüscher TF, Rubanyi GM, Aarhus LL, Vanhoutte PM (1986) Serotonin reduces coronary flow in isolated hearts of the SHR. J Hypertension 4 (Suppl 5):148–150
34. Lüscher TF, Romero JC, Vanhoutte PM (1986) Bioassay of endothelium-derived vasoactive substances in the aorta of normotensive and spontaneously hypertensive rats. J Hypertension 4 (Suppl 6):81–83
35. Lüscher TF, Vanhoutte PM (1986) Endothelium-dependent contractions to acetylcholine in the aorta of the SHR. Hypertension 8:344–348
36. Lüscher TF, Vanhoutte PM, Raij L (1987) Antihypertensive therapy normalizes endothelium-dependent relaxations in salt-induced hypertension of the rat. Hypertension 9 (Suppl III): 193–197
37. Lüscher TF, Raij L, Vanhoutte PM (1987) Effect of hypertension and its reversal on endothelium-dependent relaxations in the rat aorta. J Hypertension 5 (Suppl 5):153–155

38. Lüscher TF, Raij L, Vanhoutte PM (1987) Endothelium-dependent responses in normotensive and hypertensive Dahl rats. Hypertension 9:157–163
39. Lüscher TF, Diederich D, Vanhoutte PM, Weber E, Bühler FR (1988) Endothelium-dependent responses in the common carotid and renal artery of normotensive and spontaneously hypertensive rats. Hypertension 11:573–578
40. Lüscher TF (1988) Endothelial vasoactive substances and cardiovascular disease. S Karger Publisher AG, Basel, pp 1–133
41. Lüscher TF Vanhoutte PM (1988) Mechanisms of altered endothelium-dependent responses in hypertensive blood vessels. in: Vanhoutte PM (ed) Relaxing and contracting factors, biological and clinical research. Humana Press, Clifton, NJ, pp 495–509
42. Lüscher TF (1989) Endothelium-derived relaxing and contracting factors: potential role in coronary artery disease. Eur Heart J 10:847–857
43. Lüscher TF (1989) Imbalance of endothelium-derived relaxing and contracting factors: a new concept in hypertension? Am J Hypertension 3:317–330
44. Lüscher TF, Aarhus LL, Vanhoutte PM (1990) Indomethacin enhances the impaired endothelium-dependent relaxations in small mesenteric arteries of the SHR. Am J Hypertension 3:55–58
45. Lüscher TF, Vanhoutte PM (1990) The endothelium: modulator of cardiovascular function. CRC Press, Florida, USA, pp 1–215
46. Mayhan WG, Faraci FM, Heistad DD (1987) Impairment of endothelium-dependent in responses of cerebral arterioles in chronic hypertension. Am J Physiol 253:H1435–H1440
47. Mayhan WG, Faraci FM, Heistad DD (1988) Responses of cerebral arterioles to adenosine diphosphate, serotonin and the thromboxane analogue U-46619 during chronic hypertension. Hypertension 12:556–561
48. Miller MJS, Pinto A, Mullane KM (1987) Impaired endothelium-dependent relaxations in rabbits subjected to aortic coarctation hypertension. Hypertension 10:164–170
49. Miyauchi T, Ishikawa T, Tomobe Y, Yanagisawa M, Kimura S, Sugishita Y, Ito I, Goto K, Masaki T (1989) Characteristics of pressor response to endothelin in spontaneously hypertensive Wistar-Kyoto rats. Hypertension 14:427–434
50. Miyauchi T, Yanagisawa M, Suzuki N, Iida K, Sugishita Y, Fujino M, Saito T, Goto K, Masaki T (1989) Venous plasma concentrations of endothelin in normal and hypertensive subjects. Circulation 80 (Suppl II):2280
51. Moritoki H, Hosoki E, Ishida Y (1986) Age-related decrease in endothelium-dependent dilator response to histamine in rat mesenteric artery. Eur J Pharmacol 126:61–67
52. Nara Y, Kihara M, Mano M, Horie R, Yamori Y (1984) Dietary effect on platelet aggregation in men with and without a family history of essential hypertension. Hypertension 6:339–343
53. Palmer RMJ, Ashton DS, Moncada S (1988) Vascular endothelial cells synthesize nitric oxide from L-arginine. Nature 333:664–666
54. Panza JA, Quyyumi AA, Epstein SE (1988) Impaired endothelium-dependent vascular relaxation in hypertensive patients (abstract). Circulation 78 (Suppl II):473
55. Rees DD, Palmer RMJ, Moncada S (1989) The role of endothelium-derived nitric oxide in the regulation of blood pressure. Proc Natl Acad Sci USA 86:3375–3378
56. Rees DD, Palmer RMJ, Hodson HF, Moncada S (1989) A specific inhibitor of nitric oxide formation from L-arginine attenuates endothelium-dependent relaxation. Br J Pharmacol 96:-418–424
57. Richard V, Tanner FC, Tschudi M, Lüscher TF (1990) Differential activation of the endothelial L-arginine pathway by bradykinin, serotonin and clonidine in porcine coronary arteries. Am J Physiol 259:H1433–H1439
58. Rinaldi G, Bohr D (1989) Endothelium-mediated spontaneous response in aortic rings of deoxycorticosterone acetate-hypertensive rats. Hypertension 13:256–261
59. Saito Y, Nakao K, Shirakami M, Jougasaki M, Yamada T, Itoh H, Mukoyama M, Arai H, Hosoda K, Suga S, Ogawa Y, Imura H (1989) Detection and characterization of endothelin-1-like immunoreactivity in rat plasma. Biochem Biophys Res Commun 163:1512–1516
60. Savitsky JP, Doczi J, Black J, Arnold JD (1978) A clinical safety trial of stroma-free hemoglobin. Clin Pharmacol Ther 23:73–80
61. Schini V, Hendrickson H, Heublein D, Burnett Jr J, Vanhoutte PM (1989) Thrombin enhances the release of endothelin from cultured porcine aortic endothelial cells. Eur J Pharmacol 165:333–334

62. Shichiri M, Hirata Y, Anao K, Emori T, Ohta K, Kimoro S, Inoue A, Marumo F (1989) Plasma endothelin levels in patients with hypertension and end-stage renal failure. Circulation 80 (Suppl II):0502
63. Shichiri M, Hirata Y, Ando K, Emori T, Ohta K, Kimoto S, Ogura M, Inoue A, Marumo F (1990) Plasma endothelin levels in hypertension and chronic renal failure. Hypertension 15:493–496
64. Sim MK, Singh M (1987) Decreased responsiveness of the aortae of hypertensive rats to acetylcholine, histamine and noradrenaline. Br J Pharmacol 90:147–150
65. Soltis EE (1987) Effect of age blood pressure and membrane-dependent vascular responses in the rat. Circ Res 61:889–897
66. Stewart DJ, Cernacek P (1989) Plasma endothelin levels are markedly elevated in cardiogenic shock. Circulation 80 (Suppl II):2329
67. Suzuki N, Miyauchi T, Tomobe Y, Matsumoto H, Goto K, Masaki T, Fujino M (1990) Plasma concentrations of endothelin-1 in spontaneously hypertensive rats and DOCA-salt hypertensive rats. Biochem Biophys Res Commun 167:941–947
68. Tanner FC, Noll G, Boulanger C, Lüscher TF (1991) Oxidized low density lipoproteins inhibit relaxations of porcine coronary arteries: role of scavenger receptor and endothelium-derived nitric oxide. Circulation (in press)
69. Tesfamariam B, Halpern W (1988) Endothelium-dependent and endothelium-independent vasodilation in resistance arteries from hypertensive rats. Hypertension 11:440–444
70. Tolins JP, Palmer RMJ, Moncada S, Raij L (1990) Role of endothelium-derived relaxing factor in regulation of renal hemodynamic responses. Am J Physiol 258:H655–H662
71. Tomobe Y, Miyauchi T, Saito A, Yanagisawa M, Kimura S, Goto K, Masaki T (1988) Effects of endothelin on the renal artery from spontaneously hypertensive and Wistar Kyoto rats. Eur J Pharmacol 152:373–374
72. Vallance P, Collier J, Moncada S (1989) Effects of endothelium-derived nitric oxide on peripheral arteriolar tone in man. Lancet 997–1000
73. Valtier D, Guicheney P, Badouin-Legros M, Meyer P (1986) Platelets in human essential hypertension: in vitro hyperreactivity to thrombin. J Hypertension 4:551–555
74. Van de Voorde J, Cuvelier C, Leusen I (1984) Endothelium-dependent relaxation effects in aorta from hypertensive rats. Arch Int Physiol Biochem 92:10–11
75. Van de Voorde J, Leusen I (1984) Endothelium-dependent and independent relaxation effects on aorta preparations of renal hypertensive rats. Arch Int Physiol Biochem 92:35–36
76. Van de Voorde J, Leusen I (1986) Endothelium-dependent and independent relaxation of aortic rings from hypertensive rats. Am J Physiol 250:H711–H717
77. Watt PAC, Thurston H (1989) Endothelium-dependent relaxation in resistance vessels from the spontaneously hypertensive rats. J Hypertension 7:661–666
78. Winquist RJ, Bunting PB, Baskin EP, Wallace AA (1984) Decreased endothelium-dependent relaxation in New Zealand genetic hypertensive rats. J Hypertension 2:536–541
79. Webb RC, Vander AJ, Henry JP (1987) Increased vasodilator responses to acetylcholine in psychosocial hypertensive mice. Hypertension 9:268–276
80. Wright CE, Angus JA (1986) Effects of hypertension and hypercholesteremia on vasodilatation in the rabbit. Hypertension 8:361–371
81. Yanagisawa M, Kurihara H, Kimura S, Mitsui Y, Kobayashi M, Watanabe TX, Masaki T (1988) A novel potent vasoconstrictor peptide produced by vascular endothelial cells. Nature 332:411–415
82. Ylä-Herttuala S, Palinski W, Rosenfeld ME, Parthasarathy S, Carew TE, Butler S, Witztum JL, Steinberg D (1989) Evidence for the presence of oxidatively modified low density lipoprotein in atherosclerotic lesions of rabbit and man. J Clin Invest 84:1086–1095

Author's address:

Thomas F. Lüscher, M. D.
Department of Medicine, Division of Cardiology
University Hospital
4031 Basel/Switzerland

Experimental induction of spasm, sudden progression of organic stenosis and intramural hemorrhage in the epicardial coronary arteries

M. Nakamura

Research Institute of Angiocardiology and Cardiovascular Clinic, Faculty of Medicine, Kyushu University, 3-1-1 Maidashi, Higashi-ku, Fukuoka, 812 Japan

Summary: Pathogenesis of the so-called "heart attack" still remains to be elucidated. The links between stable effort angina and unstable or acute myocardial infarction, and between asymptomatic and spontaneous angina are all missing. In medicine presently, pathophysiology of ischemic heart disease is considered a consequence of i) the progression of atherosclerotic narrowing of the coronary artery, and ii) dynamic and transient obstruction (coronary spasm), but these mechanisms are traditionally believed to be unrelated. This article demonstrates various experimental evidence indicating that these two mechanisms are related. And, this review article describes how to produce experimental coronary spasm in the presence of atherosclerosis, similar to that seen in patients with variant angina, and that coronary spasm can produce sudden progression of coronary atherosclerotic obstruction due to intramural hemorrhage. Establishment of various animal models to elucidate mechanisms related to various stages of ischemic heart disease are needed.

Key words: Animal model; ischemic heart disease; coronary spasm; intramural hemorrhage; autacoid

1. Requirement of an animal model of coronary arterial spasm

As early as the 19th century, coronary arterial spasm was thought to be a major cause of angina pectoris. Between the 1920s and 1960s, clinico-pathological studies and later coronary angiographic studies revealed that a common cause of events leading to angina pectoris was an increase in myocardial oxygen demand in the presence of advanced coronary atherosclerotic obstruction (35, 57, 86). In 1971, at the National Heart and Lung Institute conference on "angina pectoris, pathophysiology, evaluation and treatment", coronary spasm was not even mentioned and the only widely accepted explanation of the cause of angina pectoris was an increase in myocardial oxygen demand (21). In 1959, Prinzmetal and co-workers found 12 cases reported in literature between 1931–1956, and they personally observed 20 patients, in whom ST-segment elevation was present during anginal attacks, at rest. They called these cases a "variant form of angina pectoris", which differed from classic angina, and they ruled out an increase in the myocardial oxygen demand as a cause of spontaneous angina. They postulated that anginal pain resulted from a temporary occlusion of the large coronary artery with severe stenosis due to a normal increase in tonus of the vessel wall (56). They avoided using the term "coronary spasm", probably because this term was then called the "resort of the diagnostically destitute" (18).

In 1971, Guazzi et al. noted that an increase in myocardial oxygen demand did not precede anginal attacks of variant angina (30). In 1975, Maseri et al. systematically studied patients with variant angina and showed that anginal attacks were always associated with a transient complete coronary occlusion which was promptly relieved by nitroglycerin (43). Their continued and expanded studies clearly demonstrated that coronary spasm occurred, not only at areas of the angiographically stenosed lesions, but also even in coronary arteries which appeared normal (44, 46).

In present day medicine, coronary spasm is accepted as a major cause of variant angina and, in some patients, of other types of angina, such as rest, rest and effort, and post myocardial infarction angina (4, 36, 46). However, the roles of spasm in the pathogenesis of unstable angina, acute myocardial infarction, and sudden cardiac death in subjects with ischemic heart disease have not been clearly identified, although association between coronary spasm and unstable angina and/or thrombotic occlusion was considered, based on clinically-related events (1, 4, 15, 45, 46, 54, 77, 85).

Extensive clinical investigations done to detect mechanisms and triggering factors related to coronary spasm and to acute ischemic syndromes have been less than fruitful, hence a suitable animal model of coronary spasm was needed. Extensive evaluation of coronary spasm in patients with vasospastic ischemic heart disease is hampered because the required procedures violate ethical practice and the patient would often be subject to risk (16, 46). On the other hand, there are drawbacks to the use of isolated coronary arteries, because hematogenic, endothelial, and neurogenic effects are not adequately preserved (2, 49). At present, coronary angiography seems to be the only available tool with which one can demonstrate effectively the occurrence of coronary spasm of the large epicardial coronary artery. Large animals, such as pigs and dogs are suitable for coronary angiographic evaluations, and we prepared a suitable model of coronary spasm in miniature pigs. In the present article, attention is focused on this animal model of coronary spasm.

2. The animal model of coronary spasm facilitates understanding of the pathophysiology of ischemic heart disease

Establishment of a suitable animal model of coronary spasm was expected to elucidate mechanisms related to spasm and to ischemic heart diesease, e.g., the relation between spasm and coronary atherosclerosis and progression to or thrombotic occlusion.

a) normal vasomotion versus coronary spasm

Coronary spasm is an active and transient hypercontraction of the large epicardial coronary arteries sufficient to cause acute myocardial ischemia; this event can be overcome by nitrates (46). MacAlpine in 1980 proposed a geometric theory emphasizing acute luminal narrowing occurring at stenotic sites as the result of "normal" vasomotion and that even a modest mural thickening may act as a lever in translating a physiologic degree of medial smooth muscle shortening into critical luminal obstructions (41). Clinical studies indicated that ergonovine or ergometrine, vasocontrictive agents used widely to induce spasm in patients with variant angina, produced about a 20% narrowing of the diameter of the epicardial large coronary artery in patients without coronary spasm (11). MacAlpine's geometric theory was not supported by quantitative measurements of coronary arterial diameter changes in patients with variant angina (25) nor in our coronary spasm model in swine with mild eccentric type atherosclerotic lesion of the epicardial large coronary artery (19). But, further studies will be needed, especially to conclude when the atherosclerotic lesion is a concentric type.

In studies on isolated coronary arteries, no quantitative or qualitative differences between hypercontraction and spasm were noted. We do have evidence that, in addition to an abnormally decreased endothelial dependent relaxation (81), an increased number of histaminergic receptors and/or augmentation of signal transduction, but not calcium sensitivity of the contractile proteins in the atherosclerotic medial muscle cell, causes histamine-induced coronary spasm in our swine model (62).

b) Coronary atherosclerosis, hypercholesterolemia and coronary spasm

Coronary spasm frequently develops at the site of the lesion in patients with variant angina, although the extent of organic stenosis varies widely. Coronary spasm occurs even in normal appearing coronary arteries, but an angiographical normal coronary artery does not mean the artery is histologically normal. A few autopsied cases of vasospastic angina have been reported and morphological characteristics responsible for coronary spasm were not clarified. Forman et al. noted an increased number of adventitial mast cells which contain histamine and other vasoactive substances, and these substances are released in response to various stimuli in patients with vasospastic angina, as compared with findings in the case of coronary artery disease and sudden death, but without spasm, or in normal adults (23). But the roles of mast cells in the pathogenesis of coronary spasm are unknown. It is not clear whether the presence of coronary atherosclerosis is a conditio sine qua non for development of coronary spasm in humans. We reported that fatal arrhythmias, complete AV block, ventricular tachycardia or fibrillation and sudden death in patients with vasospastic angina did not depend on the presence of a significant coronary stenosis, but that the rate of myocardial infarction was significantly higher angiographically in patients with a significant coronary stenosis – 90% or greater than that in patients with a lesser degree stenosis or with normal appearing vessels at angiography (52).

In our early studies on the miniature swine model of coronary spasm, coronary spasm was provoked in the presence of a localized mild atherosclerosis by giving histamine and/or serotonin parenterally, as shown in Fig. 1 (65, 66). In five of 36 consecutively examined pigs, coronary spasm was provoked by the simple administration of histamine, under conditions of normocholesterolemia (Fig. 2). Post-mortem examinations revealed the presence of spontaneous atherosclerosis at the site of the spasm (19). A close

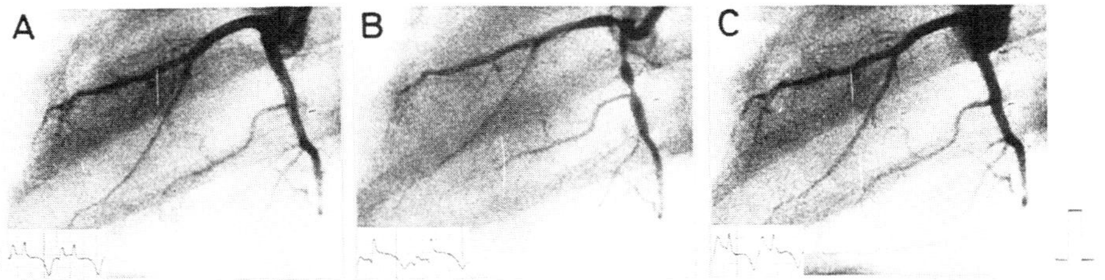

Fig. 1 A–C. Coronary arteriograms in miniature swine fed an atherogenic diet. **A** Before and **B** after intracoronary administration of histamine (200 μg) in the presence of cimetidine administered intravenously in doses of 60 mg/kg. **C** After intravenous administration of nitroglycerin in doses of 20 μg/kg. Coronary artery spasm, with associated electrocardiographic ST-segment elevation in the precordial lead, was provoked at multiple sites in the circumflex branch of the left coronary artery where skip-lesions of coronary atherosclerosis were observed histologically, in accord with the sites of spasm (65). (Reprinted by permission of the American Association for the Advancement of Science.)

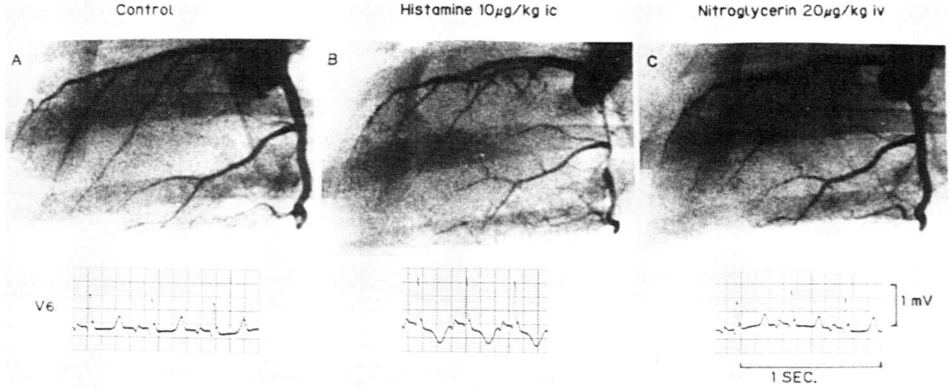

Fig. 2 A–C. Coronary angiograms and electrocardiograms obtained at control **A**, after histamine **B**, and after nitroglycerin **C** from a representative pig with spontaneous atherosclerosis (19). Tubular type vasoconstrictionis evident along the major trunk of the left circumflex coronary artery after intracoronary administration of 10 μg/kg histamine. The angiogram obtained after nitroglycerin shows no organic lesion in either the left anterior descending or circumflex coronary arteries. Electrocardiogram recorded at V_6 shows ST depression after histamine (**B**). (Reprinted by permission of the American Heart Association.)

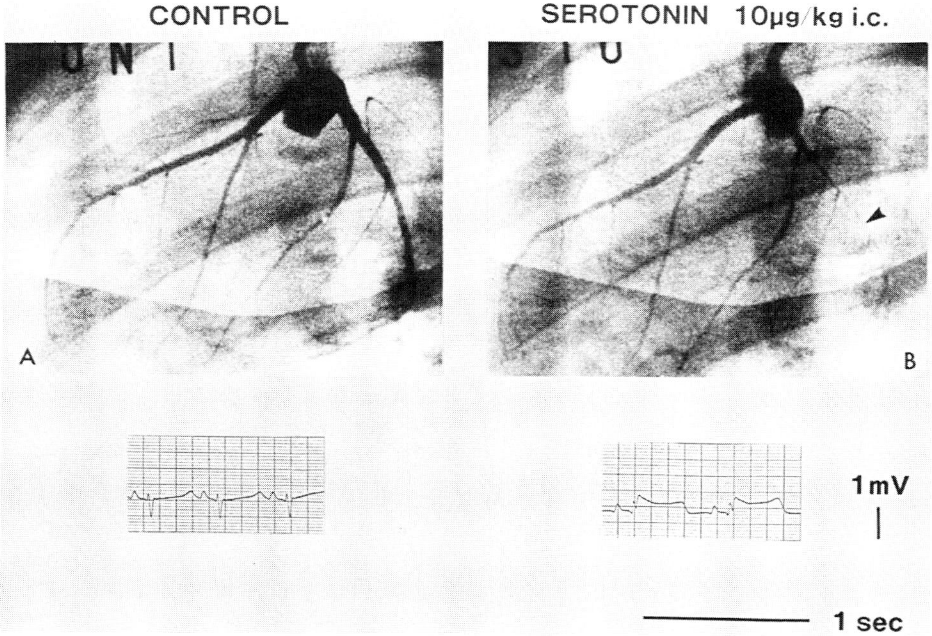

Fig. 3 A, B. Left coronary angiograms (left anterior oblique projection) oft control **A** and provocation of serotonin-induced coronary spasm **B**. Subtotal stenosis was noted along the left circumflex coronary artery. Arrow indicates the severe spastic site. During coronary spasm, ECG-ST elevation was recorded (51). (Reprinted by permission of the American Heart Association.)

topographical correlation was found between the site of spasm and atherosclerosis. In ongoing studies in this swine model with a moderate coronary atherosclerosis, we found that serotonin given intracoronarily provoked a typical coronary spasm at the site of the localized coronary atherosclerosis in association with transient myocardial ischemia which was relieved spontaneously or after nitroglycerin, as shown in Fig. 3 (51). In another study in which an atherogenic diet containing high fat, high cholesterol, and cholate, was fed, endothelial denudation was carried out on miniature swine; an average of 355 mg/dl of plasma cholesterol was maintained for several months. Contrary to expectations, we found a diffuse hypercontraction of, not only the denuded site, but also of the non-denuded site of the epicardial coronary artery, as induced by histamine or serotonin, but focal spasm and/or an acute myocardial ischemia was absent, probably because early atherosclerotic lesions had occurred at multiple sites of the coronary arteries in addition to severe hypercholesterolemia (72).

We also found that coronary spasm can be readily provoked by giving serotonin or ergonovine, and that hyperventilation accelerated the serotonin-induced spasm in the miniature swine with normocholesterolemia, at the XX-ray-irradiated site, an area where the concentric type of coronary atherosclerosis usually occurs (53).

These findings suggest that atherosclerotic changes are more pertinent than hypercholesterolemia as an initiating cause of localized coronary spasm. However, the type of atherosclerotic lesions prone to lead to a coronary spasm remains unknown.

The dog is a useful species for coronary angiography studies, and coronary physiology in the dog has been thoroughly studied. In our studies on dogs, endothelial denudation, with or without feeding a diet containing high cholesterol, produced angiographic evidence of a focal hypercontraction induced by ergonovine (34). However, the degree of luminal narrowing of the epicardial coronary arteries was insufficient and inconsistent to cause acute myocardial ischemia. Thus, this dog model does not fulfill the valid definition of coronary spasm, in contrast to the cases of atherosclerotic miniature swine.

c) Experimental induction of a sudden progression of organic stenosis and intramural hemorrhage by coronary spasm

Acute myocardial infarction frequently occurs in patients with variant angina in the area supplied by the spastic coronary artery, particularly in cases of a significant stenosis (45, 46, 52, 56). Clinical observations suggested that coronary spasm may result in a coronary thrombotic occlusion (1, 15, 45, 54, 77, 85). Maseri et al. found evidence at autopsy of thrombotic material overlying atheroma in a patient with coronary spasm. They suggested that coronary spasm resulted in a coronary thrombosis (45).

Others discounted the significant role of spasm in the pathogenesis of acute myocardial infarction, because restoration of the coronary flow with nitroglycerin in patients with an acute myocardial infarction is infrequent (40, 58, 70). However, Zellinger et al. reported a case where thrombosis was angiographically demonstrated in a vessel which had recently undergone episodes of coronary spasm. They suggested that the failure of nitroglycerin infused into the occluded coronary artery to restore coronary flow at the time of angiography does not exclude an earlier spastic contribution to development of thrombotic occlusion (85). Thus, the hypothesis that acute myocardial infarction develops as a result of coronary spasm remains an open question.

Lesions in coronary atherosclerosis which are potential causes of acute myocardial infarction are progressive luminal narrowing with rupture of the atheromatous plaque and thrombosis, or with hemorrhage in the plaque (63). None of these lesions has been experimentally demonstrated, except for the work done by Constantinides, who demonstrated thrombosis associated with intraplaque hemorrhage of the aorta and coronary arteries by giving pressor substances such as hypertensin or serotonin, in addition to Russel's viper venom, all potent thrombogenic substances, to intermittent hyperlipemia rabbits (14). However, extensive studies on coronary atherosclerosis and myocardial infarction were not described.

We have also found that in the moderately atherosclerotic miniature swine fed a diet containing high fat, 2% cholesterol, and 1.1% cholate, in addition to endothelial denudation and two administrations of x-ray irradiation, serotonin given intracoronarily five times in a dose of 10 μg/kg each time, produced a transient 25 min total or subtotal occlusion. These pigs were killed 40 min after the final provocation of spasm and morphological studies revealed the intramural hemorrhage to be limited to the spastic site (51). Microscopical examination revealed fresh intramural hemorrhage and sudden progression of coronary stenosis at the site of hemorrhage. Electron microscopy showed intercellular bridges, squeezing of the endothelial cells and adhesion of leukocytes at the severely spastic site. These events suggest a cause-effect relation between coronary spasm and disarrangement such as intraplaque hemorrhage and the resultant progression of coronary stenosis, factors considered to relate to the causal lesions seen in cases of acute myocardial infarction. Further studies on the causal relation between coronary spasm and coronary obstructions such as thrombosis and acute myocardial infarction are now in progress. Acute myocardial infarction was induced in pigs with a prolonged severe coronary spasm (38). Thus, we believe that our swine model of coronary spasm is useful for studying the pathogenesis of ischemic heart disease and further for screening drugs to treat patients with vasospastic angina.

d) Spasm and hypercontraction of coronary artery in normal animals

Gensini et al. seem to have been the first to angiographically demonstrate diffuse coronary spasm, in normal dogs by giving pitressin intravenously after pretreatment with acetylcholine (26). Perez et al. obtained angiographical evidence of a transient and complete occlusion of the epicardial coronary artery with a topical administration of potassium and serotonin adsorbed to ion exchange gels placed on the surface of the coronary arteries in open-chest normal dogs (55). They reported that other constrictors, such as norepinephrine and angiotensin, failed to evoke coronary spasm (55). Although membrane depolarization and contraction by high concentrations of potassium are widely used in studies on the isolated coronary artery, a high concentration of potassium in the plasma or in the adventitial tissues of the large epicardial coronary arteries in patients with vasospastic angina is unlikely. The only possibility is that intramyocardial small vessels in the ischemic myocardium may be surrounded by extracellular high concentrations of potassium. Other investigators demonstrated that thio-thromboxane A_2 (84), a thromboxane A_2 analogue, or the potassium channel blocker tetraethylammonium (33) given into the coronary circulation of normal rabbits in vivo or in the isolated heart caused diffuse coronary spasm. However, in our atherosclerotic miniature swine, thio-thromboxane A_2 and phenylephrine failed to provoke coronary spasm and caused only diffuse hypercontraction up to 30% luminal reduction (67). Indomethacin (2 mg/kg) or prostacyclin (50 ng/kg min^{-1}) failed to prevent the histamine-induced coronary artery spasm in our swine model (67). Thus, the imbalance between thromboxane A_2 and prostacyclin probably cannot explain the occurrence of coronary spasm in our pig model.

Studies on normal cats showed a transient decrease in coronary flow, electrocardiographic ST changes and increase in coronary resistance by giving pictrotoxin, a drug known to block the central nervous GABA ergic system (64). Hypothalamus stimulation in normal monkeys (48), cats (47), and rats (31) induced ischemia-like electrocardiographic changes, arrhythmia, and/or reduction in the mean luminal diameter of the coronary arteries. However, these studies did not include angiographic findings and do not suffice to prove provocation of coronary spasm of the epicardial large coronary artery. We found that the potent vasoconstrictor agent, leucotrien (71), a 5-lipoxygenase metabolite of arachidonic acid and endothelin (50), a vasoactive peptide present in culture medium of endothelial cells, did not provoke coronary spasm of the large epicardial coronary artery, but did cause severe hypercontractions of the small coronary arteries that resulted in acute myocardial ischemia, regardless of the presence or absence of atherosclerosis. These hypercontractions of the small coronary arteries differ from the coronary spasm that occurs in patients with variant angina. Hypercontraction of the resistant coronary arteries is difficult to define angiographically, particularly in case of small animals. The coronary spasm induced in normal animals seems to be unsuitable for study on the roles of coronary spasm in the progression of organic atherosclerosis, intraplaque hemorrhage, and coronary thrombotic occlusion in the presence of atherosclerosis.

f) Neural effects on experimentally induced coronary spasm

Clinical studies suggested that an increased α-adrenergic nerve activity plays an important role in the occurrence of variant angina (59, 82). However, other clinical studies discounted the importance of adrenergic stimulation in the pathophysiology of coronary spasm (10, 60, 78). The lack of elevation of plasma catecholamines at the onset of anginal attack (60), and failure of the α-adrenergic blockers phentolamine and prazosin to reduce anginal attacks in patients with variant angina were noted in a double-blind randomized trial (10, 78).

Clinical investigations demonstrated that muscarinic agonists, such as pilocarpine, methacholine, and acetylcholine given parenterally provoked coronary spasm in patients with variant angina (20, 73, 79, 83), and the pretreatment of atropine prevented the provocation of spasm by pilocarpine or acetylcholine (79, 83). But, the atropine study does not prove the role of parasympathetic activation, since atropine blocks most muscarinic receptors in various cells (8, 29). The experimental provocation of coronary spasm by stimulation of autonomic nerves has not been reported. Stimulation of the hypothalamus or the administration of substances acting on the central nervous system in intact animals caused ischemia-like ST/T-changes electrocardiographically, but angiographic evidence was not obtained to confirm these events (31, 47, 48, 64).

Coronary spasm can persist even following total cardiac denervation or plexetomy in patients with variant angina, although the rate of spontaneous anginal attack was reduced in some cases (3, 5, 7, 12). Coronary spasm provoked by ergonovine proved to be independent of neural control extrinsic to the heart, since the response to ergonovine was the same in heart transplant recipients lacking extrinsic neural control and in patients with normally innervated hearts (11).

In our swine model of coronary atherosclerosis, the coronary spasm provoked by histamine in situ was reproduced in vitro at the same site of the coronary artery in the

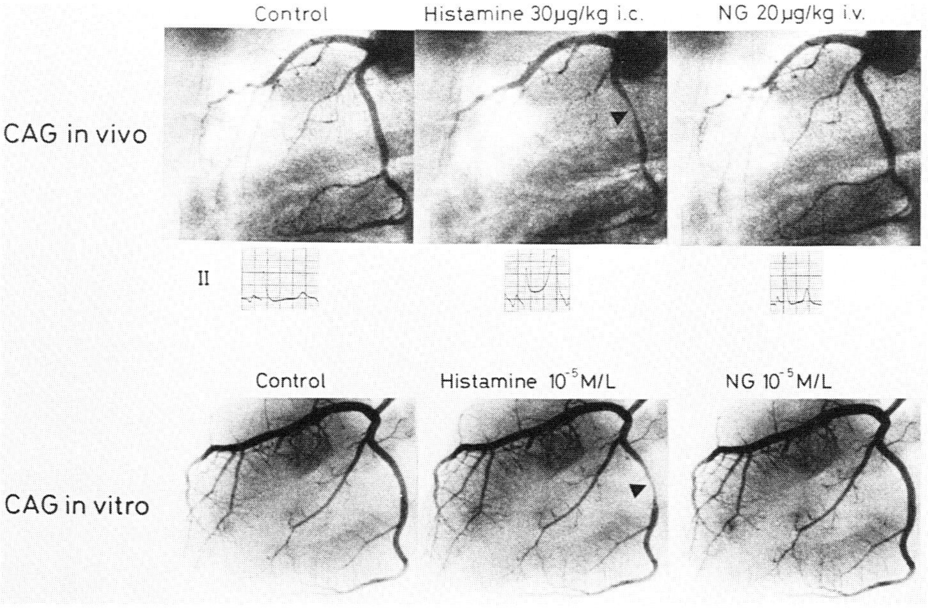

Fig. 4. Representative coronary angiograms in the miniature pig, in vivo (upper panel) and in vitro (lower panel) (80). Arrow indicates the site of coronary spasm. ECG lead II was recorded in vivo. The estimated concentration of histamine 10 µg/kg in bolus intracoronary administration was maximally 5.2×10^{-5} M/l. CAG = coronary arteriography. NG = nitroglycerin. (Reprinted by permission of the American Heart Association.)

isolated pig heart perfused by crystalline solution, as shown in Fig. 4 (80). These results may rule out the major contribution of neural effects on provocation of coronary spasm, in this swine model.

g) Autacoids, platelets, cyclic flow reduction, and coronary spasm

Autacoids, such as histamine induce coronary spasm in patients with variant angina (27). Ergonovine has been widely used to provoke coronary spasm in patients with a suspected vasospastic angina, and ergonovine-induced coronary spasm was reported to resemble spontaneously occurring spasm (17, 44). In animal studies, ergonovine or ergometrine could be classified mainly as a serotonin agonist (6) and α-adrenergic receptor stimulation was discounted (6, 32).

In our swine model with moderately advanced coronary atherosclerosis produced by x-ray irradiation, cholesterol feeding, and endothelial denudation, serotonin consistently provoked a typical coronary spasm, as shown in Fig. 3 (51).

Coronary sinus plasma from patients with coronary artery disease constricted the isolated canine coronary artery and only the serotonin antagonist, methiothepin, prevented this constriction. However, plasma from patients with no coronary artery disease evoked only an endothelium-dependent relaxation (61). The difference in the concentration of serotonin between coronary sinus and aorta was greater in patients with coronary heart disease compared with patients without significant coronary artery disease (76). These results suggest a close relation between the vasoconstrictor activity and the existence of significant coronary artery disease. Cohen demonstrated experimentally that aggregating platelets contract the isolated canine coronary artery and that the serotonin released accumulates in the coronary adrenergic endings, and upon release from nerves as a false transmitter, the amine can activate the serotonergic receptor on smooth muscle cell and reverse the action of the adrenergic nerve from dilator to constrictor (13). However, it is still unclear whether an enhanced platelet activity and/or serotonin are the causes of coronary spasm. Clinical investigation indicated that the serotonin S_2 antagonist (Ketanserin) did not significantly decrease the frequency of anginal attack in patients with vasospastic angina (9, 24).

Cyclic reduction of coronary flow in a mechanically constricted coronary artery of anesthetized dogs was described by Uchida et al. as a model of coronary spasm (74), since cyclic changes of ST elevation were often seen in patients with variant angina (46). They claimed that this cyclic flow reduction was caused by coronary spasm, because coronary dilators, such as nitroglycerin, papaverine, and nicorandil prevented this cyclic flow reduction and nicotinic acid with no antiplatelet aggregating actions diminished the cyclic flow reduction (75). On the contrary, Foltz et al. claimed that this cyclic flow reduction was caused by platelet aggregation, because aspirin (35 mg/kg) intravenously administered abolished this cyclic flow reduction and histologic sections of the narrowed coronary artery showed an amorphous mass in the area of the lumen when coronary flow was reduced (22). This cyclic flow reduction model in dogs has been used to examine effects of drugs on unstable angina (28), probably because there is a notion that unstable angina is a consequence of platelet activation and vasoconstriction at sites of complex coronary lesion and endothelial injury. Golino et al. reported that both LY 53857 and SQ 29548, specific serotonin S2 and thromboxane receptor antagonists respectively, abolished cyclic flow variations, probably due to blocking the vasoconstrictive action of serotonin and thromboxane released from the aggregating platelets at the mechanically stenosed sites (28). This slowly developing platelets aggregation model requiring the presence of a fixed severe stenosis (60–80%) does not resemble the acute, reversible coronary spasm which occurs in patients with variant angina and in whom the coronary artery was often angiographically normal. But it will be useful as an animal model to study the pathogenesis of unstable angina and to elucidate interrelations between platelet aggregation and spasm or hypercontraction. Kurgan et al. demonstrated that reduction in the luminal diameter by about 50%, with no decrease in flow of the carotid arteries by the periarterial application of $CaCl_2$ led to an endothelial desquamation, platelet adhesion, thrombus formation, and leucocyte adhesion at the site of the hypercontraction (39). However, the concentration of $CaCl_2$ applied directly to the adventitia was 0.5 M, a concentration which may cause, not only constriction, but also damage to the arterial wall, as evidenced by deposition of calcium precipitation. Platelet adhesion and thrombosis were absent in severe coronary spasm maintained for 25 min in our pig model (51) or in case of the coronary spasm induced in dogs by a topical application of high concentration of potassium and serotonin by Peretz et al. (55).

h) Similarities and dissimilarities in coronary spasm in our swine model and in patients with variant angina

In Goettingen-type miniature swine with various stages of coronary atherosclerosis, coronary spasm could be provoked by giving histamine, serotonin, and ergonovine, in association with acute myocardial ischemia, ventricular fibrillation and sudden death. These findings are similar to those seen in patients with variant angina. Coronary spasm was provoked at the angiographically normal appearing site where atherosclerotic lesions were found histologically in almost all pigs. The coronary spasm provoked by histamine was accelerated by pretreatment with the H_2 blocker, cimetidine. Clinically, the administration of cimetidine sometimes led to the occurrence of coronary spasm (68). Acute myocardial ischemia produced by the coronary spasm provoked by histamine and/or ergonovine in the swine model was relieved by nitroglycerin similar to events seen in patients with variant angina. Further, intraplaque hemorrhage and the progression of coronary organic stenosis, both considered causal lesions of acute myocardial infarction, could be produced by the induction of coronary spasm (51), as suggested by clinical observations (16, 42, 46, 69). Our preliminary results show that a degree of constriction of the coronary artery in the swine model by intracoronary administration of acetylcholine was greater in the small arteries than in the large epicardial coronary arteries. Coronary spasm provoked by serotonin in our moderately advanced model of coronary atherosclerosis was prevented mostly by ketanserin, a S_2-antagonist. However, anginal pain in patients with variant angina could not be prevented by the administration of ketanserin (9, 24).

In patients with variant angina, coronary spasm with or without chest pain occurs spontaneously. We have not demonstrated spontaneous spasm in our pig model, except in preliminary experiments in which a rigorous balloon endothelial denudation, such as a percutaneous transluminal coronary angioplasty, caused a spontaneous hypercontraction with up to 70% of luminal reduction, which subsided within 30 min (37). But this spontaneous hypercontraction was prevented by pretreatment with adequate amounts of heparin (37). In patients with variant angina, anticoagulants, such as heparin, are not given routinely to prevent coronary spasm. In light of all the aforementioned evidence, our atherosclerotic swine model of coronary spasm is indeed useful for elucidating the pathophysiology of coronary spasm, as well as other related ischemic events, although some dissimilarities between coronary spasm in our animal model and in patients with vasospastic angina, were found.

3. Conclusion

Coronary spasm is indeed an important factor in the pathogenesis of various stages of ischemic heart disease in humans. The mechanisms and definition of coronary spasm remain open to debate, as do the roles of coronary spasm in the pathogenesis of unstable angina and acute myocardial infarction.

In this article, the coronary spasm produced in experimental animals was reviewed and events related to be better understanding pathophysiology of coronary spasm in humans were discussed. Similarities and dissimilarities between our swine model of coronary spasm and the coronary spasm which occurs in patients with variant angina were discussed.

Acknowledgments. The author acknowledges grant support from the Ministry of Education, Science and Culture, and from the Ministry of Health and Welfare of Japan. Gratitude is extended to M. Ohara for helpful comments and to I. Tomizuka for secretarial services.

References

1. Benacerraf A, Scholl JM, Achard F, Tonnelier M, Lavergne G (1983) Coronary spasm and thrombosis associated myocardial infarction in a patient with nearly normal coronary arteries. Circ 67:1147–1150
2. Bertrand ME, Lablanche JM,Rousoeau MF, Warembourg Jr HH, Stankowak C, Soots G (1980) Surgical treatment of variant angina: use of plexectomy with aortocoronary bypass. Circ 61:877–882
3. Bertrand ME, Lablanche JM, Tilmant PY, Ducloux G, Warembourg Jr HH, Soots G (1981) Complete denervation of the heart (autotransplantation) for treatment of severe, refractory coronary spasm. Am J Cardiol 47:1375–1378
4. Bertrand ME, Lablanche JM, Tilmant PY, Thieuleux FA, Delforge MR, Carre AG, Asseman P, Berzin B, Libersa C (1982) Frequency of provoked coronary arterial spasm in 1089 consecutive patients undergoing coronary arteriography. Circ 65:1299–1306
5. Betrin A, Pomar JL, Bourassa MG, Grondin CM (1983) Influence of partial sympathetic denervation on the results of myocardial revascularization in variant angina. Am J Cardiol 51:661–667
6. Brazenor RM, Angus JA (1981) Ergometrine contracts isolated canine coronary arteries by serotonergic mechanism; no role for alpha adrenoceptors. J Pharm Exp Therap 218:530–536
7. Buda AJ, Fawles RE, Schroeder JS, Hunt SA, Cipriano PR, Stinson EB, Harrison DC (1981) Coronary artery spasm in the denervated transplanted human heart. Am J Med 70:1144–1149
8. Burnstock G (1988) Local purinergic regulation of blood pressure in "Vasodilation: Vascular smooth muscle, peptides, autonomic nerves, and endothelium" (ed by Vanhoute PM). Raven Press Ltd, New York, 1–14
9. Caterin RD, Capeggiani C, L'Abbate A (1984) A doubleblind, placebo-controlled study of ketanserin in patients with Prinzmetal's angina; evidence against a role of serotonin in the genesis of coronary vasospasm. Circ 69:889–894
10. Chierchia S, Davies G, Berkenboom G, Crea F, Crean R, Maseri A (1984) α-Adrenergic receptors and coronary spasm; an elusive link. Circ 69:8–14
11. Cipriano PR, Guthaner DF, Orlick AE, Ricci DR, Wexler L, Silverman JF (1979) The effects of ergonovine maleate on coronary arterial size. Circ 59:82–89
12. Clark DA, Quint RA, Mitchell RL, Angell WW (1977) Coronary artery spasm: medical management, surgical denervation and autotransplantation. J Thoracic Cardiovas Surg 73:332–339
13. Cohen RA (1985) Platelet-induced neurogenic coronary constriction due to accumulation of the false neurotransmitter, 5-hydroxytryptamine. J Clin Inv 75:286–292
14. Constantinides P (1965) Experimental atherosclerosis in the rabbit, in "comparative atherosclerosis – The morphology of spontaneous und induced atherosclerotic lesions in animals and its relation to human disease". Ed by Roberts Jr JC, Straus R, Cooper MS, Hoefer Medical Div Harper & Row Publisher, New York, Evanston and London, 276–290
15. Conti RC, Feldman RL (1985) Acute myocardial infarction; thoughts about pathogenesis and treatment. Modern Concept Cardiov Dis 54:35–38
16. Crevey BJ, Owen SF, Pitt B (1981) Irreversible coronary occlusion related to administration of ergonovine. Circ 64:853–856
17. Curry RC, Pepine Jr CJ, Sabom MB, Conti CR (1979) Similarities of ergonovine-induced and spontaneous attacks of variant angina. Circ 59:307–312
18. Daley R (1957) The autonomic nervous system in its relation to some forms of heart and lung diesease. Brit Med J II:173–179
19. Egashira K, Tomoike H, Yamamoto Y, Yamada A, Hayashi Y, Nakamura M (1986) Histamine-induced coronary spasm in regions of intimal thickening in miniature pigs; roles of serum cholesterol and spontaneous or induced intimal thickening. Circ 74:826–837
20. Endo M, Hirosawa K, Kaneko N, Hase K, Inoue Y, Konno S (1976) Prinzmetal's variant angina; coronary arteriogram and left ventriculogram during anginal attack induced by methacholine. N Engl J Med 294:252–255

21. Epstein SE, Redwood DR, Goldstein RE, Beiser GD, Rosing DR, Glancy DL, Reis RL, Stinson EB (1971) Angina pectoris; pathophysiology evaluation and treatment. Ann Int Med 75:263–296
22. Folz JD, Crowell Jr EB, Powe GG (1977) Platelet aggregation in partially obstructed vessels and its elimination with aspirin. Circ 54:365–370
23. Forman MB, Oates JA, Robertson D, Robertson RM, Roberts II. LJ, Virmani R (1985) Increased adventitial mast cells in a patient with coronary spasm. N Engl J Med 313:1138–1141
24. Freedman SB, Chierchia S, Rodriguez-Plaza L, Bugiardini R, Smith G, Maseri A (1984) Ergonovine induced myocardial ischemia; no role for serotonergic receptors. Circ 70:178–183
25. Freedman B, Richmond DR, Kelley DT (1982) Pathophysiology of coronary artery spasm.Circ 66:705–709
26. Gensini GG, Giorgi S di, Murad-Netto S, Black A (1962) Arteriographic demonstration of coronary artery spasm and its release after the use of a vasodilator in a case of angina pectoris and in the experimental animal. Angiology 13:550–553
27. Ginsburg R, Bristow MR, Kantrowitz N, Baim DS, Harrison DC (1981) Histamine provocation of clinical coronary artery spasm; implications concerning pathogenesis of variant angina pectoris. Am Heart J 102:819–822
28. Golino P, Ashton JH, Buja LM, Rosolowsky M, Taylor AL, McNatt J, Campbell WB, Willerson JT (1989) Local platelet activation causes vasoconstriction of large epicardial canine coronary arteries in vivo, thromboxane A_2 and serotonin are possible mediators. Circ 79:154–166
29. Goyal RK (1989) Muscarinic receptor subtypes: Physiology and clinical implications. N Engl J Med 321:1022–1029
30. Guazzi M, Polese A, Fiorentini C, Magrini F, Bartorelli C (1971) Left ventricular performance and related hemodynamic changes in Prinzmetal's variant angina pectoris. Br Heart J 33:84–94
31. Gutstein WH, Anversa P, Beghi C, Kiu G., Pacanovsky D (1984) Coronary artery spasm in rat induced by hypothalamus stimulation. Atheroscl 51:135–142
32. Holtz J, Held W, Sommer O, Kuhne G, Bassenge E (1982) Ergonovine induced constriction of epicardial coronary arteries in conscious dogs; α-adrenoreceptors are not involved. Basic Res Cardiol 77:278–291
33. Iwaki M, Mizobuchi S, Nakaya Y, Kawano K, Niki T, Mori H (1987) Tetraethylammonium induced coronary spasm in isolated perfused rabbit heart; a hypothesis for the mechnism of coronary spasm. Cardiov Res 21:130–139
34. Kawachi Y, Tomoike H, Maruoka Y, Kikuchi Y, Araki H, Ishii Y, Tanaka K, Nakamura M (1984) Selective hypercontraction caused by ergonovine in the canine coronary artery under conditions of induced atherosclerosis. Circ 69:441–450
35. Keefer CS, Resnik WH (1928) Angina pectoris; a syndrome caused by anoxemia of the myocardium. Arch Intern Med 41:769–807
36. Kaiwaya Y, Torii S, Takeshita A, Nakagaki O, Nakamura M (1982) Postinfarction angina caused by coronary arterial spasm. Circ 65:275–280
37. Kuga T, Ohara Y, Hata H, Hirakawa Y, Tomoike H, Nakamura M (1990) Mechanism of hypercontraction of the coronary artery after endothelial denudation. Jap Circ J (suppl) No 0813 (abstract in Japanese)
38. Kuga T, Tagawa A, Tomoike H, Nakamura M (1990) Abrupt onset of coronary spasm progresses organic stenosis and prolonged coronary spasm induces acute myocardial infarction. Jap Circ J (suppl) No 0814 (abstract in Japanese)
39. Kurgan A, Gertz SD, Wajinberg RS (1983) Intimal changes associated with arterial spasm induced by periarterial application of calcium chloride. Exp Mol Pathol 39:176–193
40. Leinbach RC, Gold HK (1982) Coronary angiography during acute myocardial infarction; a search for spasm. Am Heart J 103:768–772
41. Mac Alpine RN (1980) Contribution of dynamic vascular wall thickening to luminal narrowing during coronary arterial constriction. Circ 61:296–301
42. Marzilli M, Goldstein S,Trirella MG, Palumbo C, Maseri A (1980) Some clinical considerations regarding the relation of coronary vasospasm to coronary atherosclerosis; a hypothetical pathogenesis. Am J Cardiol 45:882–886
43. Maseri A, Minno R, Chierchia S, Marchesi C, Pesola A, L'Abbate A (1975) Coronary artery spasm as a cause of acute myocardial ischemia in man. Chest 68:625–632

44. Maseri A, L'Abbate A, Pesola A, Ballestra AM, Marzilli M, Naltinti G,Severi S, De Nes DM, Parodi O, Biagini A (1977) Coronary vasospasm in angina pectoris. Lancet I:713–717
45. Maseri A, L'Abbate A, Baroldi G, Chierchia S, Marzilli M, Ballestra AM, Severi S, Parodi O, Biagini A, Distante A, Pesola A (1978) Coronary vasospasm as a possible cause of myocardial infarction; a conclusion derived from the study of "preinfarction" angina. N Engl J Med 299:1271–1277
46. Maseri A, Chierchia S (1982) Coronary artery spasm; demonstration, definition, diagnosis and consequences. Progr Cardiovas Dis 25:169–192
47. Melville KI, Blum B, Shister H, Silver MD (1963) Cardiac ischemic changes and arrhythmias induced by hypothalamic stimulation. Am J Cardiol 12:781–791
48. Melville KI, Garvey HL, Shister HE, Knaack J (1969) Central nervous system stimulation and cardiac ischemic changes in monkeys. Ann NY Acad Sci 156:241–260
49. Morrison AD, Berwick L, Ori L, Winegrad AI (1976) Morphology and metabolism of aortic intima-media preparation in which an intact endothelium is preserved. J Clin Invest 57:650–660
50. Muramatsu K, Tomoike H, Ohara Y, Egashira S, Nakamura M, Effects of endothelin on coronary circulation; hypercontraction of the small coronary artery is responsible for myocardial ischemia (submitted)
51. Nagasawa K, Tomoike H, Hayashi Y, Yamada A, Yamamoto T, Nakamura M (1989) Intramural hemorrhage and endothelial changes in atherosclerotic coronary artery after repetitive episodes of spasm in x-ray irradiated hypercholesterolemic pigs. Circ Res 65:272–282
52. Nakamura M, Takeshita A, Nose Y (1987) Clinical characteristics associated with myocardial infarction, arrhythmias and sudden death in patients with vasospastic angina. Circ 75:1110–1116
53. Ohara Y, Tagawa H, Kuga T, Tomoike H, Nakamura M (1989) Augmentation of serotonin-induced coronary constriction in respiratory or metabolic alkalosis in miniature pigs. Circ 80 (suppl II):II-234 (abstract)
54. Oliva PB, Breckinridge JC (1977) Arteriographic evidence of coronary arterial spasm in acute myocardial infarction. Circ 56:336–374
55. Perez JE,Saffitz JE, Gutierrez FA, Henry PD (1983) Coronary artery spasm in intact dogs induced by potassium and serotonin. Circ Res 52:423–431
56. Prinzmetal M, Kennamer R, Merliss R, Wada T, Bor N (1959) Angina pectoris I. A variant form of angina pectoris. A preliminary report. Am J Med 27:375–388
57. Proudfit WL, Shirey EK, Sones FM (1966) Selective cine coronary arteriography; correlation with clinical findings in 1,000 patients. Circ 33:901–910
58. Rentrop P, Blanke H, Karsch KR, Kaiser H, Kostering H, Leitz K (1981) Selective intracoronary thrombolysis in acute myocardial infarction and unstable angina pectoris. Circ 63:307–317
59. Ricci DR, Orlick AE, Cipriano PR, Guthaner DF, Harrision DC (1979) Altered adrenergic activity in coronary arterial spasm; insight into mechanism based on study of coronary hemodynamics and the electrocardiogram. Am J Cardiol 43:1073–1079
60. Robertson D, Robertson RM, Niew AS, Oates JA, Friesinger GC (1979) Variant angina pectoris; Investigation of indexes of sympathetic nervous system function. Am J Cardiol 43:1080–1085
61. Runbanyi GM, Frye RL, Holmes DR, Vanhoutte PM (1987) Vasoconstrictor activity of coronary sinus plasma from patients with coronary artery disease. J Am Coll Cardiol 9:1243–1249
62. Satoh S, Tomoike H, Mitsuoka W, Egashira S, Tagawa H, Kuga T, Nakamura M. Smooth muscles from the spastic coronary artery segments show hypercontractility to histamine. Am J Physiol (in press)
63. Scotti TM, Hackel DB (1985) Heart; Anderson's Pathology Chapter 16. Edited by John M Kissane 8th Edition. The CV Mosby Company, St Louis, Toronto, Princeton 560–662
64. Segal SA, Pearle DL, Gillis RA (1981) Coronary spasm produced by picrotoxin in cats. Europ J Pharmacol 76:447–451
65. Shimokawa H, Tomoike H, Nabeyama S, Yamamoto H, Araki H. Nakamura M, Ishii Y, Tanaka K (1983) Coronary artery spasm induced in atherosclerotic miniature swine. Science 221:560–562

66. Shimokawa H, Tomoike H, Nabeyama S, Yamamoto H, Ishii Y, Tanaka K, Nakamura M (1985) Coronary artery spasm induced in miniature swine; angiographic evidence and relation to coronary atherosclerosis. Am Heart J 110:300–310
67. Shimokawa H, Tomoike H, Nabeyama S, Yamamoto H, Nakamura M (1985) Histamine-induced spasm not significantly modulated by prostanoids in a swine model of coronary artery spasm. J Am Coll Card 6:321–327
68. Shimokawa H, Okamatsu S, Taira Y, Nakamura M (1987) Cimetidine induces coronary artery spasm in patients with vasospastic angina. Canad J Cardiol 3:177–182
69. Singh RN (1984) Progression of coronary atherosclerosis; clues to pathogenesis from serial coronary arteriography. Br Heart J 52:451–461
70. Spann JF (1983) Changing concepts of pathophysiology, prognosis and therapy in acute myocardial infarction. Am J Med 74:877–886
71. Tomoike H, Egashira K, Yamada A, Hayashi Y, Nakamura M (1987) Leukotriene C4- and D4-induced diffuse peripheral constriction of swine coronary artery accompanied by ST elevation on the electrocardiogram; angiographic analysis. Circ 76:480–487
72. Tomoike H, Hayashi Y, Egashira K, Yamada A, Nakamura M (1989) Effects of atherogenic diets on serum content of cholesterol, histamine-induced coronary constriction and morphological changes of the coronary artery. Jap Circ J 53:900 (abstract)
73. Torii S, Araki Y, Sagara T, Kakimura S, Kanaya H, Naito S, Nakagaki O (1974) Provocation of coronary spasm by subcutaneous administration of pilocarpine. Heart 6:338–346 (in Japanese)
74. Uchida Y, Yoshimoto N, Murao S (1975) Cyclic fluctuations in coronary blood pressure and flow induced by coronary artery constriction. Jap Heart J 16:454–464
75. Uchida Y (1979) Cyclic reduction in coronary flow. Circ 46:332
76. Van den Berg EK, Schmitz JM, Benedict CR, Malloy CR, Willerson JT, Dehmer GJ (1989) Transcardiac serotonin concentration is increased in selected patients with limiting angina and complex coronary lesion morphology. Circ 79:116–124
77. Vincent GM, Anderson JL, Marshall HW (1983) Coronary spasm producing coronary thrombosis and myocardial infarction. N Engl J Med 309:220–223
78. Winniford MD, Filipchuk N, Hillis LD (1983) Alpha-adrenergic blockade for variant angina; a long term double blind randomized trial. Circ 67:1185–1188
79. Yamamoto M, Katayama S (1968) Angina pectoris induced by marked vagotonic state. Jap Circ J 32:1856 (abstract)
80. Yamamoto Y, Tomoike H, Egashira K, Kobayashi T, Kawasaki T, Nakamura M (1987) Pathogenesis of coronary artery spasm in miniature swine with regional intimal thickening after balloon denudation. Circ Res 60:113–121
81. Yamamoto Y, Tomoike H, Egashira K, Nakamura M (1987) Attenuation of endothelium-related relaxation and enhanced responsiveness of vascular smooth muscle to histamine in spastic coronary arterial segments from miniature pigs. Circ Res 61:772–778
82. Yasue H, Touyama M, Kato H. Tanaka S, Akiyama F (1976) Prinzmetal's variant form of angina as a manifestation of alpha-adrenergic receptor-mediated coronary artery spasm; documentation by coronary arteriography. Am Heart J 91:148–155
83. Yasue H, Horio Y, Nakamura N, Fujii H, Imoto N, Sonoda R, Kugiyama K, Obata K, Morikami Y, Kimura T (1986) Induction of coronary artery spasm by acetylcholine in patients with variant angina; possible role of the parasympathetic nervous system in the pathogenesis of coronary artery spasm. Circ 74:955–963
84. Yui Y, Sakaguchi K, Susawa T, Hattori R, Takatsu Y, Yui N, Kawai C (1987) Thromboxane A_2 analogue induced coronary artery vasoconstriction in the rabbit. Cardiov Res 21:119–123
85. Zellinger AB, Abramowitz BM, Schick EC, Ryan TJ (1982) Variant angina culminating in coronary thrombosis and myocardial infarction. Chest 82:188–190
86. Zoll PM, Wessler S, Blumgart HL (1951) Angina pectoris; a clinical and pathological correlation. Am J Med 11:331–357

Author's address:

M. Nakamura, M.D., D. Med. Sci.
"Nakamura-Gakuen" Graduate School of Nutritional Science,
5-7-1, Befu, Jonan-ku, Fukuoka 814, Japan

Endothelial dysfunction in hypercholesterolemia is corrected by L-arginine

J. P. Cooke [1], J. Dzau [1], and A. Creager [2]

[1] Division of Cardiovascular Medicine, Falk Cardiovascular Research Center, Stanford University School of Medicine, Stanford, California, and
[2] Division of Vascular Medicine, Brigham and Women's Hospital, Harvard Medical School, Boston

Summary. Hypercholesterolemia attenuates endothelium-dependent vasorelaxation and augments the responses to vasoconstrictor agents. Both effects are largely due to a reduction in the release of endothelium-derived relaxing factor. Since endothelium-derived relaxing factor is now known to be nitric oxide derived from the metabolism of L-arginine, we hypothesized that the abnormal vascular response in hypercholesterolemia could be corrected by supplying the precursor to EDRF, L-arginine. In a series of studies, we have found that conduit and resistance vessels of hypercholesterolemic animals demonstrate endothelial dysfunction which is reversed after exposure to high concentrations of exogenous L-arginine. The experiments suggest that hypercholesterolemia induces a reversible dysfunction of arginine availability or metabolism.

Key words: Endothelium; hypercholesterolemia; endothelium-derived relaxing factor; arginine

Introduction

There is now abundant evidence that the endothelium-derived relaxing factor (EDRF) described by Furchgott and Zawadski in 1980 is nitric oxide or a labilenitroso compound that liberates nitric oxide (1–7). It is also apparent that EDRF is derived from the metabolism of L-arginine (5–7). The endothelium releases EDRF in response to a wide variety of physical and chemical stimuli (8–13). A number of agonists that directly induce contraction of vascular smooth muscle also release EDRF from the endothelium (10–13). In this manner, the endothelium exerts a braking influence on the action of many vasoconstrictors.

In hypercholesterolemic animals and man, endothelium-dependent vasodilation is reduced and vasoconstriction to a number of agonists is augmented (14–20). Presumably, both abnormalities are due to a reduced synthesis and/or release of EDRF, as suggested by previous bioassay studies (16). We hypothesized that normal vascular reactivity could be restored in vessels from hypercholesterolemic animals by supplying the precursor for EDRF, L-arginine. This article reviews three studies in which we tested and confirmed the hypothesis that the endothelial dysfunction induced by hypercholesterolemia may be corrected by L-arginine (21–23).

L-arginine normalizes reactivity of the basilar artery of Hypercholesterolemic rabbit

New Zealand white rabbits (n = 41) were fed normal rabbit chow or chow containing 2% cholesterol for 10 weeks. Subsequently, the animals were sacrificed and the basilar artery

These investigations were supported in part by Grants-in-Aid from the American Heart Association (JPC, MAC). Dr. Creager is a recipient of an NHLBI Research Career Development Award removed for study. Isolated basilar arteries were mounted in an arteriograph filled with oxygenated physiologic saline solution at 37° C. The proximal end of the vessel was cannulated by glass capillary tubing for perfusion with physiologic saline delivered by a pressure-servo system to maintain luminal pressure at 60 ± 2 mm Hg. The distal end of the vessel was clamped, allowing luminal perfusate to exit through the small perforating branches. Changes in vessel diameter were monitored by a video system consisting of an inverted microscope, video camera, and video monitor. The images were recorded and stored on VHS tape. Midplane transverse diameters were measured with a caliper directly applied to the video screen. Absolute calibration was obtained using a micrometer grid placed at the level of the vessel. All drugs were added to the external bath except for acetylcholine, which was administered intraluminally by the pressure-servo syringe. L-arginine or D-arginine was administered simultaneously both intra- and extra-luminally.

Vessels were exposed to increasing concentrations of 5-hydroxytryptamine. After the vasoconstriction stabilized at the maximum dose, increasing concentrations of acetylcholine were added to the perfusate. Subsequently, the vessels were rinsed with fresh physiologic saline solution over a 45-min period. When the vessel diameter had returned to baseline dimensions, the vessels were then exposed to increasing concentrations of endothelin or potassium chloride. When the response stabilized to the maximum concentration of the vasoconstrictor, the vessels were relaxed by increasing concentrations of verapamil. In some studies, the vessels were first incubated with L-arginine (10^{-3} M) or D-arginine (10^{-3} M) for 45 min. To determine if L-arginine affected basal vessel tone or active tension (induced by 5-hydroxytryptamine), measurements of vessel diameter were made before and during administration of L-arginine in some tissues.

These experiments revealed that endothelium-dependent vasodilation was attenuated in vessels from hypercholesterolemic animals. The sensitivity to acetylcholine was

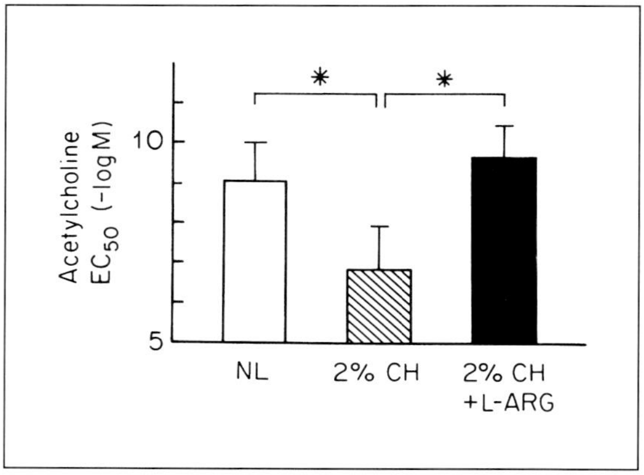

Fig. 1. Sensitivity to acetylcholine chloride is reduced in hypercholesterolemic rabbits, but restored by L-arginine. The sensitivity to acetylcholine was characterized by determining the EC_{50} (concentration of drug inducing a half-maximal vasodilation expressed as -log M) for each dose-response curve. In comparison to the animals fed a normal diet (open bar) the animals fed a high cholesterol diet (hatched bar) have a reduced sensitivity to acetylcholine chloride as reflected by the EC_{50} value. However, when vessels from hypercholesterolemic animals are perfused in vitro with L-arginine (solid bar), the sensitivity to acetylcholine chloride is normalized, as reflected by the EC_{50} value. (* Values are significantly different, $p < 0.01$, by analysis of variance followed by a Newman-Keuls test.)

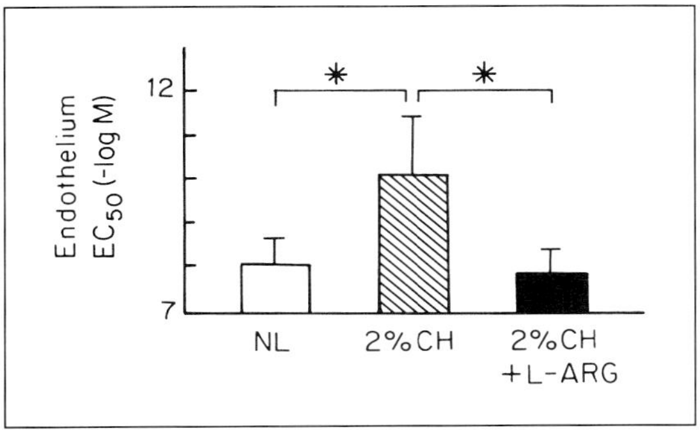

Fig. 2. The sensitivity to endothelin is augmented by hypercholesterolemia, and normalized by L-arginine. In all groups, the sensitivity to endothelin was characterized by determining the EC_{50} (the dose of drug inducing a half-maximal vasoconstriction). In comparison to vessels from animals fed a normal diet (open bar), those from animals fed a high cholesterol diet (hatched bars) had an increased sensitivity to endothelin, as reflected by the EC_{50} value. However, when isolated vessels from hypercholesterolemic animals were perfused in vitro with L-arginine (solid bar) the sensitivity to endothelin was normalized. (* Values are significantly different by analysis of variance, followed by a Newman-Keuls test, $p < 0.01$.)

reduced, although the maximal response was unaffected (Fig. 1). Conversely, vasodilation to verapamil (which is endothelium-independent), was unaffected by hypercholesterolemia. Therefore, the impairment in endothelial-mediated vasodilation was not due to an inability of the vascular smooth muscle to relax.

Vasoconstrictor responses were enhanced in vessels from hypercholesterolemic animals. The sensitivity to endothelin and that to potassium chloride was enhanced. There was pronounced leftward shift in the concentration of endothelin required to produce a half-maximal vasodilation (Fig. 2). Maximum vasoconstriction to endothelin and that to potassium chloride was unaffected. Conversely, the maximum vasoconstriction to serotonin was increased, although the sensitivity (EC_{50}) to 5-hydroxytryptamine was unaffected.

Prior exposure to L-arginine (but not D-arginine) normalized vascular reactivity in the basilar artery from hypercholesterolemic rabbits. The sensitivity to acetylcholine chloride was normalized (Fig. 1). Vasoconstrictor responses to endothelin and those to serotonin were also normalized. The maximum vasoconstriction to serotonin was not different from control in those vessels treated with L-arginine. Similarly, the sensitivity to endothelin was reduced when vessels from hypercholesterolemic animals were pretreated with L-arginine (Fig. 2).

Additional studies revealed that L-arginine did not induce vasodilation directly. Vasodilation was not observed to L-arginine under resting conditions or when the vessel was precontracted by 5-hydroxytryptamine.

L-arginine augments hindlimb vasodilation to acetylcholine in cholesterol-fed rabbits

In a second investigation, we demonstrated that intravenous infusions of L-arginine, but not D-arginine, could normalize endothelium-dependent responses in the hindlimb of the cholesterol-fed rabbit (22). New Zealand white rabbits (n = 28) were fed normal rabbit chow or that containing 2% cholesterol for 8 weeks. Subsequently, the animals were anesthetized and the right femoral artery and vein catheterized. The femoral vein catheter was used for administration of saline infusions containing L-arginine, D-arginine, or vehicle control. The arterial catheter was advanced retrograde to a position proximal to the aortic bifurcation so as to infuse vasoactive drugs into the contralateral femoral artery. The arterial catheter was attached to a pressure transducer and arterial pressure was determined prior to and following administration of drugs. An electromagnetic flow probe was placed about the left femoral artery and coupled to a calibrated flow meter. Acetylcholine chloride or sodium nitroprusside were administered intra-arterially via a constant infusion pump (0.2 ml/min) at doses of 0.3, 0.9, 3 and 9 μg/kg/min, each dose for 2 min. Two min were allowed to elapse between each dose so as to re-establish basal hindlimb blood flow prior to the next dose. The order of administration of acetylcholine and nitroprusside was randomized according to a Latin-square design. After infusion of these vasoactive drugs, physiologic saline was infused (0,2 ml/min) that contained L-arginine (10 mg/kg/min), D-arginine (10 mg/kg/min), or vehicle control. After 20 min of the intravenous infusions, basal hindlimb blood flow was measured. Subsequently, the L-arginine infusion was continued for another 50 min during the intra-arterial administration of acetylcholine or sodium nitroprusside, as detailed above.The dose of L-arginine was found to increase serum arginine levels from 0.1 mM to3 mM when measured after 70 min of the L-arginine infusion. Hindlimb blood flow measurements were made after each dose of vasoactive drug. Following completion of this in vivo protocol, some of these animals were sacrificed and their thoracic aortae harvested for in vitro studies of vascular reactivity [see below; (23)].

Baseline mean arterial pressure, heart rate, hindlimb blood flow, and hindlimb vascular resistance were not different in the cholesterol-fed rabbits. However, the hindlimb

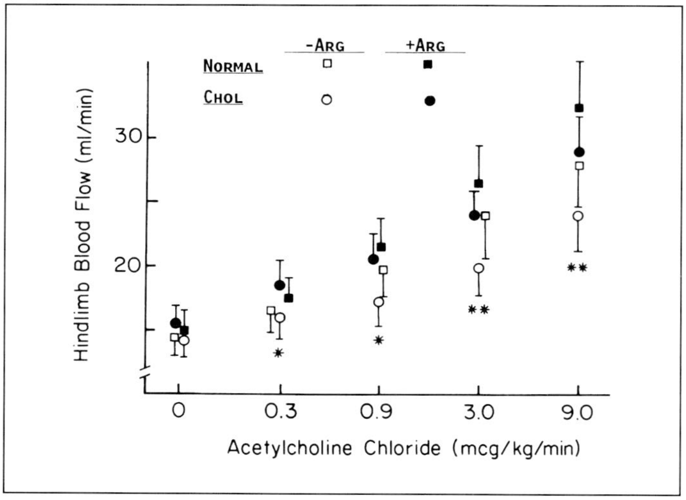

Fig. 3. Hindlimb vasodilation induced by acetylcholine chloride is reduced by hypercholesterolemia and restored by L-arginine. Hindlimb blood flow was measured during infusions of acetylcholine in normal animals receiving saline infusion (□), or saline infusion containing L-arginine (■); and in hypercholesterolemic animals receiving saline saline infusion (○), or saline infusion containing L-arginine (●). (* Hindlimb blood flow response is significantly different from that of normal animals, $p<0.05$.)

blood-flow response to acetylcholine was blunted in the hypercholesterolemic rabbits receiving the saline infusion (Fig. 3). In the hypercholesterolemic rabbits receiving L-arginine, the response to acetylcholine was significantly improved. In contrast, the response to acetylcholine in the normal animals receiving L-arginine was not different from those receiving the saline infusion alone (Fig. 3).

Basal hindlimb blood flow was not affected by the infusion of L-arginine. The hindlimb blood-flow response to sodium nitroprusside was not different between the control and hypercholesterolemic animals, and was also not affected by L-arginine. Intravenous infusions of D-arginine did not potentiate the response to acetylcholine in the hypercholesterolemic animals.

L-arginine normalizes reactivity of the thoracic aorta of hypercholesterolemic rabbit

Following the in vivo study outlined above, the animals were sacrificed with an overdose of sodium pentobarbital and the thoracic aortae removed for in vivo studies of vascular reactivity (23). The thoracic aortae were cut into vascular rings for study in the organ chamber. To study vasodilating agents, vascular rings were contracted by an EC_{50} dose of norepinephrine; when the contraction had stabilized, the rings were exposed to increasing concentrations of the vasodilator.

Endothelium-dependent relaxations to acetylcholine were impaired in the thoracic aortae from hypercholesterolemic animals receiving the saline infusion. In contrast, the thoracic aorta from hypercholesterolemic animals receiving the arginine infusion exhibited endothelium-dependent relaxations which were not different from the control animals. The intravenous infusion of L-arginine increased the sensitivity and potentiated the maximal relaxation to acetylcholine in the thoracic aortae from hypercholesterolemic animals. Conversely, endothelium-dependent relaxation to sodium nitroprusside in the hypercholesterolemic animals was unaffected by the intravenous infusion of L-arginine. In the animals fed a normal diet, there were no differences in the sensitivities or maximal relaxations to acetylcholine in thoracic aortae from animals receiving the saline infusion containing vehicle, or that containing L-arginine.

Discussion

The salient findings of these three investigations are: 1) hypercholesterolemia impairs endothelium-dependent vasodilation in conduit and resistance vessels of the rabbit; 2) hypercholesterolemia heightens the response to vasoconstrictor agents; 3) L-arginine, but not its inactive enantiomer, D-arginine, normalizes endothelium-dependent vasodilation, as well as the vasoconstrictor responses to endothelin and those to serotonin; 4) L-arginine did not affect endothelium-dependent vasodilation in the conduit or resistance vessels of rabbits fed a normal diet; 5) L-arginine did not affect endothelium-independent vasodilation to verapamil or to sodium nitroprusside in conduit or resistance vessels of hypercholesterolemic rabbits.

Endothelium-derived relaxing factor (EDRF) is thought to be nitric oxide or a labile nitroso compound which liberates nitric oxide, and is believed to be derived from the metabolism of L-arginine (1–7). It is released by a wide variety of stimuli to induce vasodilation or to exert a braking influence on vasoconstrictor agonists such as serotonin or endothelin (8–13).

Hypercholesterolemia is known to interfere with endothelium-dependent modulation of vascular reactivity. Isolated vessels from hypercholesterolemic swine, rabbits, and monkeys exhibit attenuated endothelium-dependent relaxation and are hyper-responsive to a number of vasoconstrictor agonists (14–20). It is likely both effects are due to an impairment of endothelial function in hypercholesterolemic animals.

The mechanism by which hypercholesterolemia impairs endothelium-dependent responses is not known. Hypercholesterolemia is known to induce intimal thickening in conduit vessels and a physical barrier to EDRF has been posited. A number of recent studies suggest this is not a satisfactory explanation. Resistance vessels of hypercholesterolemic animals do not develop intimal thickening, but do manifest endothelial dysfunction (18, 24). Moreover, endothelium-dependent vasodilation in vessels from normal animals may be attenuated by exposure to cholesterol in vitro within minutes (25, 26).

It is more likely that hypercholesterolemia reduces the synthesis and/or release of EDRF. This has been suggested by Verbeuren and colleagues, who used a bioassay system to demonstrate that the perfusate from the thoracic aortae of hypercholesterolemic rabbits had less relaxing activity than that from normal animals (16). If the abnormal vascular reactivity in hypercholesterolemic animals is due to a reduction in the synthesis and/or release of EDRF, it may be possible to normalize vascular responses by supplying the precursor of EDRF. Normally, L-arginine does not affect endothelium-dependent vasorelaxation, suggesting that the intracellular stores of L-arginine are sufficient to saturate the enzyme responsible for EDRF synthesis (27–30). However, under certain conditions, exogenous L-arginine is required to normalize endothelium-dependent relaxation. Bovine aortic endothelial cells deficient in L-arginine are cultured in medium, they release little EDRF, as detected by bioassay and chemiluminescence studies; when L-arginine is administered to the cells, normal amounts of EDRF are released from these cells (5). Antagonists of EDRF synthesis attenuate endothelium-dependent relaxations in vitro; normal relaxations are restored using exogenous L-arginine (6, 7). Intravenous administration of L-N-monomethylarginine increases vascular resistance, and vessels harvested from these animals exhibit attenuated endothelium-dependent relaxation and reduced release of nitric oxide; exogenous L-arginine corrects these abnormalities (28–30). Endothelium-dependent vasorelaxation is markedly reduced in isolated vessels after prolonged exposure to calcium ionophore, presumably due to overutilization of intracellular L-arginine stores; after incubation with exogenous L-arginine this abnormality is corrected (31).

For these reasons, it is not unreasonable to propose that administration of exogenous L-arginine may correct the endothelial impairment induced by hypercholesterolemia. Indeed, other strategies have been successfully employed to prevent or reverse the endothelial defect. In animals fed a high cholesterol diet, impairment of endothelium-dependent vasodilation may be prevented by co-administration of fish oil, or an inhibitor of HMG coA reductase (32, 33). Abnormal endothelial responses in atherosclerotic monkeys may be reversed by a low-cholesterol diet (34).

Therefore, we attempted to normalize endothelium-dependent responses in conduit and resistance vessels of hypercholesterolemic animals, either by intravenous infusions of L-arginine or by in vitro exposure to L-arginine. Our investigations reveal that the abnormal endothelium-dependent vasorelaxation and heightened sensitivity to vasoconstrictor agents that are seen in vessels from hypercholesterolemic animals may be corrected by administration of L-arginine. This effect is stereospecific, since D-arginine had no affect. Endothelium-dependent vasorelaxation in vessels from normal animals was unaffected by L-arginine, confirming the results of other investigators (27–30). Finally, L-arginine did not affect endothelium-independent vasorelaxation in hypercholesterolemic animals, suggesting that its effect was due to an action on the endothelium rather than a direct effect on vascular smooth muscle.

Nitric oxide is not only a potent vasodilator, but it is also an anti-platelet and anti-proliferative agent (35–37). Therefore, a reduction in the release of EDRF by hypercholesterolemia would not only alter vascular reactivity, but may promote platelet aggregation as well as intimal proliferation of vascular smooth muscle cells. This dysfunction of the endothelium would thus promote the development and progression of atherosclerosis in hypercholesterolemic man. Indeed, we find that the forearm blood-flow response to intra-arterial methacholine is reduced in young hypercholesterolemic subjects, suggesting that endothelial dysfunction predates clinical evidence of atherosclerosis (20). Interestingly enough, in preliminary studies, we found that intravenous administration of L-arginine normalizes the forearm blood-flow response to methacholine in hypercholesterolemic man (unpublished data). If the result of these investigations may be extrapolated, exogenous administration of L-arginine (i.e., in the form of dietary supplements) might represent a therapeutic adjunct in the treatment and/or prevention of atherosclerosis.

References

1. Furchgott RF, Zawadzki JV (1980) The obligatory role of endothelial cells in the relaxation of arterial smooth muscle by acetylcholine. Nature 288:373–376
2. Palmer RMJ,Ferridge AG, Moncada S (1987): Nitric oxide release accounts for the biological activity of endothelium-derived relaxing factor. Nature 327:524–526
3. Ignarro LJ, Burns RE, Buga GM, Wood KS (1987) Endothelium-derived relaxing factor from pulmonary artery and vein possesses pharmacologic and chemical properties identical to those of nitric oxide radical. Circ Res 61:866–879
4. Furchgott RF (1988) Studies on relaxation of rabbit aorta by sodium nitrite: the basis for the proposal that the acid-activatable inhibitory factor from bovine retractor penis is inorganic nitrite and the endothelium-derived relaxing factor is nitric oxide. In: Vanhoutte PM (ed), Vasodilatation. New York, Raven Press, pp 427–435
5. Palmer RMJ, Ashton DS, Moncada S (1988) Vascular endothelial cells synthesize nitric oxide from L-arginine. Nature 333:664–666
6. Palmer RM, Rees DD, Ashton DS, Moncada S (1988) L-arginine is the physiological precursor for the formation of nitric oxide in endothelium-dependent relaxation. Biochem Biophys Res Commun 153:1251–1256
7. Schmidt HH, Nau H, Wittfoht W, Gerlach J, Prescher KE, Klein MM, Niroomand F, Bohm E (1988) Arginine is the physiological precursor of endothelium-derived nitric oxide. Eur J Pharmacol 154:213–216
8. Lüscher TF, Cooke JP, Houston DS, Neves RJ, Vanhoutte PM (1987) Endothelium-dependent relaxations in human arteries. Mayo Clin Proc 72:601–606
9. Cooke JP, Stamler JS, Andon N, Davies PF, Loscalzo J (in press) Flow stimulates endothelial cells to release a nitrovasodilator that is potentiated by reduced thiol. Am J Physiol
10. Cocks TM, Angus JA (1983) Endothelium-dependent relaxation of coronary arteries by noradrenaline and serotonin. Nature 305:627–630
11. Katusic ZS, Shepherd JT, Vanhoutte PM (1984) Vasopressin causes endothelium-dependent relaxations of the canine basilar artery. Circ Res 55:575–579
12. Houston DS, Shepherd JT, Vanhoutte PM (1985) Adenine nucleotides, serotonin, and endothelium-dependent relaxations to platelets. Am J Physiol 248:H389–H395
13. Warner TD, Mitchell JA, Nucci de G, Vane Jr (1989) Endothelin-1 and endothelin-3 release EDRF from isolated perfused arterial vessels of the rat and rabbit. J Cardiovasc Pharmacol 13(suppl 5):585–588

14. Shimokawa H, Tomoike H, Nabeyama S, Yamamoto H, Araki H, Nakamura M, Ishii Y, Tanaka K (1983) Coronary artery spasm induced in atherosclerotic miniature swine. Science 221:560–562
15. Heistad DD, Armstrong MLI, Marcus ML, Piegors DJ, Mark AL (1984) Augmented responses to vasoconstrictor stimuli in hypercholesterolemic and atherosclerotic monkeys. Circ Res 54:711–718
16. Verbeuren TH, Jordaens FH, Zonnekeyn LL, VanHove GE, Coene MC, Herman AG (1986) Effect of hypercholesterolemia on vascular reactivity in the rabbit. Circ Res 58:552–564
17. Yamamoto Y, Tomoike H, Egashira K, Nakamura M (1987) Attenuation of endothelium-related relaxation and enhanced responsiveness of vascular smooth muscle to histamine in spastic coronary arterial segments from miniature pigs. Circ Res 61:772–778
18. Yamamoto H, Bossaller C, Cartwright J Jr, Henry PD (1988) Videomicroscopic demonstration of defective cholinergic arteriolar vasodilation in atherosclerotic rabbit. J Clin Invest 81:1752–1758
19. Shimokawa H, Kim P, Vanhoutte PM (1988) Endothelium-dependent relaxation to aggregating platelets in isolated basilar arteries of control and hypercholesterolemic monkey. Circ Res 63:604–612
20. Creager MA, Cooke JP, Mendelsohn ME, Callagher SJ, Coleman SM, Loscalzo J, Dzau VJ (1990) Impaired vasodilation of forearm resistance vessels in hypercholesterolemic humans. J Clin Invest 86:228–234
21. Rossitch E, Alexander E III, Black PM, Cooke JP (in press) L-arginine normalizes endothelial function in cerebral vessels from hypercholesterolemic rabbits. J Clin Invest
22. Girerd XJ, Hirsch AT, Cooke JP, Dzau VJ, Creager MA (1990) L-arginine augments endothelium-dependent vasodilation in cholesterol fed rabbits. Circ Res 67:1301–1308
23. Cooke JP, Andon NA, Girerd XJ, Hirsch AT, Creager MA (in press) Arginine normalizes cholinergic relaxation of hypercholesterolemic rabbit thermic aorta. Circulation
24. Osborne JA, Siegman MJ, Sedar AW, Mooers SU, Lefer AM (1989) Lack of endothelium-dependent relaxation in coronary resistance arteries of cholesterol-fed rabbits. Am J Physiol 256 (Cell Physiol 25):C591–C597
25. Andrews HE, Bruckdorfer KR, Dunn RC, Jacobs M (1987) Low-density lipoproteins inhibit endothelium-dependent relaxation in rabbit aorta. Nature 327:237–239
26. Tomita T, Ezaki M, Miwa M (1990) Rapid and reversible inhibition by low density lipoprotein of the endothelium-dependent relaxation to hemostatic substances in porcine coronary arteries. Circ Res 66:18–27
27. Thomas G, Vargas R, Wroblewska B, Ramwell PW (1989) Role of the endothelium and arginine peptides on the vasomotor response of porcine internal mammary artery. Life Sci 44:1823–1830
28. Aisaka K, Gross SS, Griffith OW, Levi R (1989) N_G-methylarginine, an inhibitor of endothelium-derived nitric oxide synthesis, is a potent pressor agent in the guinea pig: does nitric oxide regulate blood pressure in vivo? Biochem Biophys Res Commun 160:881–886
29. Amezcua JL, Palmer RMJ, De Souza BM, Moncada S (1989) Nitric oxide synthesized from L-arginine regulates vascular tone in the coronary circulation of the rabbit. Br J Pharmacol 97:1119–1124
30. Rees DD, Palmer RMJ, Moncada S (1989) Role of endothelium-derived nitric oxide in the regulation of blood pressure. Proc Natl Acad Sci USA 86:3375–3378
31. Gold ME, Wood KS, Buga GM, Byrns RE, Ignarro LJ (1989) L-arginine causes whereas L-argininosuccinic acid inhibits endothelium-dependent vascular smooth muscle relaxation. Biochem Biophys Res Commun 161:536–543
32. Shimokawa H, Vanhoutte PM (1988) Dietary cod-liver oil improves endothelium-dependent responses in hypercholesterolemic and atherosclerotic porcine coronary arteries. Circ 78:1421–1430
33. Osborne JA, Lento PH, Siegfried MR, Stahl GL, Fusman B, Lefer AM (1989) Cardiovascular effects of acute hypercholesterolemia in rabbits: reversal with lovastatin treatment. J Clin Invest 83:465–473
34. Harrison DG, Armstrong ML, Freiman PC, Heistad DD (1987) Restoration of endothelium-dependent relaxation by dietary treatment of atherosclerosis. J Clin Invest 80:1808–1811

35. Stamler JS, Mendelsohn ME, Amarante P, Smick D, Andon N, Davies PF, Cooke JP, Loscalzo J (1989) N-acetylcysteine potentiates platelet inhibition by endothelium-derived relaxing factor. Circ Res 65:789–795
36. Radomski MW, Palmer RMJ, Moncada S (1987) Comparative pharmacology of endothelium-derived relaxing factor, nitric oxide and prostacyclin in platelets. Br J Pharmacol 92:181–187
37. Garg UC, Hassid A (1989) Nitric oxide-generating vasodilators and 8-bromo-cyclic guanosine monophosphate inhibit mitogenesis and proliferation of cultured rat vascular smooth muscle cells. J Clin Invest 83:1774–1777

Author's address:
John P. Cooke, M.D., Ph. D.
Falk Cardiovascular Research Center
Stanford University Medical Center
300 Pasteur Drive
Stanford, CA 94305, USA

Endothelial function in the clinical setting

Assessment of coronary vasomotor tone in humans

H. Wollschläger, A. M. Zeiher, H. Drexler, and H. Just

Medizinische Universitätsklinik, Abteilung Innere Medizin III, Kardiologie, Freiburg

Summary: The assessment of endothelium-mediated modulation of coronary vasomotor tone in the intact human circulation under physiologic conditions requires very precise determination of both epicardial artery diameters, reflecting effects within the conduit vessels, as well as coronary blood flow, reflecting effects within the resistance vasculature during cardiac catherization. In the present report, the accuracy and limitations of quantitative approaches to assess arterial dimensions from coronary angiograms are discussed. Using state-of-the-art image-processing techniques and x-ray imaging, epicardial artery diameter changes within the range of 8–10% can be reliably detected by quantitative coronary angiography. In addition, advances in interventional techniques do provide a means to selectively assess intracoronary blood-flow velocities using intracoronary Doppler catheters. Combining epicardial artery diameter measurements and intracoronary blood-flow velocity parameters allows for a reasonably accurate instantaneous estimate of coronary arterial blood flow. The advantages and limitations of the intracoronary Doppler technique compared to other techniques are discussed.

Key words: Coronary vasomotor tone, endothelium-mediated modulation; quantitative, image-processing techniques; intracoronary blood-flow velocity

Introduction

The endothelium plays an important role in the active modulation of coronary vasomotor tone [7]. A number of contributions in this volume illustrate the pathophysiological relevance of coronary vascular reactivity for the regulation of coronary blood flow in the experimental setting. The extrapolation of these experimental findings to the clinical situation may have important diagnostic and therapeutic implications.

However, the detection and quantification of vascular reactivity in the intact human coronary circulation is much more difficult. Especially, precise measuring devices such as electromagnetic flow meters in the experimental setting can be applied in man only intraoperatively, e. g., during bypass surgery.

Because caution must be exercised in extrapolating the experimental data to the human coronary circulation, methods should be developed in the intact coronary circulation.

These methods have to be applied safely under routine clinical conditions and should have a high degree of accuracy and reproducibility.

The present paper reviews in brief the currently available techniques to assess coronary vasomotor tone in the clinical setting.

Assessment of epicardial artery dimensions

The first parameter necessary for the assessment of coronary vascular tone is the precise measurement of coronary dimensions from routine angiograms.

Several methods for the quantification of vessel diameters have been developed [8]. Most of these methods are based on automated contour-detection of coronary arteries using digital image-processing and geometric edge-differentiation techniques (Fig. 1).

For this purpose, videodigitized cineframes or digitally acquired images are stored in an image-analysis system. After delineation of a centerline within the vessel segment to be measured, the computer automatically generates a number of scanlines perpendicular to the centerline. The first and second derivative functions of the densogram along each scanline are then computed, and the contour point is defined between the local extrema of the first and second derivative functions. Thereafter, a number of refinement steps and contour smoothing procedures are applied.

Phantom measurements under ideal x-ray conditions have shown the high accuracy and reproducibility of this contour-detection technique [9].

However, under clinically relevant x-ray conditions, the automated contour-detection has several potential limitations. Overlapping of the vessel segment with the spine or diaphragm or location of the vessel in a high-contrast region, e. g., at the border of the cardiac silhouette with adjacent lung tissue, may lead to a considerable reduction of the reliability of the contour-detection algorithm.

This problem is of special concern when the diameter measurements (expressed in pixel data) have to be converted into absolute measurements using a scaling device.

Usually, the coronary catheter or a grid are used as reference, introducing potential sources of error:

1) the contour detection has to be performed twice: at the site of the vessel, as well as at the site of the catheter; and,
2) out-of-plane positioning of the catheter and the vessel can lead to different radiological magnification.

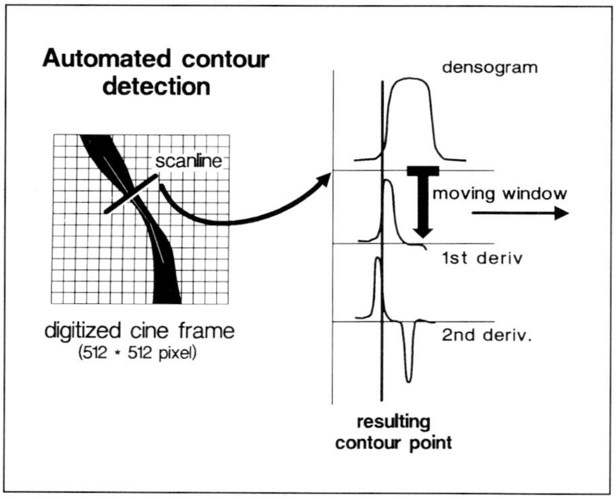

Fig. 1. Schematic graph of the automatic contour detection process from digital cine frames. (For details see text.)

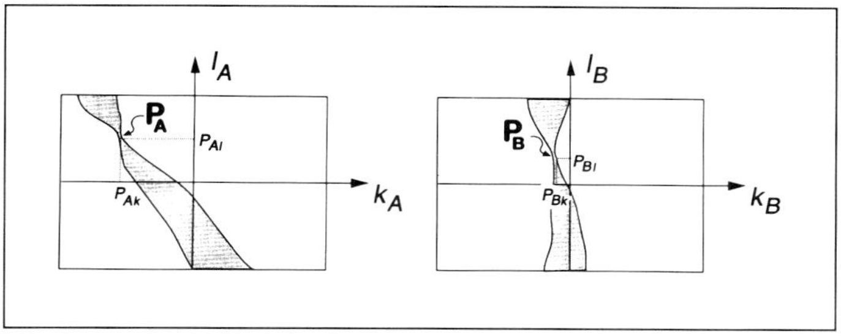

Fig. 2. Calculation of "local" coordinate systems (k and l) on the image intensifier entrance fields of the biplane x-ray system (A and B). The point of interest (center of a stenosis or radiopaque tip of the Doppler catheter) is identified in two simultaneous views (P_A and P_B) and the coordinates P_{AK}, P_{AL} and P_{BK}, P_{BL} are determined.

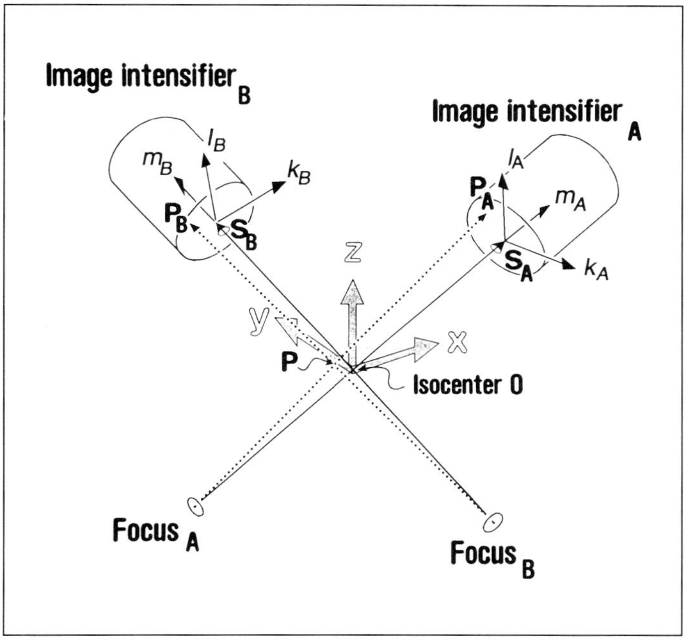

Fig. 3. Calculation of the exact radiological magnification factor II. The spatial position of the point of interest P is calculated in a "global" three-dimensional coordinate system (z, y, z) around the isocenter O of a biplane x-ray system. Knowing the angulation data of the biplane views, the projections of P (P_A and P_B) onto the "local" coordinate systems (k, l, m; where m = focus image intensifier distance) are transformed into the "global" coordinate system. The exact radiological magnification factor is calculated by the quotient of the distances: $focus_{A/B}$–$P_{A/B}$ and $focus_{A/B}$–P.

These sources of potential errors may be cumulative in an unpredictable manner!

Therefore, we developed a method for the conversion of diameter measurements, expressed in pixels, into absolute dimensions, without the need for a scaling device [14]. Using a biplane, multidirectional x-ray system, the exact spatial position of any vessel segment of interest can be calculated in a three-dimensional (3D) coordinate system around the constant isocenter of the x-ray gantry from simultaneous biplane views.

In these two images, the projections of one point of interest, e. g. the center of a stenosis or a branching point of the vessel or the radiopaque tip of a small catheter in the vessel have to be defined (Fig. 2).

Knowing the geometric properties of the x-ray system [13] and the angulation data of that projection, the spatial position of the point of interest can be determined (Fig. 3): from the known distances, i. e., focus-II and focus-point of interest, the exact radiological magnification factor of that special point can be calculated, allowing the conversion of pixels into absolute dimensions without a scaling device.

Thus, the calculation of the radiological magnification factor eliminates two of the three potentially cumulative sources of error in absolute quantification, and allows for the estimation of the accuracy and reliability of automatic contour detection under clinically relevant x-ray conditions.

Studies measuring the diameters of coronary catheters with known dimensions in routine angiograms revealed an absolute error between true and measured values of $4.0 \pm 2.9\%$ (mean ± 1 SD). The reproducibility of the measurements (coefficient of variation) was $2.2 \pm 1.1\%$ (mean ± 1 SD).

Assuming a 95% confidence interval, a diameter change of 8–10% in interventional studies is necessary to reliably discriminate true biological phenomena from errors due to measurement variability!

Thus, quantitative coronary angiography using automated edge-detection and calculation of the exact radiological magnification factors does provide a reasonably accurate method to study vascular reactivity of epicardial coronary arteries during cardiac catheterization.

Estimation of coronary blood flow

The second relevant parameter in measurement of variations of coronary vascular tone in humans is the estimation of coronary blood flow.

Several techniques have been applied to measure blood flow in the human coronary circulation. However, all of these methods have some important limitations:

The *coronary sinus thermodilution technique* [3] shows only a limited reliability, due to the slow time-constant which precludes the assessment of rapid changes of coronary flow. In addition, this technique is quite insensitive, because large changes in flow are necessary. Furthermore, regional changes of blood flow cannot be assessed, which is essential in the presence of coronary artery disease.

Although the *gas clearance methods* [5] (e. g., the Argon Method) allow for the calculation of flow/g tissue, these techniques are also limited by long time-constants and the lack of regional assessment of flow.

The *densitometric techniques* [6] using digital image-processing after radiographic contrast injection are theoretically promising, however, many assumptions are necessary in the native human coronary circulation, and the use of dye as coronary dilator in most studies shows only small ratios of flow increase. Newer approaches like *PET* [1] *or Cine-*

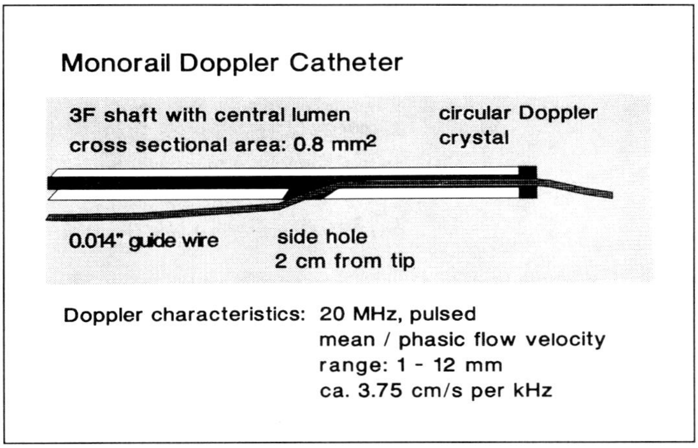

Fig. 4. Schematic drawing of the tip of the monorail Doppler catheter.

CT [10] potentially allow for the assessment of flow in different myocardial layers, but the experience with these techniques is limited so far.

Based on the experience with interventional techniques in invasive cardiology, especially with PTCA, the insertion of small devices into the human coronary system is possible without substantial increase of risk.

The *intracoronary Doppler catheter* [11] is such an interventional device and has several advantages compared to the above mentioned methods:

- selective measurements can be performed,
- rapid changes can be detected and, therefore,
- serial interventions can be performed during one study.

However, the most important disadvantage is that only the blood-flow velocity, but not blood flow is measured.

In addition, Doppler-derived measurements only provide relative flow-velocity measurements, expressed as the Doppler shift in kHz. Therefore, the Doppler technique is best suited for interventional studies, where each patient serves as his own control.

The Doppler system used in our laboratory [15] (Fig. 4) consists of a circular Doppler crystal, which is mounted at the tip of a 3F infusion catheter.

The Doppler is a pulsed 20 MHz device which allows for the registration of mean and phasic flow velocity.

The Doppler catheter is advanced into the coronary vessel via a .014 inch fully flexible guide wire through an 8F guiding catheter, using conventional PTCA equipment and technique.

The steerability of the guide-wire allows insertion even into peripheral vessel segments.

Careful positioning and adjustment of the operational range of the Doppler cather is essential to provide an optimal stable signal.

The internal lumen of the Doppler catheter can be used for subselective infusion of drugs to assess vascular reactivity. In contrast to other Doppler catheters, the Monorail Doppler catheter is equipped with a side hole 2 cm proximal of the catheter tip. Therefore, the local drug effects can be assessed at the catheter tip [15].

Since the Doppler technique provides only relative flow-velocity measurements, interventions have to be performed to alter coronary blood flow. This can be obtained by atrial pacing, dynamic exercise [4], or pharmacological stimulation with i.v. dipyridamole. More importantly, the subselective intracoronary infusion of adenosine or papaverine [12] induces alterations in coronary blood flow without any systemic hemodynamic effects, this allowing repeated measurements during one study.

Because the Doppler technique allows only for the assessment of blood-flow velocity, the cross-sectional area of the vessel segment has to be taken into account to assess changes in blood flow. This can be accomplished by calculating a flow index using the mean Doppler derived blood-flow velocity prior to contrast injection multiplied with the vessel cross-sectional area determined by quantitative angiography. Because the Doppler crystal is radiopaque, its location in simultaneous biplane images can be detected easily, providing the point of interest for the calculation of the exact radiological magnification factor. The vessel cross-sectional area is calculated from the measured diameters in the two views, assuming an elliptical shape of the vessel. Using the intracoronary infusion of the smooth muscle relaxant papaverine, the coronary flow reserve can be calculated from the quotient: peak flow index after intervention divided by resting flow index.

Validation studies in our laboratory revealed a high reproducibility of repeated measurements of coronary flow reserve ($r = 0.91$) [2]. However, it should be kept in mind that changes in cross-sectional area may affect blood-flow velocity recordings due to altered flow profiles and different angles of the interrogating ultrasound beam.

There is a potential risk for complications if an interventional device is inserted into the coronary arteries and left in place for about 30–45 min. To avoid thrombotic complications, a total of 12500 units heparin are given prior to the investigation. In addition, the Doppler catheter is constantly perfused with heparinized saline.

In our experience with more than 100 investigations, we have seen one thrombotic complication with intermittent occlusion of the vessel at the site of an about 50% stenosis. The vessel was successfully reopened after intracoronary application of urokinase and subsequent PTCA.

Thus, the combination of intracoronary Doppler derived flow velocity measurements and angiographically determined arterial dimensions allows for a reasonably accurate assessment of relative blood flow changes in the intact human coronary circulation.

In the absence of hemodynamically significant, flow-limiting epicardial artery stenosis, coronary blood-flow changes reflect alterations in vasomotor tone of the coronary resistance vessels. Thus, whereas quantitative coronary angiography enables the assessment of changes in vasomotor tone of epicardial arteries, simultaneously measuring the intracoronary Doppler flow velocity permits the evaluation of vasomotor changes of the coronary resistance vasculature.

References

1. Bergman SR, Fox KAA, Geltman EM, Sobel BE (1985) Positron emission tomography of the heart. Progr Cardiovasc Dis 18:165
2. Drexler H, Zeiher AM, Wollschläger H, Meinertz T, Just H, Bonzel T (1989) Flow-dependent coronary artery dilation in humans. Circulation 80:466–474
3. Ganz W, Tamura K, Marcus HS, Donoso R, Yoshida S, Swan HJC (1971) Measurement of coronary sinus blood flow by continuous thermodilution in man. Circulation 44:181
4. Hess OM, Felder L, Gaglione A, Buechi M, Vassalli F, Jiang Z, Grimm J, Krayenbühl HP (1991) Coronary vasomotion and coronary flow reserve during exercise. Bas Res Cardiol 86 (Suppl 2):193–201
5. Klocke FJ (1976) Coronary blood flow in man. Progr Cardivasc Dis 19:117

6. Mancini GBJ, Higgins DB (1985) Digital subtraction anigiography: a review of cardiac applications. Progr Cardiovasc Dis 18:111
7. Pohl U, Holtz J, Busse R, Bassenge E (1986) Crucial role of endothelium in the vasodilator response to increase flow in vivo. Hypertension 8:37–44
8. Reiber JHC, Kooijman CJ, Slager CJ, Gerbrands JJ, Schuurbiers JCH, Boer A den, Wijns W, Serruys PW (1984) Computer assisted analysis of the severity of obstructions from coronary cineangiograms: a methodological review. Automedica 5:219
9. Reiber JHC, Serruys PW, Kooijman CJ, Wijns W, Slager CJ, Gerbrands JJ, Schuurbiers JCH, Boer A den, Hugenholtz PG (1985) Assessment of short-, medium-, and long-term variations in arterial dimensions from computer-assisted quantitation of coronary cineangiograms. Circulation 71:280
10. Rumberger JA, Feiring AJ, Higgins CR, Lipton MJ, Ell SR, Marcus ML (1987) Use of ultrafast CT to quantitate myocardial perfusion: a preliminary report. J Am Coll Cardiol 9:59
11. Wilson RF, Laughlin DE, Ackell PH, Chilian WM, Holida MD, Hartley CJ, Armstrong ML, Marcus ML, White CW (1985) Transluminal subselective measurement of coronary artery blood flow velocity and vasodilator reserve in man. Circulation 72:82
12. Wilson RF, White CW (1985) Intracoronary papaverine: an ideal coronary vasodilator for studies of the coronary circulation in conscious humans. Circulation 73:444
13. Wollschläger H, Lee P, Zeiher AM, Solzbach U, Bonzel T, Just H (1986) Derivation of spatial information from biplane multidirectional coronary angiograms. Med Progr Technol 11:57
14. Wollschläger H, Lee P, Zeiher AM, Solzbach U, Bonzel T, Just H (1986) Improvement of quantitative angiography by exact calculation of radiological magnification factors. In: Computers in Cardiology 1985. IEEE Computer Society Press, Washington DC, pp 483–486
15. Zeiher AM, Drexler H, Wollschläger H, Saurbier B, Just H (1989) Coronary vasomotion in response to sympathetic stimulation in humans: importance of the functional integrity of the endothelium. J Am Coll Cardiol 14:1181–1190

Authors address:

Dr. H. Wollschläger
Med. Univ.-Klinik
Hugstetter Straße 55
W-7800 Freiburg, FRG

Coronary vasomotion and coronary flow reserve during exercise

O. M. Hess, L. Felder, A. Gaglione, M. Buechi,
F. Vassalli, Z. Jiang, J. Grimm, and H. P. Krayenbuehl

Department of Internal Medicine, Medical Policlinic, Cardiology,
University Hospital, Zürich, Switzerland

Summary: Coronary vasomotion and coronary blood flow are important determinants of myocardial perfusion in patients with coronary artery disease. New digital angiographic techniques allow to study, not only the dimensions of a stenotic lesion (quantitative coronary arteriography), but also coronary flow reserve (parametric imaging). In a preliminary study both techniques were combined and coronary dimensions, as well as coronary flow reserve were determined in 15 patients (seven normals and eight patients with coronary artery disease) at rest, 45 s after 10 mg i.c. papaverine, during two levels of supine bicycle exercise, as well as 5 min after 1.6 mg sublingual nitroglycerin.

Our results show that with modern digital subtraction techniques, not only stenosis geometry, but also coronary flow reserve can be determined at rest and during exercise conditions.

Key words: Quantitative coronary arteriography; parametric imaging; coronary vasomotion; coronary flow reserve; papaverine; supine bicycle exercise; coronary artery disease; myocardial ischemia

Introduction

The gold standard for the assessment of coronary artery disease has been in the past and still is coronary arteriography. More recently, digital subtraction techniques have been used to assess coronary anatomy and to determine coronary flow reserve (2, 5, 12). In a preliminary study, the effect of papaverine and supine bicycle exercise on coronary dimensions and coronary flow reserve has been evaluated in 15 patients with either normal or stenotic coronary arteries, using a combination of quantitative coronary arteriography and parametric imaging.

Patients and methods

Fifteen patients with a mean age of 48 years (range: 33–64 years) were included in the present analysis. Seven patients had normal coronary arteries (group 1) and eight patients had coronary artery disease (group 2). Two of the eight patients in group 2 had one-vessel disease and six had two-vessel disease. Coronary arteriography was carried out for diagnostic purposes, because of a history of chest pain or previous myocardial infarction and/or ST-segment depression of more than 0.1 mV during upright bicycle exercise. Left ventriculography was performed in all patients and left ventricular biplane ejection fraction amounted to 58% (range: 48–68%; lower limit of normality 57%).

---

* Supported by a grant of the Swiss National Science Foundation, Bern

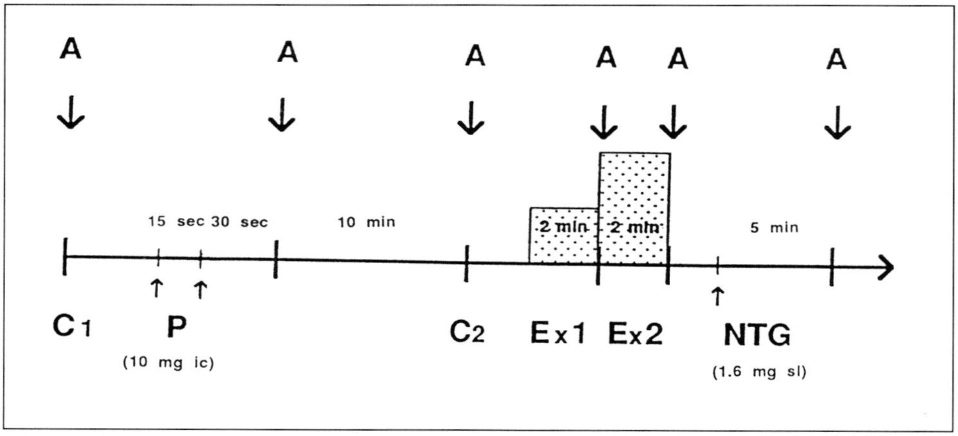

Fig. 1. Study protocol for measuring coronary luminal area and coronary flow reserve in 15 patients with either normal or stenotic coronary arteries. Biplane coronary arteriography (A) was carried out at rest (c1), 45 s after 10 mg intracoronary papaverine injection (P), after a second control run (C 2), during a first (Ex 1) and a second exercise level (Ex 2), as well as 5 min after sublingual administration of 1.6 mg nitroglycerin (NTG)

Study protocol

Biplane coronary arteriography was carried out at the end of diagnostic coronary arteriography. Eight ml of a nonionic contrast material (Jopamiro 370) were injected into the left coronary artery at a flow rate of 4 ml/s using in ECG-triggered power injector (Contrac, Siemens-Albis AG, Zürich). First, baseline coronary arteriography was performed (Fig. 1) then 10 mg papaverine was injected over 15 s into the left coronary artery and 30 s later coronary arteriography was repeated. After papaverine injection, transient ST-wave and T-wave changes were observed in all patients, but no arrhythmias were detected. After an interval of 10 min the patient's feet were attached to the bicycle ergometer and exercise was begun at a level of 50 to 75 watts, which was increased every 2 min in increments of 25 to 50 watts. Maximal workload averaged 103 watts in group 1 and 107 watts in group 2, respectively. Coronary arteriography was carried out at the end of each exercise level and 5 min after 1.6 mg nitroglycerin administered sublingually at the end of the exercise test. There were no complications related to the procedure in any of the 15 patients.

Quantitative coronary arteriography

Quantitative evaluation of biplane coronary arteriograms was performed using a semiautomatic system which has been described previously (1, 6, 9). Briefly, the system is based on a 35-mm film projector (Tagarno A/S, Horsens, Denmark), a slow-scan CCD-camera for image digitation that was developed at the Institute of Biomedical Engineering in Zurich, and a computer work-station (Apollo DN 3000, Apollo Computer AG, Wangen, Switzerland) for image storage and processing. Calibration was performed by the isocenter technique which is based on two fixed reference points in the center of the

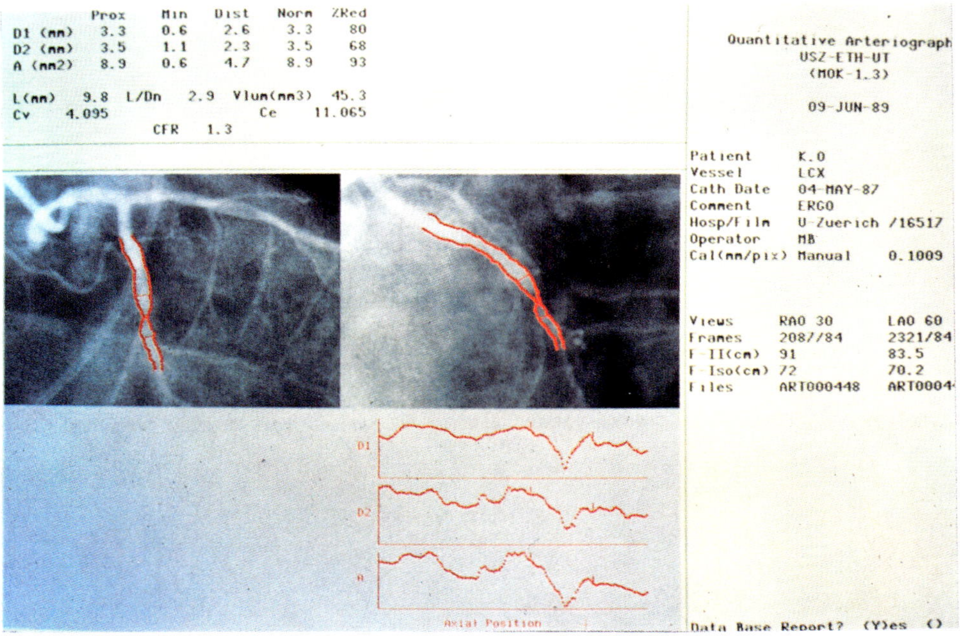

Fig. 2. Representative coronary angiogram under exercise conditions in biplane projection in a patient with severe stenosis of the left circumflex coronary artery. The contour of the circumflex artery is traced automatically by the computer and the diameter for both projections (D 1, D 2) and for the coronary luminal area (A) is displayed graphically

two image intensifiers (1, 6, 9). Contour detection (Fig. 2) was carried out in biplane projection in 11 of 15 patients, but in four patients (=26%) data were analyzed in monoplane projection because of overlying vessels or because the analyzed vessel was orthogonal to one of the two projections (= foreshortening). Interobserver and intraobserver variabilities have been reported to be small for this system, ranging between 2% and 4% (1).

Parametric imaging

Coronary flow measurements were carried out on an image processing system with a modified 35-mm film projector (model XR-35, Vanguard Corp., Melville, New York) and a high resolution (2048 × 2048 × 12) photodiode camera (Eikonixscan model 78/99, Eikonix Corp., Bedford, Massachusetts, USA). After digitation, images were processed on a VAX 750 computer (Digital Equipment Corp., Maynard, Massachusetts, USA) and stored, averaged, and subtracted on a DeAnza IP8500 (Gould Inc., San Jose, California, USA) image-processing system. Relative coronary blood flow was determined in a circular region of interest (249 pixels) in the perfusion zone of the left anterior descending coronary artery and the left circumflex coronary artery. Six to seven end-diastolic frames (one per cardiac cycle) were digitized in the left anterior oblique projection at rest, after papaverine injection, was well as during a first and second ex-

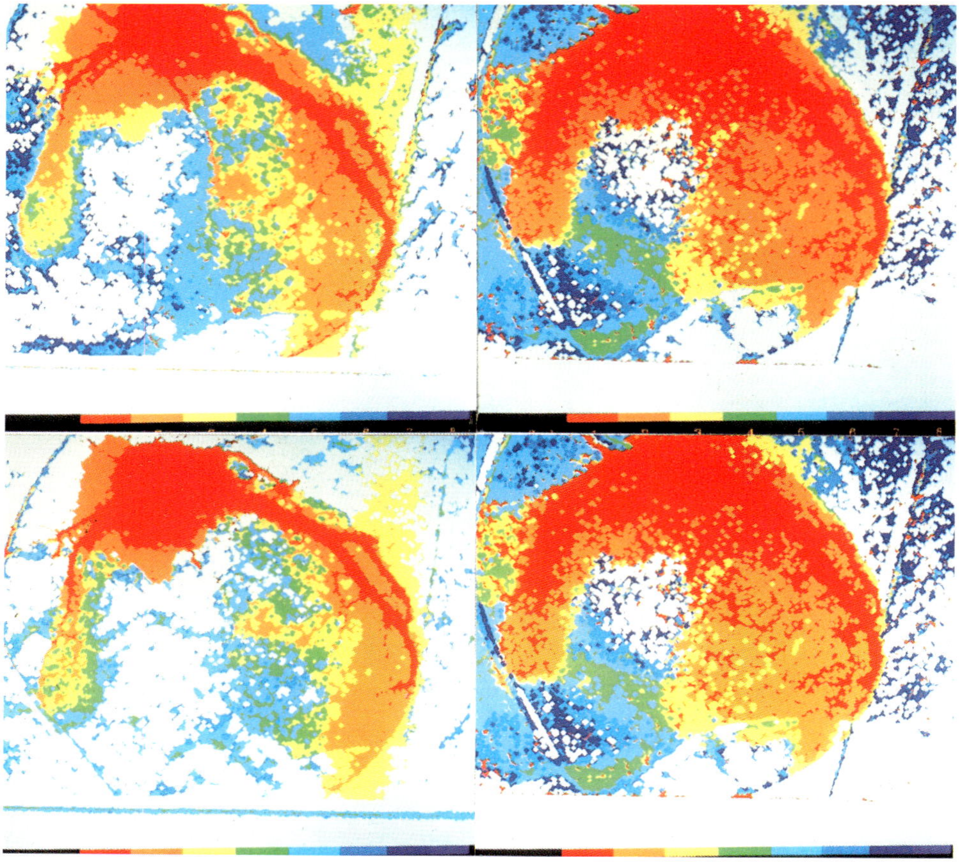

Fig. 3. Representative parametric images for a patient with normal coronary arteries. Images are shown at rest (C 1; upper left panel), after 10 mg intracoronary papaverine (P; upper right panel), after a second control run (C 2, lower left panel), as well as during exercise (Ex 2; lower right panel). The subtracted images are color-coded, i.e., the contrast which appears in the first image is red, in the second image orange, in the third image yellow, etc. (For further explanation see text)

ercise level. The first image before contrast material injection served as a mask for image subtraction. The subtracted images were color-coded, i.e., the contrast which appeared in the first image was red, in the second image orange, in the third yellow, etc. (Fig. 3). From these color-coded images the mean appearance time in the two regions of interest were calculated. The mean appearance time was defined as the time interval from the beginning of the injection (ECG-triggered injection) to the time point where half of peak contrast density was reached (8, 10).

Regional coronary blood flow was calculated as the ratio between maximal contrast (CD) and the mean appearance time (AT): FI = CD/AT, where FI = flow index (1/s) Coronary flow reserve (CFR) was determined as the flow index after papaverine injection or during exercise (h: hyperemia) divided by the flow index at rest (r) (Fig. 3):

$$CFR = \frac{CD_h AT_r}{AT_h CD_r}.$$

Statistics

Statistical comparisons were carried out by a two-way analysis of variance for repeated measurements. Coronary flow reserve after papaverine and during exercise was compared by paired Student's *t*-test.

Results

1. Quantitative coronary arteriography (Fig. 4): Quantitative evaluation of coronary vasomotion was performed for the proximal and sital portion of the normal vessel in the control group, as well as for the proximal and distal portion of the nonstenotic vessel in group 2. Similarly, minimal luminal area of the stenotic vessel segment was determined in group 2. Data are reported in percent of coronary luminal area at rest.

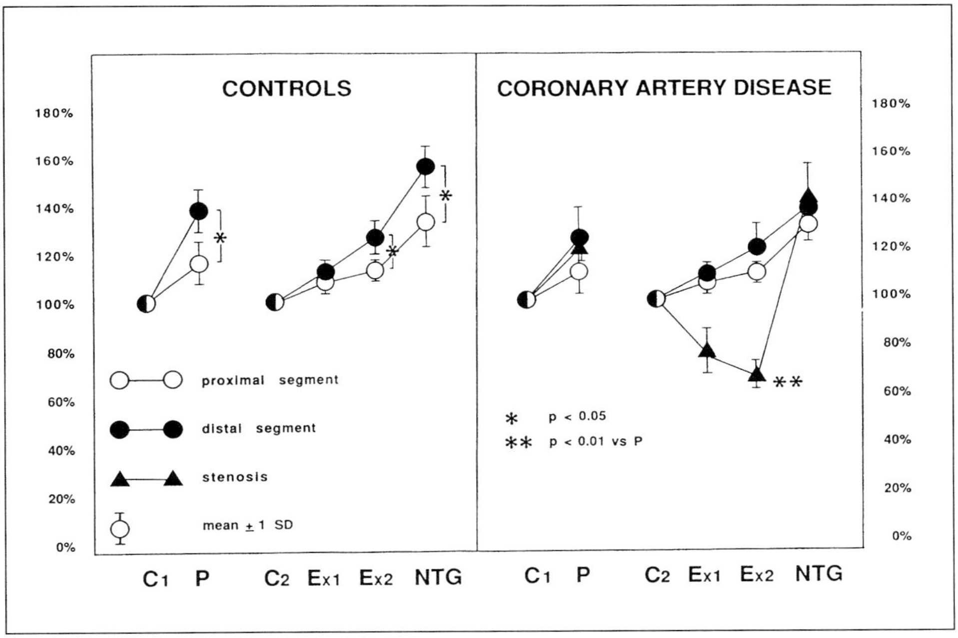

Fig. 4. Coronary luminal areas for the normal proximal and distal epicardial arteries in group 1 (= controls), as well as for the nonstenotic proximal and distal epicardial arteries and the stenotic arteries in group 2 (= coronary artery disease). Data are given at rest (C 1, C 2), after intracoronary papaverine injection (P), during exercise (Ex 1, Ex 2), and after sublingual administration of nitroglycerin (NTG). (For further explanation see text)

Normal and nonstenotic vessel segments: Both proximal and distal vessel segments showed coronary vasodilation after intracoronary papaverine injection. However, distal segments dilated significantly more in group 1 than 2. During exercise both proximal and distal segments elicited coronary vasodilation, which was significantly more pronounced for the distal than proximal vessels in group 1 (distal +37% vs +16% proximal, $p<0.05$), but not in group 2 (distal +25% vs +12% proximal, NS). After sublingual administration of nitroglycerin, both proximal and distal segments dilated significantly in both groups, but vasodilation of the distal vessel segments was significantly more pronounced than that of the proximal vessels in group 1 (distal +54% vs +32% proximal, $p<0.05$), but not in group 2 (distal +35% vs +30% proximal, NS).

Stenotic vessel segments: Intracoronary administration of papaverine was associated with coronary vasodilation of the stenotic vessel segment (+21%, NS vs the nonstenotic vessel segment), whereas during exercise the stenotic segment showed coronary vasoconstriction (−30%). However, exercise-induced stenosis narrowing was reversible after administration of sublingual nitroglycerin (+41%).

2. Parametric imaging: (Fig. 5)
Coronary flow reserve (papaverine/rest) in group 1 and in the region perfused by the stenotic coronary artery in group 2 was 2.5 and 2.1, respectively (NS).During exercise (Ex 1) coronary flow reserve (Ex 1/rest) was significantly lower than after papaverine administration in group 2, but not in group 1. During the second exercise level (Ex 2) flow reserve increased to 3.1 in group 1 and was significantly larger than during Ex 1, but was not different from papaverine injection. In group 2 flow reserve remained unchanged during Ex 1 and Ex 2 and was significantly lower (1.3) than after papaverine injection (2.1).

Discussion

The goal of modern imaging techniques in the assessment of coronary artery disease is not only to provide information on the anatomy of coronary stenoses, but also to give an answer on their functional significance. Digital angiographic systems allow to assess coronary anatomy with high temporal and spatial resolution and new intracoronary Doppler flow probes help to determine coronary flow velocity and coronary flow reserve within the major branches of the coronary tree (3, 11, 13). The disadvantage of the Doppler flow technique is related to the fact that only regional coronary flow velocity can be measured and that intracoronary probing is associated with a certain risk for vessel dissection, especially under high flow situations and exaggerated motions of the coronary arteries such as during dynamic exercise. Thus, the ideal technique for assessing coronary anatomy and flow reserve would be digital coronary arteriography because this technique allows to determine coronary anatomy and regional coronary flow reserve under resting and exercise conditions (2, 5, 8, 10, 12). The purposeof the present study is to describe our preliminary experiences with a combination of quantitative coronary arteriography and parametric imaging for assessing coronary anatomy and coronary flow reserve in a small group of patients with either normal or stenotic coronary arteries.

Coronary vasomotion and coronary flow reserve

Intracoronary administration of papaverine was associated with a significant increase in coronary luminal area which was more pronounced for the small distal than the large proximal epicardial arteries. At the same time, coronary blood flow increased significantly after papaverine injection. The increase in coronary luminal area appears to be flow mediated via the release of the endothelium-derived relaxing factor (= EDRF) as suggested recently by Drexler and coworkers (3). Papaverine is associated with a decrease in peripheral vascular resistance with a 3- to 5-fold increase in blood flow and only a minimal effect directly on the epicardial coronary arteries. The flow-dependent increase in coronary luminal area is slightly more pronounced for the distal than the proximal epicardial arteries in control patients, but not for the angiographically normal arteries in patients with coronary artery disease. The differences observed in controls might be explained by a higher coronary vasomotor tone of the distal epicardial arteries (11); in patients with coronary artery disease no such differences seem to exist between the proximal and distal epicardial arteries.

Supine bicycle exercise was associated with coronary vasodilation of the normal and nonstenotic vessel segments, but with coronary vasoconstriction of the stenotic segments (Fig. 4). This opposite response of the normal and stenotic arteries has been attributed to several mechanisms such as a passive collapse of the disease-free vessel wall within the stenosis (= Venturi mechanism), an insufficient production of the endothelium-derived relaxing factor of the atherosclerotic wall, an increased response to α-adrenergic stimulation during exercise and enhanced platelet aggregation due to turbulent coronary blood flow with release of vasoconstrictive substances (4). Exercise-induced stenosis narrowing might, however, be associated with important consequences because aggravation of a preexisting stenotic lesion during exercise might further impair coronary flow reserve. The effect of this phenomenon on coronary flow reserve has been evaluated in the present study and has been compared to the data obtained after maximal vasodilation with papaverine in order to assess the clinical importance of the two interventions for assessing the functional significance of a stenotic lesion. After papaverine injection coronary flow reserve was normal in group 2 with an area stenosis of 77% (range 61 to

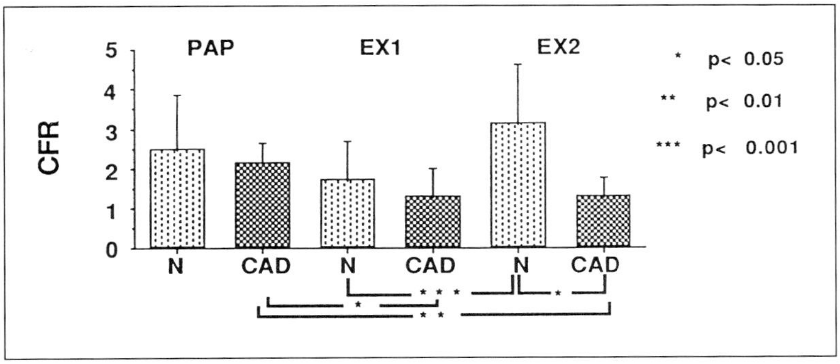

Fig. 5. Coronary flow reserve (CFR) for patients with normal (N) and stenotic coronary arteries (CAD). Coronary flow reserve is calculated after papaverine injection (PAP), during the first (Ex 1) and second (Ex 2) exercise level. There is no difference between the two groups after papaverine injection, but coronary flow reserve is significantly lower under the second exercise level in patients with coronary artery disease than in control patients

91%). However, in the presence of exercise-induced stenosis, narrowing coronary flow reserve cannot be increased normally (Fig. 5) and the stenotic lesion can become flow-limiting and impair coronary flow reserve. It has to be realized that other factors such as an increase in coronary vascular (intrinsic) resistance, a decrease in coronary driving pressure, or an increase in extracoronary resistance can be responsible for the reduction in coronary flow reserve during exercise. Intrinsic coronary vascular resistance might have been increased during exercise, as it has been shown experimentally, that in the presence of myocardial ischemia, coronary vessels retain a certain dilator reserve which can only be recruited pharmacologically (7). Coronary driving pressure was smaller during exercise because mean aortic pressure was significantly smaller at the same workload in group 2 (110 mmHg) than 1 (126 mmHg). Extracoronary vascular resistance might have been increased during exercise because left ventricular end-diastolic pressure increased, probably as a result of myocardial ischemia (mean pulmonary artery pressure increased during exercise in group 2 from 21 to 42 mmHg and in group 1 from 20 to 34 mmHg). Thus, coronary flow reserve is affected by several mechanisms under physiologic situations and might be completely different under clinical situations such as papaverine- or exercise-induced hyperemia.

Clinical implications

The combination of quantitative coronary arteriography and parametric imaging allows the assessment of a stenotic lesion at rest and during exercise conditions. Based on these techniques it can be demonstrated that coronary vasomotion and coronary flow reserve are greatly dependent on the physiologic stimulus of hyperemia and might be completely different after papaverine- or exercise-induced hyperemia. Thus, an appraisal of the clinical impact of a coronary stenosis based solely on pharmacologically induced hyperemia might be misleading, because other pathophysiologic mechanisms such as exercise-induced vasoconstriction, increased coronary (intrinsic) resistance, enhanced extracoronary vascular resistance, and decreased coronary driving pressure might be important for the regulation of coronary perfusion and vasomotor tone in situations of clinical ischemia, such as during exercise.

References

1. Büchi M, Hess OM, Kirkeeide RL, Suter Th, Muser M, Osenberg HP, Niederer P, Anliker M, Gould KL, Krayenbühl HP (1990) Validation of a new automatic system for biplane quantitative coronary arteriography. Int J Cardiovasc Imaging 5:93–103
2. Cusma JT, Toggart EJ, Folts JD, Peppler WW, Hangiandreou NJ, Lee C, Mistretta CA (1987) Digital subtraction angiographic imaging of coronary flow reserve. Circulation 75:461–472
3. Drexler H, Zeiher AM, Wollschläger H, Meinertz T, Just H, Bonzel T (1989) Flow-dependent coronary artery dilation in humans. Circulation 80:466–474
4. Gage JE, Hess OM, Murakami T, Ritter M, Grimm J, Krayenbühl HP (1986) Vasoconstriction of stenotic coronary arteries during dynamic exercise in patients with classic angina pectoris: reversibility by nitroglycerin. Circulation 73:865–876
5. Hess OM, McGillem MJ, DeBoe SF, Pinto IMF, Gallagher KP, Mancini GBJ (1990) Determination of coronary flow reserve by parametric imaging. Circulation 82:1438–1448
6. Hess OM, Büchi M, Kirkeeide RL, Niederer P, Anliker M, Gould KL, Krayenbühl HP (1990) Potential role of coronary vasoconstriction in ischaemic heart disease: effect of exercise. Eur Heart J 11 (Suppl B):58–64

7. Heusch G (1989) Koronare Vasomotion bei Myokardischämie. Z Kardiol 78:485–499
8. Hodgson JMcB, LeGrand V, Bates ER, Mancini GBJ, Aueron FM, O'Neill WW, Simon SSB, Beauman GJ, LeFree MT, Vogel RA (1985) Validation in dogs of a rapid digital angiographic technique to measure relative coronary blood flow during routine cardiac catheterization. Am J Cardiol 55:188–193
9. Kirkeeide RL, Gould KL (1984) Cardiovascular imaging: coronary artery stenosis. Hosp Pract 19:160–175
10. Mancini GBJ, Higgins CB (1985) Digital subtraction angiography: a review of cardiac applications. Prog Cardiovasc Dis 18:111–141
11. Marcus ML, Wilson RF, White CW (1987) Methods of measurement of myocardial blood flow in patients: a critical review. Circulation 76:245–253
12. Vogel RA (1985) The radiographic assessment of coronary blood flow parameters. Circulation 72:460–465
13. Wilson RF, Marcus ML, White CW (1987) Prediction of the physiologic significance of coronary arterial lesions by quantitative lesion geometry in patients with limited coronary artery disease. Circulation 75:723–732

Author's address:

Otto M. Hess, M.D.
Medical Policlinic
Cardiology
University Hospital
8091 Zürich/Switzerland

Coronary hemodynamic determinants of epicardial artery vasomotor responses during sympathetic stimulation in humans

A. M. Zeiher and H. Drexler

Medizinische Klinik III, University of Freiburg, FRG

Summary: Sympathetic stimulation by cold-pressor testing induces a complex interplay between adrenergic receptor stimulation, humoral and local metabolic factors, and alterations in coronary perfusion pressure. Since the endothelium importantly modulates the effect of neurohumoral stimulation, we evaluated the coronary hemodynamic determinants of epicardial artery vasomotor responses to cold-pressor testing in 12 normal patients with intact endothelial function, and in 20 patients with early atherosclerosis, demonstrating a dysfunctional endothelium. Endothelial function was assessed by intracoronary infusion of the endothelium-dependent dilator acetylcholine. Vasomotor responses were examined by quantitative coronary angiography and continuous intracoronary flow velocity measurements using a Doppler catheter. All coronary artery segments demonstrating a dilator response to intracoronary acetylcholine also vasodilated in response to cold-pressor testing by $19.7 \pm 8.2\%$ (mean $\pm$ 1 SD). In contrast, all arteries with evidence of atherosclerosis demonstrated a vasoconstrictor response during cold pressor testing with an area reduction by $18.4 \pm 7.5\%$. The systemic hemodynamic variables heart rate and mean aortic pressure increased by comparable amounts in both groups of patients during cold pressor testing, indicating comparable increases in myocardial workloads. There was a significant positive relation between increases in blood flow and changes in arterial luminal area. Increases in blood flow were closely related to increases in mean aortic pressure in normal epicardial vessels, but this relation was blunted in vessels with a dysfunctional endothelium. Estimated shear stress changes within the epicardial conductance vessels were significantly lower in normal compared to atherosclerotic arteries.

Thus, the increase in coronary blood flow is an important hemodynamic determinant of epicardial artery dilation in normal arteries during cold pressor testing. On the other hand, the vasodilator response limits increases in shear stress for a given increase in blood flow. In contrast, the failure of atherosclerotic arteries to dilate, despite increased myocardial demands, exaggerates increases in local shear stress in relation to changes in flow.

Key words: Endothelium; cold-pressor testing; coronary atherosclerosis; acetylcholine; coronary vasomotor tone

Introduction

Sympathetic stimulation by cold pressor testing induces a complex interplay between adrenergic receptor stimulation, humoral and local metabolic factors, and alterations in coronary perfusion pressure. The normal response to sympathetic stimulation in the absence of increased metabolic workloads is vasoconstriction [10]. If sympathetic stimulation is associated with increased myocardial work (e. g., during cold pressor testing), the increases in sympathetic tone compete with the effects of metabolically mediated increases in blood flow [40]. Increased blood flow stimulates vasodilation of large epicardial coronary arteries [9, 17], and this response depends on the presence of an intact endothelium [30]. Experimental studies suggested that vasodilation in response to increased blood flow is mediated by the signal of shear stress on the endothelium [21, 29] to release endothelium-derived relaxing factor(s) [30, 32]. A number of studies [14, 15, 28, 41] have demonstrated that in humans the normal response to sympathetic stimulation in combination with increased myocardial work is dilation of epicardial conductance vessels. Moreover, we have shown that the epicardial artery vasomotor response to cold pressor testing is intimately related to the integrity of endothelial function in human coronary artery disease [2, 23, 42] and may thus alter the epicardial artery vasomotor response to sympathetic stimulation by impairing shear stress-mediated vasodilation during increased blood flow.

Thus, it was the purpose of the present study to examine the coronary hemodynamic determinants of epicardial artery vasomotor responses to sympathetic stimulation by cold-pressor testing. In addition, we tested the hypothesis that there is a relation between estimated shear stress and coronary artery dilation, which is altered in the presence of a dysfunctional endothelium in patients with coronary atherosclerosis. For this purpose, epicardial vessels were classified according to the presence to the endothelium-dependent stimulator acetylcholine.

Methods

Classification of patients

Thirty-two patients undergoing routine diagnostic cardiac catheterization were studied. These patients were classified into two groups based on their history, the presence or absence of atherosclerosis on the diagnostic coronary angiogram, and – most importantly – on their epicardial artery vasomotor response to the intracoronary infusion of increasing dosages of the endothelium-dependent dilator acetylcholine. Patients with unstable angina, recent myocardial infarction, and clinical evidence of heart failure were excluded.

Written informed consent was obtained from all patients before the study. The study protocol had been approved by the Ethics Committee of the University of Freiburg.

Group I: normal patients. Twelve patients with angiographically normal coronary arteries served as normal subjects. All patients demonstrated a dilator response on the intracoronary infusion of acetylcholine (10^{-8} to 10^{-6} M) and had no risk factors for coronary artery disease. The mean age of these patients was 49.6 years (three woman, nine men). All subjects had angiographically normal, smooth coronary arteries without luminal irregularities, and no evidence of segmental wall motion abnormalities on their left-ventricular cineangiograms. The cause for referral for diagnostic coronary angiography was atypical chest pain in 10 patients, and intermittent left bundle branch block in two patients.

Group II: patients with coronary artery disease: Twenty patients with angiographic evidence of coronary atherosclerosis, but without hemodynamically significant lesions (<30% diameter reduction) within the left anterior descending coronary artery were studied. Their mean age was 51.8 years (nine women, 11 men).

Study design

Vasoactive therapy was discontinued at least 24 h prior to cardiac catherization. No patient received β-adrenergic blockers within 48 h before the study. Diagnostic coronary angiography was performed by a standard percutaneous femoral approach using the Judkins technique. After the completion of diagnostic catheterization, additional 5000 units of heparin were given intravenously and an 8F guiding catheter (Schneider, Zuerich, Switzerland) was introduced into the left main coronary artery. A 3F Monorail-Doppler catheter (Schneider, Zürich, Switzerland) with a 20 MHz pulsed Doppler crystal was advanced into the left anterior descending artery via a 0.014 inch guide wire. The Doppler catheter was carefully positioned to obtain a stable flow-velocity signal. Before introducing the Doppler catheter into the guiding catheter, the flow-velocity recordings were referenced to zero and calibrated. Five minutes after the control angiogram, cold-pressor testing was performed by immersion of the patient's hand and forearm in ice water for 90 s.

Ten min after cold pressor testing, acetylcholine was selectively infused into the left anterior descending artery via the Doppler catheter. Increasing dosages were used to achieve estimated final blood concentrations in the coronary bed of 10^{-8} M, 10^{-7} M, and 10^{-6} M (assuming a blood flow of 80 ml/min) at an infusion rate of 2 ml/min, lasting 3 min for each concentration.

Throughout the study, phasic and mean intracoronary blood flow velocity, heart rate, and aortic pressure (via the guiding catheter) were continuously measured. Serial injections of nonionic contrast material (Ultravist, Schering AG, Berlin, FRG) into the hand were performed during control, at the end of cold pressor testing, at recontrol after cold pressor test, and at the end of each acetylcholine-infusion period. Prior to completion of the study, 0.25 mg nitroglycerin was injected into the left main stem via the guiding catheter, followed by a final angiogram to assess the vasodilatory capability of the coronary arteries.

Quantitative coronary angiography

Coronary angiography was performed using a simultaneous biplane multidirectional isocentric x-ray system (Siemens Bicor, Erlangen, FRG), and cineangiograms were obtained at a frame rate of 25 frames/s. For quantitative analysis, end-diastolic cine frames were videodigitized and stored in the image-analysis system (Mipron I, Kontron Electronics, Eching, FRG) in a 512 × 512 matrix with an 8-bit gray scale.

The method of quantitative coronary angiography by automatic contour-detection has been extensively described [9, 38, 41, 42, 45]. Four to six, 8-mm straight segments without branching vessels of the proximal left anterior descending artery (the vessel under study) were measured. A series of diameter measurements were obtained for each scanline for the length of the arterial segment, and displayed in graph form, which showed diameter versus segment length, and the mean diameter value was calculated. Whenever possible, measurements were performed in both views of the biplane images using the radiopaque tip of the Doppler catheter for identification of corresponding vessel segments, and the vessel's cross-sectional area was calculated from both views, assuming an elliptical shape.

Derived parameters

For estimation of directional changes in coronary blood flow, a coronary flow index was calculated by multiplying the mean Doppler-derived blood-flow velocity with the computed cross-sectional area of the vessel segment. Wall shear stress was estimated assuming a straight tubular vessel segment using the equation provided by Milnor [26]: shear stress $= 4 \times n \times Q/r^3$, where n denotes blood viscosity, Q denotes flow index, and r denotes the mean radius of the measured vessel segment. Since the application of this equation requires making a number of assumptions, only changes from control values were calculated with each patient serving as his own control. Consequently, changes in shear stress can be approximated from the changes in local intracoronary flow velocity and diameter of the analyzed segment.

Statistical analysis

All data are expressed as mean ± SD. Statistical comparisons were made by analysis of variance for repeated measures, followed by the Student Newman Keuls test. Differences between groups were evaluated by analysis of variance followed by the Bonferroni-modified *t*-test. Statistical significance was assumed if a null hypothesis could be rejected at the 0.05 probability level.

Results

All coronary artery segments demonstrating a dilator response to intracoronary acetylcholine (group I) also vasodilated in response to cold-pressor testing by 19.7 ± 8.2% (mean ± 1 SD) from a control value of 7.6 ± 2.7 mm^2 luminal area to 9.1 ± 3.2 mm^2. In contrast all arteries with evidence of atherosclerosis demonstrated a vasoconstrictor response during cold-pressor testing with an area reduction by 18.4 ± 7.5% from 6.3 ± 1.9 mm^2 to 5.2 ± 1.8 mm^2. Thus, the responses to cold-pressor testing exactly mirrored the vasomotor responses to the endothelium-dependent agonist acetylcholine. All analyzed segments dilated in response to intracoronary nitroglycerin, indicating a preserved vasodilator capability of the measured segments.

The systemic hemodynamic variables heart rate and mean aortic pressure increased by comparable amounts in both groups of patients during cold-pressor testing. In the normal group, heart rate increased by 12 ± 9.4% and mean aortic pressure by 18.5 ± 6.5%, whereas in the group of patients with atherosclerosis, heart rate was augmented by 13.9 ± 6.5% and mean aortic pressure by 20.5 ± 9.7% during cold-pressor testing. Thus, the cold-pressor test-induced increases in myocardial workloads were not significantly different between both groups.

However, whereas the coronary blood flow index increased by 58.8 ± 16.7% in the normal group, cold-pressor test-induced increases in coronary blood flow indices were significantly blunted in patients with atherosclerosis (19.1 ± 31.5%, $p < 0.05$ vs normal group). Figure 1A illustrates that in normal epicardial arteries there was a significant linear relation between increases in coronary blood flow and increases in epicardial artery luminal area. A similar, but statistically weak relation between increases in blood flow indices and changes of epicardial artery luminal area was observed in patients with atherosclerosis (Fig. 1B), indicating that increases in coronary blood flow tended to decrease the vasoconstrictor response of atherosclerotic epicardial conductance vessels during cold-pressor testing.

Moreover, there was a statistically significant relation between increases in mean aortic pressure and changes in coronary blood flow indices in the normal group (Fig. 2A), which was completely abolished in patients with atherosclerosis and endothelial dysfunction in response to acetylcholine (Fig. 2B). Thus, despite increases in driving

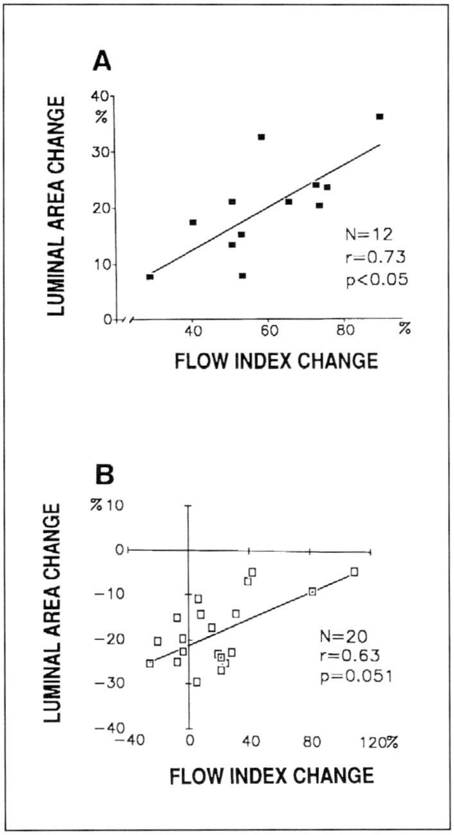

Fig. 1. Relation between percent changes in coronary blood-flow indices and epicardial artery luminal area in response to cold-pressor testing: A) in normal patients with intact endothelial function, and B) in patients with atherosclerosis and a dysfunctional endothelium.

pressure and myocardial demand, coronary blood flow indices did not adequately increase in patients with evidence of endothelial dysfunction of their epicardial arteries, suggesting an impairment in coronary blood flow regulation during cold-pressor testing.

Estimated shear stress in the proximal left anterior descending artery increased by $21.3 \pm 8.1\%$ in the normal group and by $60.8 \pm 31.7\%$ in the group of patients with atherosclerosis ($p < 0.05$). Thus, despite a larger increase in coronary blood flow, shear stress changes within the epicardial conductance vessels were significantly less in normal compared to atherosclerotic arteries. When shear stress changes were expressed in relation to changes in coronary blood flow indices, the ratio was 0.77 ± 0.08 in normal arteries compared to 1.38 ± 0.18 in atherosclerotic arteries ($p < 0.01$). Thus, the vasodilation of normal epicardial arteries had the effect of limiting increases in shear stress for a given increase in blood flow. In contrast, the vasoconstrictor response of atherosclerotic epicardial arteries considerably exaggerated increases in shear stress in relation to changes in blood flow (Fig. 3).

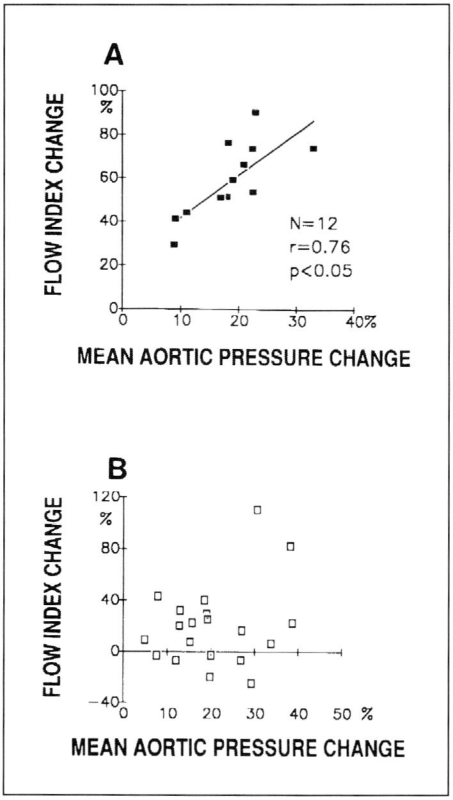

Fig. 2. Relation between percent changes in mean aortic pressure and coronary blood-flow indices in response to cold-pressor testing: A) in normal patients with intact endothelial function; and B) in patients with atherosclerosis and a dysfunctional endothelium.

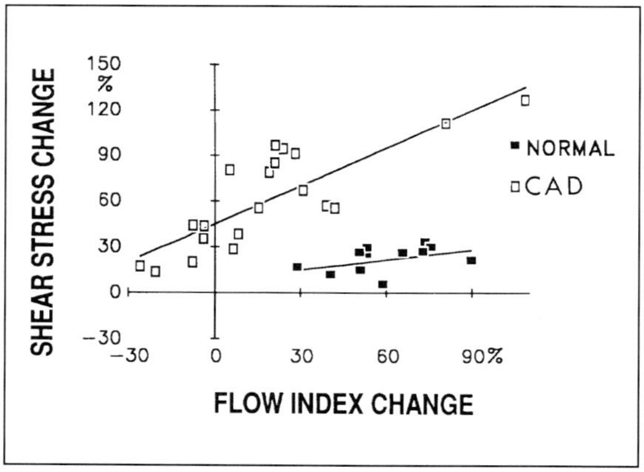

Fig. 3. Relation between percent changes in coronary blood-flow indices and estimated shear stress in response to cold-pressor testing in normal patients with intact endothelial function (filed symbols), and in patients with atherosclerosis and a dysfunctional endothelium (open symbols).

Discussion

The present investigation demonstrates that the increase in coronary blood flow is an important hemodynamic determinant of epicardial artery dilation in normal coronary arteries with intact endothelial function. The close correlation between relative increases in local coronary blood flow and luminal area changes of normal epicardial conductance vessels suggests that increases in local shear stress importantly contribute to the observed vasodilator response with increases in shear stress for any given increase in blood flow. In epicardial arteries of patients with evidence of atherosclerosis and a dysfunctional endothelium, increases in coronary blood flow tended to decrease the vasoconstrictor response, thereby indicating that flow-dependent dilatory mechanisms may have been still operating, but could not prevent the vasoconstrictor response. However, the failure of dilation in atherosclerotic artery segments with dysfunctional endothelium produced an increase in shear stress nearly double that observed in the normal segments, indicating that atherosclerosis impairs the normal control of epicardial artery shear stress in response to sympathetic stimulation. In addition, the relation between changes in mean aortic pressure and coronary blood flow were completely abolished in atherosclerotic epicardial arteries.

Mechanism of cold-pressor test-induced vasodilation

Previous studies from our laboratory [41], as well as other reports [14, 28] have shown that intracoronary β-adrenergic receptor blockade does not abolish coronary vasodilation after sympathetic stimulation in normal subjects, indicating that β-adrenergic receptor stimulation is not the major determinant of coronary vasodilator responses to cold-pressor testing. However, substantial flow-mediated vasodilation has been reported in normal coronary arteries of humans in vivo [7, 9], and this flow-dependent vasodilation was closely related to local increases in coronary blood flow [42], indicating that shear stress may, at least in part, contribute to the observed dilatory response of epicardial conductance vessels in response to increases in blood flow. The results of the present study extend these findings to the effects of sympathetic stimulation associated with increased myocardial demands by demonstrating that in normal arteries with intact endothelial function flow-mediated vasodilation counteracts the direct sympathetic vasoconstrictor effects.

The vasoconstrictor response of atherosclerotic arteries with dysfunctional endothelium observed in the present study is in line with a number of previous reports illustrating that atherosclerosis augments vasoconstrictor responses of epicardial arteries to sympathetic stimulation [14, 15, 28, 35, 41]. Atherosclerosis has been shown to impair vasodilator responses to a number of endothelium-dependent stimuli [2, 12]. Flow-dependent dilation was reduced or even completely blunted in atherosclerotic human coronary arteries in vivo [7, 9, 36]. Thus, impaired flow-mediated vasodilation in the presence of a dysfunctional endothelium may leave sympathetic constrictor effects unopposed, resulting in a constrictor response during cold-pressor testing, despite increased myocardial demands. However, the present study demonstrated that, even in atherosclerotic vessel segments, increases in blood flow tended to reduce the amount of cold-pressor test-induced vasoconstriction, indicating that flow-dependent dilatory mechanisms might still have been operating, despite a constrictor response to acetylcholine. The vasomotor response to acetylcholine depends on the net effect between endothelial muscarinic receptor stimulation to release endothelium-derived relaxing factor(s) and its direct constrictor effects upon the vascular smooth muscle [1, 13]. Constrictor effects from acetylcholine were observed very early in the development of atherosclerosis in the intact human coronary circulation [37, 39, 42]. However, in vitro studies revealed a reduced, but still measurable, stimulated EDRF activity of atherosclerotic arteries [3].

In addition, flow-dependent epicardial artery dilation has been shown to be well preserved in patients without angiographically visible atherosclerotic lesions, despite a constrictor response to acetylcholine [43], but it became progressively impaired with progression of atherosclerotic disease [7, 42]. Thus, in the absence of a concomitant vasoconstrictor stimulus, increases in blood flow may still elicit vasodilation, indicating preservation of the effects of EDRF released through the signal of shear stress, even in vessel segments, which demonstrate a blunted, stimulated, receptor-mediated release of EDRF activity in response to acetylcholine [43]. The vasoconstrictor responses to cold-pressor testing observed in atherosclerotic arteries [28, 41, 42], therefore, do not necessarily imply that endothelium-mediated dilation is completely abolished, but might rather indicate that concomitant vasoconstrictor stimuli override any potential dilatory stimuli in the presence of a dysfunctional endothelium.

Mechanisms of cold-pressor test-induced vasoconstriction

The exact nature of the vasoconstrictor stimuli remains to be determined. Recent studies from our laboratory demonstrated that local α-adrenergic receptor blockade did not prevent cold-pressor test-induced vasoconstriction of atherosclerotic arteries [44], making direct α-receptor mediated vasoconstriction a very unlikely mechanism. However, we cannot exclude the possibility that in atherosclerosis vasoconstriction may be related to the impairment of α_2-adrenoceptor (present on the endothelial cells)-mediated endothelium-dependent vasorelaxation [4]. Vasodilation in response to increases in driving pressure and flow through the signal of shear stress on the endothelium would provide a dilator feedback to oppose the constrictor feedback of the myogenic response to increased intraluminal pressure. The results of the present study indicate that the close relation between changes in mean aortic pressure and coronary blood flow observed in epicardial arteries with intact endothelial function is abolished in patients with evidence of endothelial dysfunction in response to acetylcholine. Thus, it is conceivable that, in the presence of a dysfunctional endothelium, an unopposed myogenic response may lead to an enhanced reactive vasoconstriction after increases in driving pressure, as has been recently described in experimental studies [16, 31]. In addition, interactions between platelets and an endothelium with a blunted, stimulated release of EDRF activity may enhance the constrictor responsiveness of the vessel. This could occur by direct sympathetic stimulation of platelet α-adrenergic receptors to release thromboxane, serotonin, or histamine (all of which are potent vasoconstrictors), or by platelet aggregation and activation at the site of endothelial injury. Numerous experimental studies [5, 18, 33, 34] have demonstrated that the endothelium prevents the vasoconstriction induced by aggregating platelets. We have also recently observed intense focal vasoconstriction of atherosclerotic epicardial arteries in response to intracoronary thrombus formation in the intact human coronary circulation in vivo [45]. Finally, one has to consider that atherosclerosis per se may promote the release of vasoconstrictor substances [19, 25] or may alter vascular smooth muscle reactivity.

Effects of shear stress

The present study indicates that epicardial vasodilation had the effect of limiting increases in shear stress for any given increase in blood flow in normal arteries. In contrast, in atherosclerosis the failure to dilate resulted in a near doubling of local estimated shear stress within the epicardial conductance vessel segment at comparable metabolic demands during cold-pressor testing. Increased shear stress induces pathologic changes in endothelial function and morphology [8, 11, 22]. A number of studies suggest that abnormal shear stress is a factor in the development of atherosclerosis [6, 20, 24]. Increased shear stress may lead to enhanced platelet activation with subsequent release of growth factors promoting vessel wall thickening and atheroma formation, especially at the site of endothelial injury.

Clinical implications

This study demonstrates that the vasodilator response of normal epicardial conductance vessels in humans, probably mediated by endothelium-dependent, flow-mediated mechanisms, provides a local feedback mechanism, which serves to control shear stress under conditions of increased driving pressure and blood flow in combination with sympathetic stimulation during cold-pressor testing. The failure of atherosclerotic arteries with dysfunctional endothelium to dilate in response to cold-pressor testing is associated with an impaired control of shear stress and may thus further perpetuate functional disturbances of the endothelium and promote the progression of atherosclerosis.

In addition, recent experimental studies indicated that the endothelium also plays an important role at the level of the resistance vasculature [27]. The loss of a control mechanism at the level of the resistance vessels may have even more important implications for blood-flow regulation and tissue perfusion during neurohumoral stimulation with simultaneously increased myocardial demands. Indeed, preliminary results in humans indicate that endothelial dysfunction of the coronary microvasculature may be associated with an altered linkage between myocardial oxygen demand and microvascular tone in the intact coronary circulation in vivo [46].

References

1. Bassenge E, Busse R (1988) Endothelial modulation of coronary tone. Progr Cardiovasc Dis 30:349–380
2. Bossaler C, Habib GB, Yamamoto H, Williams C, Wells S, Henry PD (1987) Impaired muscarinic endothelium-dependent relaxation and cyclic guanosine 5-monophosphate formation in atherosclerotic human coronary artery and rabbit aorta. J Clin Invest 79:170–174
3. Chester AH, O'Neil GS, Moncada S, Tadjkarimi S, Yacoub MH (1990). Low basal and stimulated release of nitric oxide in atherosclerotic epicardial coronary arteries. Lancet II:897–900
4. Cocks TM, Angus JA (1983) Endothelium-dependent relaxation of coronary arteries by noradrenaline and serotonin. Nature 305:627–630
5. Cohen RA, Shepherd JT, Vanhoutte PM (1983) Inhibitory role of the endothelium in the response of isolated coronary arteries to platelets. Science 221:273–274
6. Cornhill JF, Roach MR (1976) A quantitative study of the localization of atherosclerotic lesions in the rabbit aorta. Atherosclerosis 23:489–501
7. Cox DA, Vita JA, Treasure CB, Fish RD, Alexander RW, Ganz P, Selwyn AP (1989) Atherosclerosis impairs flow-mediated dilation of coronary arteries in humans. Circulation 80:458–465

8. Dewey CF, Bussolari SR, Gimbrone MA, Davies PF (1981) The dynamic response of vascular endothelial cells to fluid shear stress. J Biomech Eng 103:177–185
9. Drexler H, Zeiher AM, Wollschläger H, Meinertz T, Just H, Bonzel T (1989) Flow-dependent coronary artery dilatation in humans. Circulation 80:466–474
10. Feigl EO (1987) The paradox of adrenergic coronary vasoconstriction. Circulation 76:737–745
11. Frangos JA, Eskin SG, McIntire LV (1985) Flow effects on prostacyclin production by cultured human endothelial cells. Science 227:1477–1479
12. Freiman PC, Mitchell GC, Heistad DD, Armstrong ML, Harrison DG (1986) Atherosclerosis impairs endothelium-dependent vascular relaxation to acetylcholine and thrombin in primates. Circ Res 58:783–789
13. Furchgott RF, Zawadzki JV (1980) The obligatory role of endothelial cells in the relaxation of arterial smooth muscle by acetylcholine. Nature 288:373–376
14. Gaglione A, Hess OM, Corin WJ, Ritter M, Grimm J, Krayenbühl HP (1987) Is there coronary vasoconstriction after intracoronary beta-adrenergic blockade in patients with coronary artery disease. J Am Coll Cardiol 10:299–310
15. Gordon JB, Ganz P, Nabel EG, Fish RD, Zebede J, Mudge GH, Alexander RW, Selwyn AP (1989) Atherosclerosis influences the vasomotor response of epicardial arteries to exercise. J Clin Invest 83:1946–1952
16. Griffith TM, Edwards DH (1990) Myogenic autoregulation of flow may be inversely related to endothelium-derived relaxing factor activity. Am J Physiol 258:H1171–H1180
17. Holtz J, Förstermann U, Pohl U, Giesler M, Bassenge E (1984) Flow-dependent, endothelium-mediated dilation of epicardial coronary arteries in conscious dogs: effects of cyclooxygenase inhibition. J Cardiovasc Pharmacol 6:1161–1169
18. Houston DS, Shepherd JT, Vanhoutte PM (1986) Aggregating human platelets cause direct contraction and endothelium-dependent relaxation of isolated canine coronary arteries: role of serotonin, thromboxane A2 and adenine nucleotides. J Clin Invest 78:539–544
19. Katusic ZS, Shepherd JT, Vanhoutte PM (1987) Endothelium-dependent contraction to stretch in canine basilar arteries. Am J Physiol 252:H671–H673
20. Ku DN, Giddens DG, Zarins CK, Glagov S (1985) Pulsatile flow and atherosclerosis in human carotid bifurcation: positive correlation between plaque location and low and oscillating shear stress. Arteriosclerosis 5:293–302
21. Lansman JB, Hallam TJ, Rink TJ (1987) Single stretch-activated ion channels in vascular endothelial cells as mechanostransducers. Nature 325:811–813
22. Levesque MJ, Liepsch D, Moravec S, Nerem RM (1986) Correlation of endothelial cell shape and wall shear stress in a stenosed dog aorta. Arteriosclerosis 6:220–229
23. Ludmer PL, Selwyn AP, Shook TL, Wayne RR, Mudge GH, Alexander RW, Ganz P (1986) Paradoxical vascoconstriction induced by acetylcholine in atherosclerotic coronary arteries. N Engl J Med 315:1046–1051
24. Lutz RJ, Cannon JN, Bischoff KB, Dedrick RL, Stiles RK, Fry DL (1977) Wall shear stress distribution in a model canine artery during steady flow. Circ Res 41:391–399
25. Miller VM, Vanhoutte PM (1985) Endothelium-dependent contractions to arachidonic acid are mediated by products of cyclooxygenase. Am J Physiol 248:H432–H437
26. Milnor WR (1982) Hemodynamics. William & Wilkins, Baltimore, pp 49–51
27. Myers PR, Banitt PF, Guerra R, Harrison DG (1989) Characteristics of canine resistance arteries: importance of endothelium. Am J Physiol 247:H603–H610
28. Nabel EG, Ganz P, Gordon JB, Alexander RW, Selwyn AP (1988) Dilation of normal and constriction of atherosclerotic coronary arteries caused by the cold pressor test. Circulation 77:-43–52
29. Olesen SP, Clapham DE, Davies PF (1988) Hemodynamic shear stress activates a K^+ current in vascular endothelial cells. Nature 331:169–170
30. Pohl U, Holtz J, Busse R, Bassenge E (1986) Crucial role of endothelium in the vasodilator response to increased flow in vivo. Hypertension 8:37–44
31. Pohl U, Lamontagne D (1991) Impaired tissue perfusion after inhibition of endothelium-derived nitric oxide. Bas Res Cardiol 86 (Suppl 2):97–105
32. Rubanyi GM, Romero JC, Vanhoutte PM (1986) Flow-induced release of endothelium-derived relaxing factor. Am J Physiol 250:H1145–49

33. Shimokawa H, Vanhoutte PM (1989) Impaired endothelium-dependent relaxation to aggregating platelets and related vasoactive substances in porcine coronary arteries in hypercholesterolemia and atherosclerosis. Circ Res 64:900–914
34. Vanhoutte PM, Houston DS (1985) Platelets, endothelium, and vasospasm. Circulation 72:-728–738
35. Vita JA, Treasure CB, Fish RD, Yeung AC, Vekshtein VI, Ganz P, Selwyn AP (1990) Endothelial dysfunction leads to increased coronary constriction to catecholamines in patients with early atherosclerosis (abstract). J Am Coll Cardiol 15:158A
36. Vita JA, Treasure CB, Ganz P, Cox DA, Fish RD, Selwyn AP (1989) Control of shear stress in the epicardial coronary arteries of humans: impairment by atherosclerosis. J Am Coll Cardiol 14:1193–1199
37. Vita JA, Treasure CB, Nabel EG, McLenachan JM, Fish RD, Yeung AC, Vekshtein VI, Selwyn AP, Ganz P (1990) Coronary vasomotor response to acetylcholine relates to risk factors for coronary artery disease. Circulation 81:491–497
38. Wollschläger H, Lee P, Zeiher AM, Solzbach U, Bonzel T, Just H (1986) Improvement of quantitative angiography by exact calculation of radiological magnification factors. Comput Cardiol: 483–486
39. Yasue H, Matsuyama K, Matsuyama K, Okumura K, Morikami Y, Ogawa H (1990) Responses of angiographically normal human coronary arteries to intracoronary injection of acetylcholine by age and segment. Circulation 81:482–490
40. Young MA, Vatner SF (1986) Enhanced adrenergic constriction of iliac artery with removal of endothelium in conscious dog. Am J Physiol 250:H892–897
41. Zeiher AM, Drexler H, Wollschläger H, Saurbier B, Just H (1989) Coronary vasomotion in response to sympathetic stimulation in humans: importance of the functional integrity of the endothelium. J Am Coll Cardiol 14:1181–1190
42. Zeiher AM, Drexler H, Wollschläger H, Just H (1991) Modulation of coronary vasomotor tone in humans: progressive endothelial dysfunction with different early stages of coronary atherosclerosis. Circulation 83:391–401
43. Zeiher AM, Drexler H, Wollschläger H, Just H (1989) Preserved flow mediated vasodilation despite acetylcholine-induced vasoconstriction in atherosclerotic coronary arteries in man (abstract). J Am Coll Cardiol 13:132A
44. Zeiher AM, Siegemund M, Wollschläger H, Drexler H (1990) Persistence of sympathetic-mediated constriction of epicardial arteries after local α-blockade in patients with coronary artery disease (abstract). Circulation 82 (suppl III):III-300
45. Zeiher AM, Schächinger V, Weitzel SH, Wollschläger H, Just H (1991) Intracoronary thrombus formation causes focal vasoconstriction of epicardial arteries in patients with coronary artery disease. Circulation (in press)
46. Zeiher AM, Drexler H, Wollschläger H, Just H (1990) Endothelial dysfunction alters the linkage of myocardial oxygen demand to microvascular tone in humans (abstract). Circulation 82 (suppl III):III-247

Authors address:
Andreas M. Zeiher, MD
Medizinische Klinik III
University of Freiburg
Hugstetter Str. 55
W-7800 Freiburg, FRG

Coronary vasospasm in humans: the role of atherosclerosis and of impaired endothelial vasodilator function

P. Ganz, F. F. Weidinger, A. C. Yeung, V. I. Vekshtein, J. A. Vita, T. J. Ryan Jr., J. M. McLenachan, and A. P. Selwyn

Brigham and Women's Hospital and Harvard Medical School, Boston, Massachusetts, USA

Importance of coronary vasoconstriction as a mechanism of myocardial ischemia

The traditional view that coronary stenoses cause myocardial ischemia by limiting increases in blood flow is now thought to be incomplete. Convincing evidence has accumulated that coronary narrowings play an active role in causing ischemia by intermittently interfering with coronary blood flow, not only among patients with the rare Prinzmetal's variant angina, but also in nearly all patients with unstable and stable forms of angina pectoris (1, 2, 6, 7, 10, 13, 31). Studies of Chierchia and colleagues (2) in patients with unstable angina demonstrated a fall in coronary sinus oxygen saturation which could not be explained by a simultaneous increase in myocardial oxygen demand. Selwyn (1981) used radionuclides to monitor myocardial perfusion in patients with stable angina during rapid atrial pacing and found a net fall in myocardial blood flow in regions distal to coronary stenosis. More recently, positron emission tomography was used to assess changes in regional myocardial perfusion in patients with stable angina using rubidium-82. These studies also demonstrated decreases in regional blood flow which accompanied ischemia triggered by exercise, cold pressor stimulation or mental stress (6, 7). Ganz and colleagues (13) in patients with unstable angina directly measured coronary stenosis resistance by simultaneously determing pressure gradients and blood flow across moderately severe coronary narrowings, and they demonstrated increases in stenosis resistance both preceding and at the onset of episodes of ischemia.

Introduction into the catheterization laboratory of quantitative methods for assessing luminal caliber has permitted a closer examination of vasomotor responses of epicardial arteries in response to external stimuli known to trigger ischemia during daily life, such as exercise, cold, mental stress and isometric exercise (1, 11, 14, 15, 23). Through the use of quantitative angiography, Gordon (1989; (14)), Nabel (1988; (23)), and Gage (1986; (11)) have demonstrated that there are important differences in the reactions of angiographically normal arteries and those containing atherosclerotic narrowings. In patients with clinically stable angina, atherosclerotic arteries generally constrict during the same stimuli (exercise, cold pressor testing) that cause dilation of arteries that are angiographically normal. This paradoxical constriction (vasospasm) of atherosclerotic narrowings likely contributes to the development of myocardial ischemia in this patient population.

Mechanism(s) of coronary vasospasm – focus of early studies

The initial focus of investigations into the mechanisms of coronary vasospasm consisted of generally futile attempts to demonstrate that there is an excess of a circulating vasoconstrictor compound in the coronary circulation. For instance, in patients with vasospastic angina, arterial and coronary sinus concentrations of norepinephrine and epinephrine obtained early in ischemia were not elevated above baseline and rose only late in ischemia (29). In addition, sympathetic nervous system function was investigated in patients with variant angina pectoris by sampling of peripheral venous norepinephrine in supine and upright postures, by measuring urinary excretion of catecholamines, and by assessing the physiologic responses to sympathetic stimuli such as the Valsalva maneuver, the isometric handgrip test, and the cold pressor test. No differences were found in these measurements in normal subjects and in patients with variant angina (28). Thus, these studies suggested that excessive sympathetic nervous system activation is not likely to be an important cause of coronary artery spasm. The weight of the evidence to date suggests that vasospastic angina also cannot be attributed primarily to an excess of the circulating constrictor agonists thromboxane A_2 and serotonin or to a deficiency of the vasodilator prostacyclin (12).

Mechanism(s) of coronary vasospasm – role of endothelium and atherosclerosis

In 1980, two seminal studies were published that helped to shift the emphasis of investigations of vasospasm away from the neurohumoral systems and instead, focused the attention on local disturbances in the arterial wall. First, Henry observed that the isolated aortas of rabbits rendered atherosclerotic by a high cholesterol diet were hypersensitive to contraction induced by ergonovine and by serotonin (19). This study suggested that the augmented vascular responsiveness can be related directly to the biology of the atherosclerotic process. This hypothesis was particularly appealing as it was paralleled by clinical observations that vasospastic angina almost invariably occurs in the setting of coronary atherosclerosis, although the degree of luminal narrowing varies widely (27). It was appreciated that even patients thought to have normal coronary arteries at angiography may at autopsy have evidence of atherosclerosis in the same segment of the vessel that was affected by vasospasm.

The second seminal observation was the demonstration by Furchgott that endothelial cells, when appropriately stimulated, release a potent vasodilator substance, named endothelium-derived relaxing factor (EDRF), which causes relaxation of the underlying vascular smooth muscle (9). Furchgott resolved a longstanding paradox that acetylcholine (Ach) was a vasodilator in vivo yet it frequently induced constriction of arterial strips in vitro. In the presence of endothelium, increasing doses of Ach produced dose-dependent relaxation of isolated strips of rabbit aorta that had been preconstricted with norepinephrine. If the endothelium had been removed, as inadvertently happened during routine handling of isolated vessels, and which Furchgott accomplished by gently rubbing the intimal surface of the arterial strip, then only constriction was induced by Ach. It was therefore suggested that Ach has two distinct and opposite actions on blood vessels: direct constriction of vascular smooth muscle and an indirect vasodilator action that is mediated by endothelium. In most intact arteries, the net effect of these two actions is vasodilation, especially at lower concentrations of Ach (i.e., $\leqq 10^{-5}$M).

It was subsequently established that release of EDRF was a mode of action of most other vasodilators including histamine, bradykinin, substance P, ATP, ADP, thrombin, and increasing blood flow. Even substances that act as vasoconstrictors can release EDRF, such as catecholamines, serotonin, and vasopressin (25). Although the net effect on blood vessels may not be vasodilation, the presence of endothelium-dependent vasodilating influence will attenuate severe constriction in these vascular beds.

Studies of endothelium-dependent relaxation to acetylcholine in humans. Effects of atherosclerosis and of coronary risk factors

With the background of the observations of Henry on the hypercontractility of atherosclerotic arteries and of Furchgott on the importance of endothelium to vasodilation, in the study of Ludmer et al. (21), we addressed the hypothesis that constrictor hyperresponsiveness of atherosclerotic human coronary arteries is caused by endothelial vasodilator dysfunction. To test this concept, acetylcholine (endothelium-dependent agent) and nitroglycerin (endothelium-independent agent) were administered directly into the left anterior descending coronary artery of patients undergoing a cardiac catheterization and vasomotor responses were assessed by quantitative angiography. Ach induced dose-dependent dilation of human epicardial coronary arteries in the majority of patients free from any evidence of atherosclerosis. As in many animal preparations with intact endothelium, this dilatation was best observed in the Ach range of 10^{-9} to 10^{-6} M. Higher concentrations, which have since been employed by some investigators, are more likely to favor constriction of presumably normal arteries. The Ach-induced dilation of human coronary arteries likely involves an endothelium-dependent mechanism, as the administration of methylene blue, an inhibitor of the actions of EDRF, abolishes this response (20).

Ludmer first demonstrated that atherosclerotic arteries paradoxically constrict in response to Ach and that this abnormal constriction may be related to disturbed endothelial vasodilator function. Arterial segments from patients with advanced coronary stenoses (greater than 70% luminal narrowing) constricted in a dose-dependent manner to increasing concentrations of Ach in the same dose range in which normal arteries dilated. The ability of these atherosclerotic segments to dilate in response to nitroglycerin, an agent that acts directly on vascular smooth muscle, was preserved, suggesting that the paradoxical response to Ach was indeed related to endothelial dysfunction.

In addition, coronary arterial segments from patients with angiographic evidence of only minor intimal irregularities also constricted to Ach. This indicates that endothelium-dependent vasodilation is impaired early in the atherosclerotic process. Such disturbances in endothelial vasodilator function have been recently shown to exist in angiographically normal arteries of patients with risk factors for the development of atherosclerosis or in arteries with a high likelihood of presence of early atherosclerosis. Thus, angiographically smooth coronary arteries in patients who have a significant narrowing in another coronary artery are likely to constrict to Ach (21, 38). Impairment of endothelium-dependent dilation has been shown to be also particularly marked at branchpoints of coronary arteries that are sites of disturbed blood-flow patterns at which atherosclerosis is particularly likely to develop. Studies of Vita (36) and Yasue (40) have shown that there is an important correlation between the presence of coronary risk factors and the response to Ach in patients with angiographically normal arteries. In the study of Vita, a constrictor response to Ach was independently associated with elevated serum cholesterol, male gender, family history of coronary artery disease, and patient age. The overall number of coronary risk factors was the best predictor of the response to Ach. In the study of Yasue, the response to Ach matched the expected distribution of occult atherosclerosis; the proximal segments were more likely to constrict to Ach than the distal segments.

Thus abnormal vasomotor responses to Ach have served as convenient functional markers of endothelial dysfunction in both early and advanced stages of atherosclerosis. This endothelial vasodilator dysfunction is likely to be an important pathophysiologic link between atherosclerosis and associated vasospasm.

Measurements of EDRF in atherosclerosis

EDRF has been shown to be nitric oxide (NO) or a closely related compound, derived from arginine. While insights into endothelium-dependent relaxation in the clinical setting have been obtained using the test agent acetylcholine, more direct assays of EDRF have not been practical in patients. However, EDRF activity can be determined in arteries with experimental atherosclerosis. Several groups of investigators have demonstrated in bioassay studies a depressed release or diminished activity of EDRF from atherosclerotic arteries in response to acetylcholine and serotonin (16, 33, 34).

Endothelial vasodilator function and patterns of responses to stimuli known to trigger myocardial ischemia during daily life

Ach, an extremely useful test agent of endothelial function, is not likely to be an important physiologic regulator of vascular tone. It is interesting, however, that the patterns of vasomotor reactions to Ach are mirrored by the reaction of smooth, irregular, and stenosed coronary arteries to the types of common stimuli that are known to trigger ischemia in daily life such as supine bicycle exercise and the cold pressor test (11, 14, 23, 41). Thus, during exercise or cold pressor stimulation, angiographically smooth arteries dilate, while arteries with evidence of early and advanced atherosclerosis paradoxically constrict. Moreover, an excellent agreement exists in the responses (dilation/constriction) of individual arterial segments to Ach and in the responses of the same segments to exercise (14) or the cold pressor stimulation (41), suggesting that endothelial function may modulate vasomotion during these activities – in health and in disease. While the responses to dynamic exercise and the cold pressor test are of great relevance to the pathophysiology of ischemia during daily life, they are difficult to interpret in light of simultaneous changes in multiple parameters such as activation of the sympathetic nervous system, augmentation of coronary blood flow, and increases in heart rate and blood pressure. With the aim of understanding the responses during these complex daily activities, vasomotion of epicardial coronary arteries has been examined in relation to each individual parameter individually, i.e., increasing blood flow and rising catecholamines.

Studies of flow-mediated dilation in humans. Effects of atherosclerosis

While the release of EDRF was initially described using pharmacologic agents that act through activation of specific membrane receptors on endothelial cells, it was subsequently shown, that mechanical stimuli, including blood flow and pulsatility, can also stimulate the release of EDRF (26, 30). Dilatation of the conduit arteries in response to increasing blood flow was first described in 1933, but the mechanism remained unknown until the recent demonstration of Bassenge and colleagues (26) that endothelial cells act as mediators of flow-dependent dilation. Mechanical removal of endothelial cells from the canine femoral artery abolished dilatation in response to increased blood flow. Use of the bioassay techniques demonstrated that EDRF and Ach release a relaxing substance with the same characteristics (30).

In humans, coronary arteries free of atherosclerosis (as judged by angiography) have also been shown to dilate in response to increased blood flow (4, 8, 24). This flow-mediated response is impaired by atherosclerosis. In these studies, increases in blood flow were induced by the administration of dilators of the resistance vessels such as adenosine and papaverine. Diameter of epicardial arteries free of angiographic evidence of atherosclerosis dilated by approximately 16% in response to a three-fold increase in blood flow (4), while arteries with even mild angiographic evidence of atherosclerosis failed to dilate or even constricted (4, 24). This impaired response to increasing blood flow may in part explain the abnormal vasomotor behavior of atherosclerotic epicardial coronary arteries during daily activities such as exercise, whereby normal arteries dilate and atherosclerotic arteries fail to dilate appropriately during exercise as the demand for blood flow increases with increased metabolic requirements.

The role of endothelial function in modulating the effects of catecholamines in the constriction of human coronary arteries

Stimuli for myocardial ischemia such as exercise and exposure to cold are associated with sympathetic (adrenergic) activation and increase in circulating catecholamine concentrations. Catecholamines exert their effects on vascular smooth muscle by α_1- and α_2-adrenergic mediated constriction and by β-adrenergic mediated dilation. Healthy endothelium is capable of modulating the constrictor effects of catecholamines by several mechanisms. Stimulation of α_2-adrenergic receptors on endothelial cells can lead to a release of EDRF. Cocks (3) demonstrated that stimulation of α_2-receptors on endothelial cells leads to release of EDRF and attenuation of the constrictor effects of norepinephrine. In addition, Martin and Furchgott observed that removal of endothelium from arterial rings markedly increased the sensitivity of arteries to constriction by phenylephrine which lacks significant α_2-agonist properties at the doses administered (22). They were able to attribute their findings to removal of the tonic dilator influence resulting from the continuous basal release of EDRF.

Vita (37) demonstrated in patients undergoing a cardiac catheterization that coronary segments exhibiting evidence of endothelial dysfunction (assessed by acetylcholine) had a constrictor response to phenylephrine at a 100-fold lower concentration than segments that had normal endothelial function. These results suggest that the endothelial dysfunction that characterizes early and advanced atherosclerosis is associated with a marked increase in sensitivity to the constrictor effects of catecholamines. These results could also in part explain the observation that atherosclerotic coronary arteries constrict during exercise, the cold pressor stimulation and other stimuli associated with elevated catecholamines.

Treatment of endothelial vasodilator dysfunction in atherosclerosis

Endothelium overlying atherosclerotic plaques is physically present, but exhibits distinct morphologic abnormalities. In experimental atherosclerosis, these atypical cells are often cuboidal rather than flat, and lack the typical orientation in the direction of blood flow (39). Similar abnormalities of the endothelial morphology have been found in human coronary arteries (5). As endothelial cells in atherosclerosis are not absent, it might be feasible to find treatments that restore their function. Such treatments could involve approaches that directly address the biology of atherosclerosis (e.g. cholesterol lowering, fish oil administration) or could more narrowly focus on restoring EDRF (e.g. administration of large amounts of the EDRF precursor arginine, administration of N-acetylcysteine to increase the potency of residual (EDRF).

Effects of cholesterol-lowering

Harrison (17), Heistad (18) and their colleagues have shown in monkeys that endothelium-dependent relaxation to acetylcholine and serotonin is impaired in diet-induced atherosclerosis (17) and that cholesterol lowering will return endothelial vasodilator function to normal in association with histologic evidence of plaque healing (i.e., the inflammatory and cellular components of lesions diminish) and without the need for complete regression of atherosclerotic plaques to occur.

In humans, the efficacy of cholesterol-lowering in restoring endothelium-dependent relaxation is not yet known. However, Vita et al. (36) have shown in patients with preclinical stages of coronary atherosclerosis that the level of serum cholesterol (and of other coronary risk factors) relates closely to the abnormal constriction elicited by the endothelium-dependent dilator agent acetylcholine.

Effects of fish oil administration

Treatment of atherosclerosis with fish oils has been of considerable interest in view of the findings of reduced rates of cardiovasular disease reported in populations consuming a diet rich in fish oil and in view of the ability of fish oils to reduce atherosclerosis in experimental models. With respect to the ability of fish oils to improve regulation of vascular tone in atherosclerosis, Shimokawa (32) demonstrated in a pig model that a brief course of dietary supplementation with fish oil reverses the impaired endothelium-dependent relaxation in experimental coronary atherosclerosis.

Vekshtein (35) and colleagues have shown in patients that fish oil administration for 6 months can restore dilation of atherosclerotic coronary arteries to acetylcholine. This improved response to acetylcholine occurred without any change in response to the endothelium-independent agent nitroglycerin, suggesting that the beneficial effect of fish oils can be attributed to improved endothelial vasodilator function.

Conclusions

Studies over the last decade have revealed that healthy endothelial cells produce a relaxing substance, EDRF, which is pivotally involved in the regulation of vascular tone. This substance is similar to the active principle of nitroglycerin, nitric oxide, and can thus be thought of as the "endogenous nitroglycerin". In human and experimental atherosclerosis, the activity of EDRF is diminished, a condition which predisposes to arterial vasospasm and thereby to myocardial ischemia. Treatments directed at restoring endothelial vasodilator function and thereby improving ischemia are being tested in the clinical setting.

References

1. Brown BG, Lee AB, Bolsen E, Dodge HT (1984) Reflex constriction of significant coronary stenosis as a mechanism contributing to ischemic left ventricular dysfunction during isometric exercise. Circulation 70:18–24
2. Chierchia S, Lazzari M, Freedman B, Brunellis C, Maseri A (1983) Impairment of myocardial perfusion and function during painless myocardial ischemia. J Am Coll Cardiol 16:1359–1373

3. Cocks TM, Angus JA (1983) Endothelium-dependent relaxation of coronary arteries by noradrenaline and serotonin. Nature 305:627–630
4. Cox DA, Vita JA, Treasure CB, Fish RD, Alexander RW, Ganz P, Selwyn AP (1989) Impairment of flow-mediated dilation coronary dilation by atherosclerosis in man. Circulation 80:-458–465.
5. Davies MJ, Woolf N, Rowles PM and Pepper J (1988) Morphology of the endothelium over atherosclerotic plaques in human coronary arteries. Br Heart J 60:459–464
6. Deanfield J, Maseri A, Selwyn AP, Ribeiro P, Cherchia S, Krikler S, Morgan M (1983) Myocardial ischemia during daily life in patients with stable angina: Its relation to symptoms and heart rate changes. Lancet 2:753–761.
7. Deanfield JE, Kensett M, Wilson RA, Shea M, Horlock P, deLandsheere CM, Selwyn AP (1984) Silent myocardial ischemia due to mental stress. Lancet 2:1001–1004.
8. Drexler H, Zeiher AM, Wollschläger H, Meinertz T, Just H, Bonzel T (1989) Flow-dependent coronary artery dilatation in humans. Circulation 80:466–474
9. Furchgott RF, Zawadzki JV (1980) The obligatory role of endothelial cells in the relaxation of arterial smooth muscle by acetylcholine. Nature 288:373–376.
10. Fuster V (1988) Insights into the pathogenesis of acute ischemic syndromes. Cirulation 77: 1213–1220.
11. Gage JE, Hess OM, Murakami T, Ritter M, Grimm J, Krayenbuehl HP (1986) Vasoconstriction of stenotic coronary arteries during dynamic exercises in patients with classic angina pectoris: reversibility by nitroglycerin. Circulation 73:865–867
12. Ganz P, Alexander RW (1985) New insights into the cellular mechanisms of vasospasm. Am J Cardiol 56:11E–15E
13. Ganz P, Abben RP, Barry WH (1987) Dynamic variations in resistance of coronary arterial narrowings in angina pectoris at rest. Am J Cardiol 59:66–70
14. Gordon JB, Ganz P, Nabel EG, Zebede J, Mudge GH, Alexander RW, Selwyn AP (1989) Atherosclerosis and endothelial function influence the coronary vasomotor response to exercise. J Clin Invest 83:1946–1952
15. Gould KL (1985) Quantification of coronary artery stenosis in vivo. Circ Res 57:341–353.
16. Guerra R, Brotherton AFA, Goodwin PJ, Clark CR, Armstrong ML, Harrison DG (1990) Mechanism of abnormal endothelium-dependent vascular relaxation in atherosclerosis. Blood Vessels (in press)
17. Harrison DG, Armstrong ML, Freiman PC, Heistad DD (1987) Restoration of endothelium-dependent relaxation by dietary treatment of atherosclerosis. J Clin Invest 80:1808–1811.
18. Heistad DD, Mark AL, Marcus ML, Piegors DJ, Armstrong ML (1987) Dietary treatment of atherosclerosis abolishes hyperresponsiveness to serotonin: Implications for vasospasm. Circ Res 61:346–351.
19. Henry PD, Yokoyama M (1980) Supersensitivity of atherosclerotic rabbit aorta to ergonovine. Mediation by a serotonergic mechanism. J Clin Invest 66:306–313
20. Hodgson JM, Marshall JJ (1989) Direct vasoconstriction and endothelium-dependent vasodilation; mechanisms of acetylcholine effects on coronary flow and arterial diameter in patients with nonstenotic coronary arteries. Circulation 79:1043–1051
21. Ludmer PL, Selwyn AP, Shook TL, Wayne RR, Mudge GH, Alexander RW, Ganz P (1986) Paradoxical vasoconstriction induced by acetylcholine in atherosclerotic coronary arteries. N Engl J Med 315:1046–1051
22. Martin W, Furchgott RF, Villani GM, Jothianandan D (1986) Depression of contractile responses in rat aorta by spontaneously released endothelium-derived relaxing factor. J Pharm Exp Therap 237:529–538
23. Nabel EG, Ganz P, Gordon JB, Alexander RW, Selwyn AP (1988) Dilation of normal and constriction of atherosclerotic coronary arteries caused by the cold pressor test. Circulation 77:43–52
24. Nabel EG, Selwyn AP, Ganz P (1990) Large coronary arteries in humans are responsive to changing blood flow: an endothelium-dependent mechanism that fails in patients with atherosclerosis. J Am Coll Cardiol 16:349–356
25. Peach MJ, Loeb AL, Singer HA and Saye J (1985) Endothelium-derived vascular relaxing factor. Hypertension 7(Suppl 1): I-94–I-100

26. Pohl U, Holtz J, Busse R, Bassenge E (1986) Crucial role of endothelium in the vasodilator response to increased flow in vivo. Hypertension 8:37–44
27. Roberts WC (1986) Morphologic cardiac findings in coronary arterial spasm. In: Conti, CR (ed) Coronary Artery Spasm. Pathophysiology, Diagnosis and Treatment. New York, Dekker, pp. 23–47
28. Robertson D, Robertson RM, Nies AS, Oates JA and Friesinger GC (1979) Variant angina pectoris: Investigation of indexes of sympathetic nervous system function. Am J Cardiol 43:-1080–1085
29. Robertson RM, Bernard Y, Robertson D (1983) Arterial and coronary sinus catecholamines in the course of spontaneous coronary artery spasm. Am Heart J 105:901–906
30. Rubanyi GM, Romero JC, Vanhoutte PM (1986) Flow-induced release of endothelium-derived relaxing factor. Am J Physiol 250:H1145–H1149
31. Selwyn AP, Forse G, Fox K, Jonathan A, Stiner R (1981) Patterns of disturbed myocardial perfusion in patients with coronary artery disease. Circulation 64:83–90
32. Shimokawa H, Lam JYT, Chesebor JH, Bowie EJW, Vanhoutte PM (1987) Effects of dietary supplemention with cod-liver oil on endothelium-dependent responses in porcine coronary arteries. Circulation 76:898–905
33. Shimokawa H, Vanhoutte PM (1989) Impaired endothelium-dependent relaxation to aggregating platelets and related substances in porcine coronary arteries in hypercholesterolemia and atherosclerosis. Circ Res 64:900–914
34. Sreeharan N, Jayakody RL, Senaratne MPJ, Thomson ABR, Kappagoda CT (1986) Endothelium-dependent relaxation and experimental atherosclerosis in the rabbit aorta. Can J Physiol Pharmacol 64:1451–1453
35. Vekshtein VI, Yeung AC, Vita JA, Nabel EG, Fish RD, Bittl JA, Selwyn AP, Ganz P (1989) Fish oil improves endothelium-dependent relaxation in patients with coronary artery disease (abstr). Circulation 80:II–434A
36. Vita JA, Treasure CB, Nabel EG, McLenachan JM, Fish RD, Yeung AC, Vekshtein VI, Selwyn AP, Ganz P (1990a) The coronary vasomotor response to acetylcholine relates to risk factors for coronary artery disease. Circulation 81:491–497
37. Vita JA, Treasure CB, Fish RD, Yeung AC, Vekshtein VI, Ganz P, Selwyn AP (1990) Endothelial dysfunction leads to increased coronary constriction to catecholamines in patients with early atherosclerosis. (abstr.) J Am Coll cardiol 15:158A
38. Werns SW, Walton JA, Hsia HH, Nabel EG, Sanz ML, Pitt B (1989) Evidence of endothelial dysfunction in angiographically normal coronary arteries of patients with coronary artery disease. Circulation 79:287–291
39. Weidinger FF, McLenachan JM, Cybulski MI, Gordon JB, Rennke HG, Hollenberg NK, Fallon JT, Ganz P, Cooke JP (1990) Persistant dysfunction of regenerated endothelium after balloon angioplasty of rabbit iliac artery. Circulation 81:1667–1679
40. Yasue H, Matsuyama K, Okumara K, Morikami Y, Ogawa H (1990) Responses of angiographically normal human coronary arteries to intracoronary injection of acetylcholine by age and segment. Possible role of early coronary atherosclerosis. Circulation 81:482–490
41. Zeiher AM, Drexler H, Wollschläger H, Saurbier B, Just H (1989) Coronary vasomotion in response to sympathetic stimulation in humans: importance of the functional integrity of the endothelium. J Am Coll Cardiol 14:1181–1190

Authors address:
P. Ganz, M.D.
Cardiovascular Division
Brigham and Women's Hospital
75 Francis Street
Boston, Massachusetts 02115
USA

Progression of coronary endothelial dysfunction in man and its potential clinical significance

H. Drexler and A. M. Zeiher

Medizinische Klinik III, University of Freiburg, Freiburg, FRG

Summary: Endothelial injury represents an important factor in the initiation of atherosclerosis and is associated with abnormal vasomotor responses (=dysfunctional endothelium) to a variety of stimuli. Therefore, the evaluation of endothelial function may provide a means to detect early vascular alteration preceeding overt atherosclerotic lesions.

To test this clinically important hypothesis, we studied the coronary vasomotor responses to three different endothelium-dependent stimuli in patients with different early stages of coronary artery disease: first, increasing doses of intracoronary infusion of acetylcholine (ACH) (10^{-8}, 10^{-7}, 10^{-6} M); second, transient increases in coronary flow causing flow-dependent dilation by injection of papaverine into the midportion of the left descending artery (exposing the proximal segment of this vessel to increased flow, but not to papaverine); and third, sympathetic stimulation by cold pressor test. Coronary diameters were assessed by repeated coronary angiography and quantitative angiography, blood flow velocity (and subsequent calculation of blood flow) was obtained by intracoronary Doppler. In normal individuals, all three stimuli elicited epicardial artery dilation. In patients with smooth coronary arteries, but hypercholesterolemia, a substantial vasoconstriction was observed in response to ACH, whereas the response to cold pressor test and increases in flow was normal, that is, vasodilation occurred. In patients with angiographically visible atherosclerosis, acethylcholine and cold pressor test exerted coronary vasoconstriction. Moreover, flow-dependent, endothelium-mediated dilation was attenuated in those patients demonstrating visible luminal irregularities in the vessel under study. In patients with hypercholesterolemia, substantial endothelial dysfunction (as assessed by attenuated blood-flow increase in response to acetylcholine) was demonstrated in the coronary microcirculation.

Thus, progression of endothelial dysfunction occurs during the early course of development of coronary atherosclerosis. Utilizing quantitative coronary angiography and the intracoronary Doppler technique, these early functional alterations can be identified safely at a stage when atherosclerotic lesions are not detectable by angiography. This may be useful in designing early effective interventions which restore endothelial function and prevent the occurrence of overt atherosclerosis.

Key words: Endothelial dysfunction; hypercholesterolemia; coronary microcirculation; flow-dependent dilation

Endothelial injury represents a critical initiating event in the pathogenesis of atherosclerosis. The modified response to injury hypothesis of atherosclerosis suggests that at least two pathways may lead to formation of initial smooth-muscle proliferation lesions. One pathway, demonstrated in hypercholesterolemia, involves monocyte and possibly platelet interactions, which in turn may stimulate fibrons-plaque formation by growth-factor release from a variety of cells (32). It is likely that hypercholesterolemia induces a subtle form of "injury" to endothelium, e.g., if endothelial cells are bathed in chronically elevated levels of LDL, rapid cholesterol exchange may emerge with plasma membrane of endothelial cells, leading to subtle elevations in cholesterol, phospholipid, and protein ratios (18). In addition, elevated levels of lipoprotein (a) may suppress the cells "sentinel" fibrinolytic mechanism, by inhibiting plasminogen binding and, hence, plasmin generation, thereby leading to a prothrombolytic tendency (15). In addition to its gradual modification of the endothelial cells with hyperlipidemic plasma as observed in atherosclerosis, LDL may instantly modify the property of the endothelial cells through its functional changes, i.e., LDL may antagonize the defense mechanism of the endothelium against various vasoconstrictors. Andrews et al. have shown that LDL reduces endothelium-dependent relaxation of the isolated rabbit aorta and diminishes the release of EDRF from cultured endothelial cells (1). Indeed, numerous experimental studies in animals of diet-induced hypercholesterolemia have demonstrated attenuation of endothelium-dependent relaxation in vivo (14, 41), as well as the augmented vasoconstrictor responses to various neurohumoral agents (22). Collectively, it is conceivable that early endothelial dysfunction represents an important link in the occurrence and progression of coronary artery disease in man. Since chronically elevated levels of LDL are associated with an increased incidence of atherosclerosis in humans, patients with established hypercholesterolemia type II may serve as an appropriate study population for investigating early functional endothelial alterations in the development of atherosclerosis.

Importantly, despite the abnormal endothelial response, morphologic endothelial injury has not been described early in cholesterol diet-induced atherosclerosis (5, 8, 13). Thus, the evaluation of endothelial function may provide a means to detect early vascular alterations preceeding obstructive atherosclerotic lesions. This would be of utmost importance for the coronary circulation, e.g., if functional abnormalities, due to endothelial dysfunction within the coronary circulation are associated with substantial changes in coronary flow, they may be involved in the development of ischemia, and hence, clinical symptoms. The early detection of endothelial dysfunction of the coronary circulation in the absence of flow-limiting stenosis, may therefore provide a clue for early interventions in order to restore the functional integrity and to induce the regression of abnormalities associated with the development of atherosclerosis.

Until recently, the investigation of endothelial function was confined to in-vitro experiments or animals research. Although our understanding of basic mechanisms has been substantially expanded by the experimental data, the functional significance of the endothelium in humans remained elusive. Ludmer et al. first demonstrated in humans that atherosclerotic arteries paradoxically constrict in response to acetylcholine and, thus, abnormal constriction may be related to impaired endothelial vasodilator function (23). In contrast, in individuals without risk factors of coronary artery disease, a modest coronary vasodilation in response to acetylcholine was observed. More recently, Hodgson et al. confirmed in humans that the net response to acetylcholine depends on the interplay between direct vasoconstriction and EDRF-mediated vasodilation (16). Pretreatment with methylene blue, an inhibitor of EDRF, potentiated epicardial artery vasoconstriction with acetylcholine (16). However, we have recently shown that acetylcholine induces dilation of resistance vessels, even in patients with coronary artery disease who demonstrated vasoconstriction of epicardial coronary arteries (11). Thus, vascular tone of the coronary resistance vessels of humans are, at least in part, under control of EDRF. The vasoconstrictor response to acetylcholine is confined to epicardial arteries, indicating that the direct vasoconstriction of acetylcholine overrides the endothelium-dependent dilation in atherosclerotic epicardial arteries.

Evaluation of progression of endothelial dysfunction in humans

To investigate the progression of endothelial dysfunction in the coronary circulation of humans, the evaluation should include patients with different degrees of coronary artery disease. To this end, we studied four groups of patients. Group I comprised normal patients with smooth coronary arteries, devoid of risk factors for atherosclerosis such as hypertension, family history, smoking or high serum cholesterol.

Since hypercholesterolemia type II represents a condition associated with early subtle endothelial injury (without morphologic alterations) and subsequent development of coronary artery disease, patients with high serum LDL-cholesterol levels and angiographically normal coronary arteries comprised group II. Patients with different degrees of overt atherosclerosis within the coronary circulation comprised group III (angiographically normal vessel under study, yet angiographic evidence of atherosclerosis elsewhere in the coronary system) and group IV (visible luminal irregularities in the vessel under study, but no flow-limiting stenosis).

Since the impairment of endothelium-dependent relaxation in hypercholesterolemia may be receptor-specific (5), it is crucial to test several vasodilator (or vasoconstrictor) stimuli. In contrast to the experimental setting, the functional assessment of endothelial function in the coronary circulation of humans in vivo has been limited to the intracoronary application of acetylcholine. More recently, other endothelium-dependent agents such as substance P (2) and serotonin (24) were utilized in humans. However, substance P is disadvantageous in that it elicits only modest vasodilator effects with a rapid development of tolerance. Yet, the contrasting effects of acetylcholine on normal vs atherosclerotic arteries facilitate the recognition of the abnormal response. Serotonin would be a very attractive agent since it presumably has pathophysiologic relevance. However, serotonin bears an increased risk of platelet activation and, subsequently, intracoronary thrombosis, thus posing a high risk in patients instrumented with intracoronary catheters.

Although acetylcholine represents an important agent to assess endothelial function in the coronary circulation in humans in vivo, the role of acetylcholine as a physiological regulator of vascular tone remains controversial. It is widely believed that acetylcholine released from parasympathic nerve endings cannot reach the endothelium to cause the release of EDRF (40). In contrast, recent studies provided some evidence that acetylcholine can activate endothelial cells from the adventitial side, indicating the acetylcholine released from cholinergic nerve endings may contribute to the vasomotor tone by an endothelium-dependent mechanism (10, 19, 38). In our study, acetylcholine was used as a means to evaluate endothelial function, irrespective of its controversial pathophysiological role.

In addition to the large number of neurohumoral substances that stimulate the release of EDRF, mechanical stimuli such as changes in shear stress do modulate EDRF-release (30, 33). Indeed, several experimental studies have shown that increases in flow are accompanied by a dilation of the conduit vessels. By injecting papaverine subselectively into the midportion of a coronary artery, a transient maximal flow can be elicited. We have recently demonstrated that using this approach, a substantial *flow-dependent* dilation emerges in the proximal coronary artery exposed to increased flow, but not to papaverine directly (12). The cold pressor test is another stimuli applicable to patients in the catheterization laboratory. We have shown that the dilation of normal and the constriction of atherosclerotic coronary arteries with the cold pressor test exactly mirrors the response to acetylcholine (43). It appears that endothelial dysfunction in coronary atherosclerosis results in a loss of normal dilator function and permits that vasoconstrictor response to sympathetic stimulation to supercede in this setting. Thus, the cold pressor test provides a useful tool to test the endothelial-dependent coronary vasomotion.

Endothelial function in different early stages of coronary atherosclerosis

Utilizing these three different endothelial-dependent stimuli, we demonstrated progressive impairment in endothelium-mediated modulation of coronary vasomotor tone with different stages of early atherosclerosis in humans (43). In patients with angiographically completely normal epicardial coronary arteries and absence of any risk factor for coronary artery disease, the vasomotor response to intracoronary acetylcholine increased blood flow and sympathetic stimulation is characterized by coronary dilation. In patients with angiographically normal coronary arteries, but significant hypercholesterolemia (LDL >180 mg%), acetylcholine elicited coronary vasoconstriction, whereas the dilator response to sympathetic stimulation with cold pressor test and flow-dependent, endothelium mediated dilation was preserved. In coronary artery disease, acetylcholine and cold pressor test caused coronary vasoconstriction. Moreover, flow-dependent endothelium-mediated dilation was attenuated in those patients demonstrating visible luminal irregularities by angiography (indicative of advanced atherosclerosis in the vessel). Patients of group I, II, and III demonstrated similar vasodilator responses to intracoronary nitroglycerin, excluding that unspecific unresponsiveness of the coronary vessels accounts for these findings in patients with abnormal reactivity to acetylcholine. The demonstration of progressive endothelial dysfunction with early stages of atherosclerosis as observed in the clinical setting (44) are in keeping with experimental studies. Cohen et al. (5) reported a selective endothelial cell-receptor mediated relaxation, suggesting that it is not the ability of the coronary artery endothelium to elaborate vasodilators. Rather the initiation of the coronary artery endothelial cell response to 5-hydroxytryptamin and substance P was affected by hypercholesterolemia in the pig (5).

Shimokawa and Vanhoutte have demonstrated that hypercholesterolemia attenuates endothelium-dependent relaxation in response to platelets and serotonin, but not to bradykinin and calcium ionophore (35). This suggests that hypercholesterolemia interferes with some, but not all receptor-mediated mechanisms for the release of EDRF.

Kolodgie et al. observed that endothelial-dependent relaxation in the hyperlipidemic Watanabe rabbit progressively decreased as the severity of the individual lesions increased (21).

In all these experimental studies, hypercholesterolemia selectively impaired receptor-mediated mechanisms for induction of endothelium-dependent relaxation. In contrast, endothelium-dependent relaxation induced to calcium ionophore A 23187 has been shown to be preserved in hypercholesterolemia. The release of nitric oxide from endothelial cells critically depends on a sustained increase of intracellular free calcium (3). Whereas A 23187 mediates the release of EDRF (= nitric oxide) and, subsequently endothelium-dependent relaxation, by directly inducing calcium influx in the endothelial cells, the receptor-mediated increase in cytosolic free calcium involves several steps. Intracellular events that link receptor stimulation to the release of EDRF include the activation of a guanosine 5′-triphosphate regulatory protein and phospholipase C, which in turn results in the generation of inositol 1, 4, 5 triphosphate and diacylglycerol. IP3 is responsible for the discharge of calcium from intracellular stores, (diacylglycerol activates proteinkinase C). In addition, receptor-mediated hyperpolarization appears to exert a sustained increase in calcium influx from extracellular space (3).

There is experimental evidence that endothelial dysfunction in the chronic regenerated stage (such as hyperlipidemia) may be associated with a dysfunctional pertussis-toxin sensible G-protein. These findings may implicate an impaired G protein mediated mechanism (limiting the generation of IP3) as an important factor involved in the attenuated endothelium-dependent relaxation in hypercholesterolemia. Although such a mechanism has been reported for serotonin only, there is evidence that acetylcholine acts via an activation of G-protein and the phosphoinosital-pathway (29). Moreover, it has been shown that LDL interferes with the phosphotidyl-inositol metabolism which may account for (or contribute to) the attenuated endothelium-dependent relaxation in hypercholesterolemia. Nevertheless, as mentioned earlier, an unspecific (and reversible?) inhibition of endothelium-dependent relaxation by hypercholesterolemic plasma cannot be excluded at present (39). Obviously, altered plasma lipid composition in hypercholesterolemia may affect endothelium-dependent dilation by different mechanisms.

It should be kept in mind, however, that the plasma levels of cholesterol achieved in these experimental studies exceeded by far those levels seen in the clinical setting.

The present clinical data demonstrate that the assessment of coronary endothelial function in patients during coronary angiography provides a functional assessment of the vascular reactivity to detect early alteration in the development of atherosclerosis beyond the simple evaluation of coronary anatomy and severity of lesions associated with advanced atherosclerosis.

Interestingly, the coronary vasomotor response to cold pressor test was normal in patients with hypercholesterolemia, in keeping with a normal vascular response to norepinephrine in the rabbit aorta with modest elevations of serum cholesterol (26). Yet, there is some evidence that hypercholesterolemia promotes exaggerated alpha-adrenergic vasoconstriction possibly by an exaggerated release of thromboxane A 2 (37).

In contrast, patients with coronary artery disease demonstrated a vasoconstrictor response to sympathetic stimulation, as reported recently (43). Although atherosclerotic lesions were not angiographically visible in the LAD of group III, an early stage of atherosclerosis with diffuse intimal thickening of the vessel wall can be anticipated. Indeed, intra-operative echocardiographic studies have demonstrated that vessel atherosclerosis may be extensive, despite lack of angiographical evidence of coronary artery disease (25). Thus, the vasoconstrictor response to cold pressor test in group III patients may reflect the notion that the LAD (vessel under study) was diseased, demonstrating a paradoxical constriction to both cold pressor test and intracoronary acetylcholine [see (44)].

Interestingly, the flow-dependent, endothelium-mediated vasodilation of large epicardial coronary arteries, appears to be a robust mechanism of vasorelaxation. We have recently demonstrated that this mechanism is impaired in atherosclerotic coronary arteries (12). The present data suggest that flow-dependent dilation remains preserved during the early stages of atherosclerosis, but deteriorates only in more advanced atherosclerotic conduit arteries. In such arteries, the vasodilative response to the endothelium-independent agent nitroglycerin was attenuated to similar extent, suggesting an overall impairment in vascular dilator capacity. It is conceivable that flow-dependent, endothelium-mediated dilation may be mediated, not only by the release of nitric oxide, but also by activation of potassium channels to hyperpolarize the endothelium and the underlying smooth muscle (6). In early stages of endothelial dysfunction, e.g., as observed in hypercholesterolemia, the synthesis and/or release appear to be reduced (7), however, the ion flux mediated hyperpolarization and subsequent relaxation of vascular smooth muscle may be preserved.

Endothelial dysfunction in the coronary microcirculation

Intracoronary acetylcholine induces a substantial increase in flow, both in humans and animals, indicating dilation of resistance vessels (11, 16, 17). Even when acetylcholine

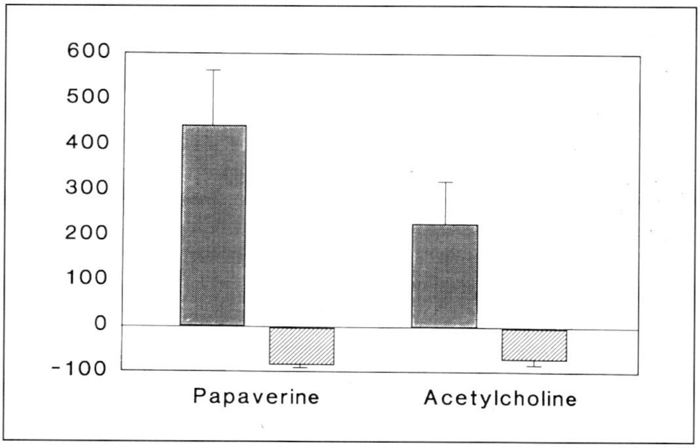

Fig. 1. Percent change in coronary blood flow (black bars) and vascular resistance (hatched bars) in response to papaverine (endothelial-independent dilator of coronary resistance vessels) and acetylcholine (endothelium-dependent, presumably by stimulating release of EDRF) in patients with normal coronary arteries without risk factors

constricts epicardial coronary arteries, vasodilation of coronary resistance vessels have been observed in patients with coronary artery disease (11, 16, 27). By comparing the blood-flow response of the endothelium-mediated dilator acetylcholine to the one elicited by the non-specific dilator of resistance vessels papaverine, the degree of endothelium-dependent arteriolar dilation can be demonstrated in comparison to a maximal arteriolar coronary dilation (Fig. 1). This approach revealed that endothelial-dependent vasodilation within the coronary microcirculation is substantially impaired in patients with hypercholesterolemia (Fig. 2). The abnormal endothelium vascular relaxation in the coronary microcirculation in patients of group III and IV was most prominent if they had elevated serum LDL-cholesterol levels (44).

Thus, hypercholesterolemia impairs endothelium-mediated dilation in the coronary microcirculation where overt atherosclerosis does not develop. It is conceivable that these abnormalities of endothelial function modify the regulation of myocardial perfusion by neurohumoral agents, such as noradrenaline, thromboxane, or serotonin. In fact, endothelial dysfunction of the coronary microvasculature may contribute to the pathogenesis of myocardial ischemia and chest pain in these patients. In this respect, recent experimental studies have shown that reactive hyperemia in the coronary circulation is significantly reduced during inhibition of NO-formation by L-NMMA (31).

It appears that the reduced peak hyperemic flow (attenuated reactive hyperemia) following inhibition of endothelium-derived nitric oxide (= EDRF) is due to reduced flow-dependent (endothelium-mediated) dilation and enhanced myogenic activity of coronary resistance vessels.

Coronary dilation of resistance vessels (which in turn regulates flow during reactive hyperemia) may be attributed to both the release of adenosine and adenosine nucleotides such as ATP and ADP besides other unidentified mechanisms. Whereas adenosine causes vasodilation via specific adenosin receptors, ATP and ADP activate purinergic receptors and thereby release nitric oxide (20). Thus, endothelial dysfunction (= reduced release of EDRF) of resistance vessels is likely to impair reactive hyperemia in the

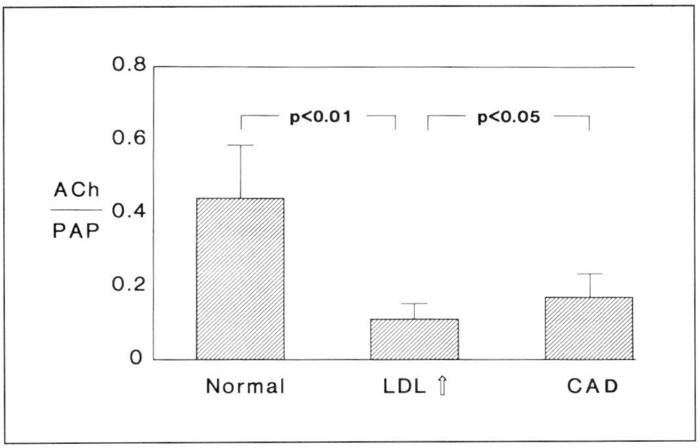

Fig. 2 Ratio of coronary blood flow during acetylcholine vs blood flow during papaverine in normal individuals, in patients with hypercholesterolemia (LDL↑) and patients with coronary artery disease (CAD). Since this ratio comprises the response to endothelial-dependent vs endothelial-independent dilation of coronary resistance vessels, it indicates endothelial dysfunction in the microvasculature of patients with hypercholesterolemia

coronary circulation secondary to the loss of ATP and ADP mediated release of EDRF. Notably, the pharmacological-induced maximal coronary flow reserve to papaverine is not affected by endothelial dysfunction.

Taken together, impaired release of EDRF does not only affect basal vascular resistance, but also affects mechanisms which are important in the control of flow adaptation to changing tissue demand. Indeed, a reduced oxygen uptake associated with increased lactate release has been observed in isolated hearts after treatment with N-nitro-L-arginine (31). Reduced endothelium-mediated coronary flow reserve may represent a contributing factor for the development of myocardial ischemia in the absence of obstructive coronary artery disease. Preliminary data from our laboratory (unpublished observation) as well as of Vogt et al. (42) suggest that endothelial dysfunction may be present in a subset of patients with normal coronary arteries and chest pain.

Aggregation of human platelets is inhibited by EDRF. Thus, functioning endothelium not only protects the underlying smooth muscle from a variety of constricting substances, but also prevents platelet aggregation. It is conceivable that endothelial dysfunction of the coronary resistance vessels facilitate platelets aggregation, which in turn is associated with the release of thromboxane and serotonin. Moreover, endothelial dysfunction of the coronary microcirculation would favor vasoconstriction to thromboxane and serotonin as recently observed in atherosclerotic primates (4, 34).

In addition, recent studies have documented that the relaxation in response, not only to acetylcholine, but also to ADP is abolished in isolated coronary resistance vessels obtained from cholesterol-fed rabbits (28). Endothelial dysfunction of the microvasculature in patients with hypercholesterolemia might therefore favor platelet adhesion and aggregation with subsequent platelet-induced contraction of coronary smooth muscle (e.g., by increased levels of thromboxane and serotonin) and thus, facilitate ischemic events. Recent studies suggest that both EDRF and endothelial and vascular smooth muscle-derived prostaglandins do modulate the coronary response to thromboxane in vivo (36). Interestingly, increased thromboxane levels in the coronary sinus blood with cold pressor test have been observed in patients with typical angina and angiographically normal coronary arteries (9).

References

1. Andrews HE, Bruckdorfer KR, Dunn RC, Jacobs M (1987) Low-density lipoproteins inhibit endothelium-dependent relaxation in rabbit aorta. Nature 327:237–9
2. Bosaller C, Hehlert-Frierich C, Jost S, Rafflenbeul W, Lichtlen P (1989) Angiographic assessment of human coronary artery endothelial function by measurement of endothelium-dependent vasodilation. Eur Heart J 10:44–48
3. Busse R, Lückhoff A, Mülsch A (1991) Cellular mechanisms controlling EDRF/NO formation in endothelial cells. Bas Res Cardiol 86 (Suppl 2):7–16
4. Chilian WM, Dellsperger KC, Layne SM, Eastham CL, Armstrong MA, Marcus ML, Heistad DD (1990) Effects of atherosclerosis on the coronary microcirculation. Am J Physiol 258:H529–39
5. Cohen RA, Zitnay KM, Haudenschild CC, Cunningham LD (1988) Loss of selective endothelial cell vasoactive functions caused by hypercholesterolemia in pig coronary arteries. Circ Res 63:903–910
6. Cooke JP, Andon N, Loscalzo J (1989) Mechanism of flow-mediated endothelium-dependent vasodilation (abstract). Circulation 80:II–124
7. Cooke JP, Dzau VJ, Creager MA (1991) Endothelial dysfunction in hypercholesterolemia is corrected by L-arginine. Bas Res Cardiol 86 (Suppl 2):173–181
8. Davies PF, Reidy MA, Goode TB, Bowyer DE (1976) Scanning electron microscopy in the evaluation of endothelial integrity of the fatty lesions in atherosclerosis. Atherosclerosis 25:125–130
9. DiDonato M, Fantini F, Maioli M, Prisco D, Rogasi PG, Neri Serneri GG (1987) Blood velocity in the coronary artery circulation: Relation to thromboxane A2 levels in coronary sinus in patients with angiographically normal coronary arteries. Catheterization and cardiovascular diagnosis 13:162–6
10. Dohi Y, Thiel MA, Bühler FR, Lüscher TF (1990) Activation of endothelial L-arginine pathway in resistance arteries. Effect of age and hypertension. Hypertension 15:170–9
11. Drexler H, Zeiher AM, Wollschläger H, Meinertz T, Just H (1989) Contrasting effects of acetylcholine on coronary conductance and resistance vessels in patients with coronary artery disease. (abstr) J Am Coll Cardiol 13:133 A
12. Drexler H, Zeiher AM, Wollschläger H, Meinertz T, Just H, Bonzel T (1989) Flow-dependent coronary artery dilatation in humans. Circulation 80:466–74
13. Faggioto A, Ross R, Harker L (1984) Studies of hypercholesterolemia in the nonhuman primates. I. Changes that lead to fatty streak formation. Arteriosclerosis 4:323–340
14. Freiman PC, Mitchell GC, Heistad DD, Armstrong ML, Harrison DG (1986) Atherosclerosis impairs endothelium-dependent vascular relaxation to acetylcholine and thrombin in primates. Circ Res 58:783–789
15. Hajjar KA, Gavish D, Breslow JL, Nachman RL (1989) Lipoprotein (a) modulation of endothelial cell surface fribinolysis and its potential role in atherosclerosis. Nature 339:303–305
16. Hodgson J, Marshall JJ (1989) Direct vasoconstriction and endothelium-dependent vasodilation. Mechanism of acetylcholine effects on coronary flow and arterial diameter in patients with nonstenotic coronary arteries. Circulation 79:1043–51
17. Horio Y, Yasue H, Okumura K, Takaoka KI, Matsuyama K, Goto K, Monoda K (1988) Effects of intracoronary injection of acetylcholine on coronary arterial hemodynamics and diameter. Am J Cardiol 62:887–891
18. Jackson RL, Gotto AM (1976) Hypothesis concerning membrane structure, cholesterol and atherosclerosis. In: Paoletti R, Gotto AM (eds) Atherosclerosis Reviews, vol 1. Raven, New York, pp 21–32
19. Kalsner S (1989) Cholinergic constriction in the general circulation and its role in coronary artery spasm. Circ Res 65:237–57

20. Kelm M, Feelisch M, Spahr R, Piper H-M, Noack E, Schrader J (1988) Quantitative and kinetic characterization of nitric oxide and EDRF released from cultured endothelial cells. Biochem Biophys Res Commun 154:236–244
21. Kolodgie FD, Virmani R, Rice HE, Mergner WJ (1990) Vascular reactivity during the progression of atherosclerotic plaque. A study in watanabe heritable hyperlipidemic rabbits. Circ Res 66:1112–1126
22. Lopez JAG, Armstrong ML, Piegors DJ, Heistad (1989) Effect of early and advanced atherosclerosis on vascular responses to serotonin, thromboxane A2, and ADP. Circulation 79:698–705
23. Ludmer PL, Selwyn AP, Shook TL, Wayne RR, Madge GH, Alexander RW, Ganz P (1986) Paradoxical vasoconstriction induced by acetylcholine in atherosclerotic coronary arteries. N Engl J Med 315:1046–51
24. McFadden E, Clarke J, Haider W, Kaski J, Davies G, Maseri A (1990) The effect of serotonin on the coronary circulation in patients (abstract). Eur Heart J 11:206
25. McPherson DD, Hiratzka LF, Lamberth WC, Brandt B, Hunt M, Kieso RA, Marcus ML, Kerber R (1987) Delineation of the extent of coronary atherosclerosis by high-frequency epicardial echocardiography. N Engl J Med 316:304–9
26. Merkel LA, Rivera LM, Bilder GE, Perrone MH (1990) Differential alteration of vascular reactivity in rabbit aorta with modest elevation of serum cholesterol. Circ Res 67:550–555
27. Newman CM, Hackett DR, Fryer M, El-Tamimi HM, Davies GJ, Maseri A (1987) Dual effects of acetylcholine on angiographically normal human coronary arteries in vivo (abstract). Circulation 76:IV–238
28. Osborne JA, Siegman MJ, Sedar AW, Mooers SU, Lefer AM (1989) Lack of endothelium-dependent relaxation in coronary resistance arteries of cholesterol-fed rabbits. Am J Physiol 256:C591–7
29. Piomelli D, Pinto A, Mullane K (1986) The mechanism of release of endothelium-derived relaxing factor by acetylcholine (abstract 79). Hypertension 8:834
30. Pohl U, Holtz J, Busse R, Bassenge E (1986) Crucial role of endothelium in the vasodilator response to increased flow in vivo. Hypertension 8:37–44
31. Pohl U, Lamontagne D (1991) Impaired tissue perfusion after inhibition of endothelium-derived nitric oxide. Basic Res Cardiol 86 (Suppl 2):97–105
32. Ross R (1986) The pathogenesis of atherosclerosis – an update. N Engl J Med 314:488–500
33. Rubanyi GM, Romero JC, Vanhoutte PM (1986) Flow-induced release of endothelium-derived relaxing factor. Am J Physiol 250:H1145–9
34. Sellke FW, Armstrong ML, Harrison DG (1990) Endothelium-dependent vascular relaxation is abnormal in the coronary microcirculation of atherosclerotic primates. Circulation 81:1586–93
35. Shimokawa H, Vanhoutte (1989) Impaired endothelium-dependent relaxation to aggregating platelets and related substances in porcine coronary arteries in hypercholesterolemia and atherosclerosis. Circ Res 64:900–14
36. Szwajkun K, Lamping KG, Dole WP (1990) Role of endothelium-derived relaxing factor and prostaglandins in reponses of coronary arteries to thromboxane in vivo. Circ Res 66:1729–37
37. Takahashi K, Kawaguchi H, Yasuda H (1989) The hypertensive response to vasopressor agents stimulates the release of thromboxane A2 in hypercholesterolaemic rabbits. Cardiovasc Res 23:788–796
38. Tesfamariam B, Halpern W (1988) Endothelium-dependent and endothelium-independent vasodilation in resistance arteries from hypertensive rats. Hypertension 11:440–4
39. Tomita T, Ezaki M, Miwa M, Nakamura K, Inoue Y (1990) Rapid and reversible inhibition by low density lipoprotein of the endothelium-dependent relaxation to hemostatic substances in porcine coronary arteries. Heat and acid labile factors in low density lipoprotein mediate the inhibition. Circ Res 66:18–27
40. Vanhoutte PM (1989) Endothelium and control of vascular function. Hypertension 13:658–67
41. Verbeuren TJ, Jordaens FH, Zonnekeyn LL, Van Hove CE, Coene MC, Herman AG (1986) Effect of hypercholesterolemia on vascular reactivity in the rabbit. Circ Res 58:552–564
42. Vogt M, Rabenau O, Motz W, Strauer BE (1989) Evidence of endothelial dysfunction in patients with angina pectoris and angiographically normal coronary arteries (abstr) Circulation 80:II–436A

43. Zeiher M, Drexler H, Wollschläger H, Saurbier B, Just H (1989) Coronary vasomotion in response to sympathetic stimulation in humans: importance of the functional integrity of the endothelium. J Am Coll Cardiol 14:1181–1190
44. Zeiher AM, Drexler H, Wollschläger H, Just H (1991) Modulation of coronary vasomotor tone in humans: progressive endothelial dysfunction with different early stages of coronary atherosclerosis. Circulation 83:391–401

Author's address:
Helmut Drexler, M.D.
Medizinische Klinik III
University of Freiburg
Hugstetter Str. 55
W-7800 Freiburg, FRG

Response of coronary arteries to nitrates, the EDRF-donor SIN-1, and calcium antagonists

W. Schulz and G. Kober

Faculty of Medicine, Johann Wolfgang Goethe-Universität Frankfurt/Main, FRG

Summary: Intracoronary drug administration is an important tool to study coronary effects without interaction of systemic effects. The difficult methodological aspects and the results of clinical trials in which the effects of vasodilating drugs were evaluated with respect to coronary dilatation are reviewed.

Major (coronary substrate, study design) and minor (measuring devices, methods of evaluation) methodological problems make it difficult to precisely evaluate pharmacological effects such as dose-response relationship, duration of action, and selective responses, and to compare the effects of different drugs. From a clinical point of view, knowledge of the maximal effect (ED_{max}) in coronary stenoses and the duration of action is essential.

NO-donors tend to act stronger than CA-channel blockers which may be attributable to their different modes of action. Among those NO-donors investigated, SIN-1 showed stronger effects than nitroglycerin. Only with SIN-1 were maximal effects obviously achieved. The additional administration of nitroglycerin or nisoldipine never led to a more prominent dilatation.

In coronary stenoses, the underlying morphology causes a wider range of responses than is seen in normal segments: deendothelialized stenoses with high coronary tone show a larger dilatation, while fully sclerotic stenoses may not react.

Key words: Coronary tone; coronary spasm; coronary vasomotion; NO-donors; calcium antagonists

Introduction

Early in this century, assumptions were increasingly made that coronary vasomotion and coronary spasms contribute to coronary heart disease. They were based on clinical and electrocardiographic observations by Osler 1910, Siegel and Feil 1931, Parkinson and Bedford 1931, Wilson and Johnston 1941, Prinzmetal et al. 1959, and Peretz 1961 (24–27, 41, 43). Angiographic confirmation of coronary spasms eliciting angina pectoris was given by Gensini 1962, Dhurandhar et al. 1972, Oliva et al. 1973, Maseri et al. 1975, and Maseri et al. 1977 (10, 15, 21–23).

The dilatation of epicardial coronary arteries following drug-therapy was first demonstrated by Gensini in 1962 (15) using intravenous isosorbide dinitrate, and by Maseri in 1975 (21) with sublingual nitroglycerin. The effects of intracoronary injections of various compounds on epicardial coronary arteries were also investigated with nitroglycerin (14), nifedipine (31), verapamil (9), gallopamil (38), and SIN-1, the active metabolite of molsidomine (35).

Some aspects with respect to the quality and quantity of the effects of different drugs on epicardial coronary segments and stenoses have since been answered. However, many other questions are still open. This paper will therefore review the current pharmacological knowledge, and highlight open questions.

Methodological aspects

The precise pharmacological characterization of coronary dilating effects – which comprises the dose-response relationship, half-life time, and selective responses – is largely dependent on the methods used. Several methodological problems impair a precise characterization and comparisons of drug effects.

Coronary substrate

The site of measurement is not standardized. With respect to clinical relevance it seems most reasonable to measure coronary stenoses. Coronary stenoses, however, show a wider range of individual reactions than normal segments according to their underlying morphology, e.g., concentric or excentric stenoses.

Study design

There is no design yet which can meet all experimental and ethical needs in the special situation of coronary arteriography. *Intraindividual* comparisons of repetitive angiograms (cross-over design) are limited by carry-over effects and the duration of the investigation. *Interindividual* investigations (parallel design) require an unrealistic high number of patients as the interindividual variability of the coronary reactions is very high.

Methods to measure coronary stenoses

In the past, investigators used simple caliper measurements from standardized projections with a subsequent correction for magnification factors based on simple calculations (20, 35). Today, highly sophisticated computerized self-contouring systems with multiple algorithms for evaluation are in use. These new methods have been validated and avoid the high inter- and intraindividual variability (7, 30), yet they are time-consuming and cannot avoid bias caused by angiograms obtained in slightly different angulations which can be essential in eccentric stenoses.

Evaluation of response

The published data differ concerning the evaluation of the coronary response. Some authors evaluate the data of all patients investigated according to "intention to treat" (36, 40). In other investigations only so-called responders are considered (19, 29).

Furthermore, the changes in coronary segments are sometimes expressed as measured diameter changes (3, 13, 32, 33), and sometimes as calculated cross-sectional-area changes (7, 28, 29).

Results of published clinical studies

Dose-response relationship

Many investigators have given different doses of various vasoactive compounds by the intracoronary route. These results from the literature for nitroglycerin, nifedipine,

Table 1. Coronary dilatation in percent following intracoronary, intravenous, sublingual, and oral administration of various antianginal drugs

CORONARY DILATATION (%)
Evaluation (E): D = diam., C = cross-sect. area, A = all patients, R = responder only
t = time of measurement after application

Investigator	Substance (mg)	E	t (min)	N=	Glob.	Normal vessels Prox.	Normal vessels Med.	Normal vessels Dist.	Stenotic vessels Prest.	Stenotic vessels Sten.	Stenotic vessels Postst.
	Nitroglycerin										
Brown	0.05IC	A, C	1′	11	46	–	–	–	–	29	–
Feldman	0.40SL	A, D	5′	34	–	16	20	25	–	–	–
			5′	41	–	–	–	–	–	6	–
Rafflenbeul	0.80IC	R, C	10′	25	–	–	–	–	–	28	–
Schulz	0.16IC	A, D	5′	80	–	7	10	12	–	24	–
	1.60IV	A, D	5′	80	–	12	14	14	–	10	–
	Nifedipine										
Rafflenbeul	20PO	R, C	5′	20	–	–	–	–	–	31	–
Schulz	0.1IC	A, D	10′	16	–	14	7	14	11	6	8
	1.0IV	A, D	10′	16	–	19	17	26	9	8	7
	Diltiazem										
Bonzel	20IV	R, D	5′	22	–	2	–	16	4	5	6
	Verapamil										
Simonetti	0.05IC	A, C	5′	3	0	–	–	–	–	–	–
	0.25IC	A, C	5′	7	5	–	–	–	–	–	–
	0.35IC	A, C	5′	6	11	–	–	–	–	–	–
	0.50IC	A, C	5′	13	20	–	–	–	–	–	–
Chew	0.145/kgIV	A, C	2′	12	7–14	–	–	–	–	–	–

diltiazem, and verapamil are given in Table 1, and for SIN-1 – the most extensively investigated compound – in Table 2. In addition in Table 1, some relevant results achieved with sublingual, oral, and intravenous application are shown. A dose-response relationship is usually characterized by ED_{min}, ED_{50} and ED_{max}. Such a precise characterization, however, has not been convincingly established for coronary effects with any drug. As may be expected from the mentioned methodological problems, the results of the different studies are in part contradictory and show a tremendous variability.

Fortunately, there is no real clinical need to precisely evaluate dose-response relationships for coronary reactions. It is, however, important to have an idea about ED_{max}, which may provide the best clinical effect for the patient in relation to side-effects.

Intracoronary doses of NO-donors (nitroglycerin, SIN-1) causing maximal dilating effects usually do not create safety problems, because even intracoronary overdoses are only low systemic doses. Calcium channel-blockers as verapamil, gallopamil, and diltiazem, however, may most likely impair SA- and AV-conduction and are in some patients not suitable for intracoronary injection, whereas nifedipine does not have negative electrophysiological effects (35).

The following intracoronary doses have been evaluated so far: SIN-1 0.125–1 mg, nitroglycerin 0.05–0.80 mg, nifedipine 0.1 mg, and verapamil 0.05–0.50 mg. Direct com-

Table 2. Coronary dilatation in percent following intracoronary administration of SIN-1, the active metabolite of molsidomine

CORONARY DILATATION (%)
Evaluation (E): D = diam., C = cross-sect. area, A = all patients, R = responder only
t = time of measurement after application

Investi-gator	SIN-1 (mg)	E	t (min)	N=	Normal vessels				Stenotic vessels		
					Glob.	Prox.	Med.	Dist.	Prest.	Sten.	Postst.
Bertrand	0.2I C	A, D	5′	6	20	–	–	–	–	–	–
	0.4I C	A, D	5′	6	67–73	–	–	–	–	–	–
	0.8 IC	A, D	5′	6	28	–	–	–	–	–	–
Bonzel	0.125IC	A, C	2′	5	36	–	–	–	45	35	52
	0.250IC	A, C	2′	5	40	–	–	–	63	45	95
	0.500IC	A, C	2′	5	77	–	–	–	95	10	15
Karsch	0.4I C	R, D	0.3′	14	–	–	–	–	–	28	–
Schulz	0.4I C	A, D	2′	17	–	9	18	26	10	32	22
	0.4I C	A, D	10′	17	–	12	18	29	17	48	38
Serruys	1.0I C	A, C	2′	10	12	LAD:11	11	9	–	16	–
						RC:14	–	17	–	–	–
	1.0I C	A, C	60′	10	8	LAD: 9	4	4	–	10	–
						R, C: 8	–	13	–	–	–
	1+1IC	A, C	62′	10	14	LAD:13	12	12	–	15	–
						RC:16	–	22	–	–	–
Sobolski	0.8I C	A, D	4′	15	–	26	40	50	–	47	–
	0.8I C	A, D	8′	15	–	25	43	26	–	24	–

Table 3. EC50-values and corresponding NO-release following various organic nitrates with cysteine and SIN-1 without cysteine (from (12)).

Organic nitrate + cysteine (5 mM)	EC_{50} value mM	Nitric oxide release (μmol/min)
ETN	0.145	0.046 ± 0.002
GTN	0.069	0.050 ± 0.005
IMDN	0.200	0.045 ± 0.003
IIDN	0.240	0.047 ± 0.004
ISDN	0.280	0.046 ± 0.002
IS-2-N	0.750	0.047 ± 0.004
IS-5-N	1.000	0.045 ± 0.003
SIN-1 (without cysteine)	0.0028	0.054 ± 0.007

parisons of the results are difficult. It seems, however, that SIN-1 shows stronger effects than nitroglycerin or calcium channel-blockers. This difference may be due either to a specific pharmacological effect or to relative overdosing of SIN-1.

SIN-1 was often given in equal or higher mg-doses than nitroglycerin. Preclinical studies, however, showed that the EC50-value for guanylate stimulation is much lower for SIN-1 (12) than for any other NO-donor (Table 3). Thus, it seems very likely that in the published clinical studies with only SIN-1 the end of the dose-response curve was reached and SIN-1, which is well tolerated, was most likely overdosed. This assumption is supported by the clinical finding that additional 0.8 mg i.c. nitroglycerin following 0.025 mg/kg SIN-1 as intracoronary infusion did not induce further coronary dilatation (16).

Pharmacological differences between NO-donors (SIN-1, nitroglycerin) and Ca-blockers (nifedipine, diltiazem, verapamil), however, may explain the weaker dilating action of Ca-channel-blockers. Again, additional 0.1 mg i.c. nisoldipine does not increase coronary dilatation following 1.0 mg i.c. SIN-1 (17).

Duration of action

It is not possible for ethical reasons to repeat coronary angiograms only for scientific purposes beyond 60 min. For longer acting drugs it may therefore be difficult to determine dynamic half-lives. Only few studies are reported, in which the duration of action has been evaluated up to 60 min. Nifedipine shows 80% of its maximal effect after 15 min (39) and SIN-1 shows approximately 75% (16) and 63% (40), respectively, of its maximal effect after 1 h. Nitroglycerin has completely lost its coronary dilating properties on normal coronary segments after 30 min (2).

Dilatation in proximal, medial, and distal segments

Increasing dilative effects from proximal (P) to medial (M) to distal (D) proportions of angiographically normal epicardial coronary arteries have been published for 0.4 mg nitroglycerin sublingually by Feldman (13) (P 16%, M 20%, D 25%), for 0.4 mg SIN-1 i.c. by Schulz (32) (P 9%, M 18%, D 26%), and 0.8 mg SIN-1 i.c. by Sobolski (42) (P 26%, M 40%, D 50%), and for 20 mg diltiazem i.v. by Bonzel et al. (3) (P 2%, D 16%). The results of Serruys and coworkers (40) with 1 mg SIN-1 i.c. were inconclusive.

Dilatation in normal coronary segments and stenoses

There are only few publications showing a simultaneous evaluation of stenotic and normal segments. Sometimes, in coronary stenoses (S), a more prominent dilatation than in nonstenotic reference vessels (R) was found: with 0.4 mg SIN-1 i.c. S: 48%, R: 18% (32) and with 4 mg molsidomine i.v. S: 50%, R: 20% (5). However, the opposite finding was also made with 0.5 mg SIN-1 i.c. (4): S: 10%, R: 95%. These opposing findings may be explained by the underlying morphologic substrate in coronary stenoses. Preclinical experiments showed that endothelium-free stenoses are hyperreactive to NO-liberating agents (8). If, however, the total circumference of the vessel is damaged by severe sclerosis, a hyporeactive response of this stenosis may be anticipated.

Dilatation of poststenotic segments and non-poststenotic reference vessels

Poststenotic segments (PS) dilate more than non-poststenotic (NPS) reference segments, which are located at the same distance from the ostium of the respective coronary artery. This was shown with 0.5 mg nitroglycerin (PS +21%, NPS +14%) (2) and with 0.4 mg

SIN-1 (PS +38%, NPS +18%) (36). This finding may be explained by a combination of a reduction of coronary tone and pressure-dependent dilatation of poststenotic segments, which usually occurs when the preceding coronary stenosis dilates.

Response rate of coronary patients showing coronary dilation

Response rates must be evaluated in representative study populations and must be based on reasonable definitions.

So far, there is only one study with a sufficient number of patients (33): in 100 consecutive patients with coronary artery disease, 0.16 mg NTG were injected by the intracoronary route. Eighty stenoses could be evaluated: In 73% (58/80) a diameter increase of more than 10% was found within coronary stenoses. Thus, a dilatation of coronary stenoses – which may be considered clinically relevant – is achieved in a high percentage of the patients with coronary artery disease.

Discussion

In the 1970s, the mode of action of antianginal compounds was not fully evaluated. Peripheral effects causing reduction in oxygen demand were well accepted; additional coronary or cardiac effects besides oxygen-saving negative inotropic effects, however, were not thought to be of importance (14).

Especially in the initial euphoria after introduction of coronary angiography (showing organic stenotic correlates in most of the patients) the possibility of coronary spasms was largely overlooked by clinicians and often denied by pathologists. Increasing experience, however, showed that changing coronary tone or superimposed coronary spasms may be the sole cause for anginal symptoms in patients with low grade organic coronary stenosis.

Various clinical studies with nitrates, SIN-1, and calcium channel-blockers have shown reduction in stenoses, which may improve the clinical situation of the patients. These studies have shown a stronger action of NO-donors compared to calcium channel-blockers, which may be attributable to their different modes of action. The sometimes opposite clinical observation, however, that in some patients only calcium channel-blockers may relieve acute coronary spasms while NO-donors are not effective cannot be properly explained, yet.

Among the NO-donors investigated, SIN-1 turned out to be more effective than nitroglycerin. This effect may be explained either by not using equipotent doses, e.g., application of SIN-1 in a dosage nearer to the maximum dilating activity compared to nitroglycerin, or this stronger action of SIN-1 may be drug-specific. Additional nitroglycerin never induced further dilatation.

Today, it is widely accepted that cardiac effects, especially drug-induced dilatation of coronary stenoses, are clinically most important (18, 1, 11, 7). But a large range of different effects in stenoses may be expected according to the underlying morphologic substrate: a concentric calcified stenosis involving the total circumference of the vessel does not dilate, whereas an eccentric, non-calcified, deendothelialized stenosis with increased basal tone can show a tremendous dilatation.

Derived from the frequency of dilatation of coronary stenoses after nitroglycerin (33) it is now evident that in far more than 50% of the patients a dilatation of stenosis by changes in vasomotor tone can be achieved. Additionally, the high frequency of "spastic" symptoms in far more than 50% of patients with coronary heart disease (37) emphasizes the clinical importance of these medically induced changes in vasomotor tone in these patients. This effect can be essential in reducing myocardial ischemia, especially in high-grade stenoses, in which a conceivable increase in flow can be anticipated even by a small decrease in the percentage of stenosis.

Acknowledgement. We are indebted to Ulla Schmidt and Tanja Milewsky for their secretarial assistance.

References

1. Berkenboom GM, Unger P, Jottrand M, Loiseau J, Pype F, Degre SG (1987) Exercise-induced angina alleviated by intracoronary SIN-1. Cardiology 74:427–435
2. Bernauer R, Schulz W, Kober G (1986) Auswirkungen von intrakoronaren Nitroglyceringaben auf die poststenotische Gefäßweite vor und nach transluminaler koronarer Angioplastie. Z Kardiol 75:19–26
3. Bonzel T, Wollschläger H, Löllgen H (1985a) Erweiterung der epikardialen Koronargefäße durch intravenöses Diltiazem bei Patienten mit koronarer Herzkrankheit. Z Kardiol 74: 238–244
4. Bonzel T (1985b) Interner Prüfbericht Cassella AG. Protokoll-Nr. 84-0276-091
5. Bonzel T, Hasenfuß G, Wollschläger H, Hug J, Just H (1988) Koronardilatierende Langzeitwirkung nach intravenöser Bolusinjektion von Molsidomin. Z Kardiol 77 (Suppl 1)
6. Brown BG, Bolson E, Frimer M, Dodge HT (1977) Quantitative coronary arteriography: estimation of dimensions, hemodynamic resistance, and atheroma mass of coronary artery lesions using the arteriogram and digital computation. Circulation 55:329–337
7. Brown BG (1983) Dilation of coronary artery stenosis: A major mechanism of the effect of nitrates. Z Kardiol (Suppl 3) 72:77–81
8. Busse R, Pohl U, Mülsch A, Bassenge E (1989) Modulation of the vasodilator action of SIN-1 by the endothelium. J Cardiovasc Pharmacol 14 (Suppl 11)81–85
9. Chew CYC, Brown BG, Singh BN, Hecht HS (1980) Mechanism of action of verapamil in ischemic heart disease: observations on changes in systemic and coronary hemodynamics and coronary vasomobility. Clin Invest Med 3:151–158
10. Dhurandhar RW, Watt DL, Silver MD, Trimble AS, Adelman AG (1972) Prinzmetal's variant form of angina with arteriographic evidence of coronary arterial spasm. Am J Cardiol 30: 902–905
11. Dirschinger J, Fleck E, Redl A, Rudolph W (1983) Regionale Myokarddurchblutung unter der Wirkung von Nifedipin in Abhängigkeit von Lumenänderung im Stenosebereich und Kollateralversorgung. Z Kardiol (Suppl 1) 72:14
12. Feelisch M, Noack EA (1987) Correlation between nitric oxide formation during degradation of organic nitrates and activation of guanylate cyclase. Eur J of Pharmacol 139:19–30
13. Feldman RL, Pepine CJ, Conti CR (1981) Magnitude of dilatation of large and small coronary arteries by nitroglycerin. Circulation 64:324–333
14. Ganz W, Markus HS (1972) Failure of intracoronary nitroglycerin to alleviate pacing-induced angina. Circulation 46:880–889
15. Gensini GG, Di Giorgi S, Murad-Netto S, Black A (1962) Arteriographic demonstration of coronary artery spasm and its release after the use of a vasodilator in a case of angina pectoris and in the experimental animal. Angiology 13:550–553
16. Jost S, Reil GH, Knop I, Rafflenbeul W, Gulba D, Hecker H, Frombach R, Lichtlen P (1989) Vasodilatatorische Effekte von SIN-1-Wirksamkeit zusätzlicher Nitroglycerin-Gaben. Perfusion 3
17. Jost S, Auricchio A, Rafflenbeul W, Gulba D, Frombach R, Hecker H, Lichtlen P (1990) Maximale Dilatation epikardialer Koronararterien mit Calcium-Antagonisten und/oder Nitroverbindungen? Z Kardiol 79 (Suppl 1):151
18. Kaltenbach M, Schulz W, Kober G (1979) Effects of nifedipine after intravenous and intracoronary administration. Am J Cardiol 44:832–838

19. Karsch KK, Niemczyk P, Voelker W, Seipel L (1984) Dynamik der kritischen Stenose bei Patienten mit instabiler Angina pectoris. Z Kardiol 73:552–559
20. Kober G, Spahn G, Becker HJ, Kaltenbach M (1974) Weite und Querschnittsfläche der großen epikardialen Koronararterien bei Herzmuskelhypertrophie. Z Kardiol 63:297–310
21. Maseri A, Mimmo R, Chierchia S, Marchesi C, Pesola A, L'Abbate A (1975) Coronary artery spasm as a cause of acute myocardial ischemia in man. Chest 68:625–633
22. Maseri A, Pesola A, Marzilli M, Severi S, Parodi O, L'Abbate A, Ballestra AM, Maltinti G, De Nes DM, Biagini A (1977) Coronary vasospasm in angina pectoris. Lancet I:713–717
23. Oliva PB, Potts DE, Pluss RG (1973) Coronary arterial spasm in prinzmetal angina. N Engl J Med 288:745–751
24. Osler W (1910) The lumleian lectures on angina pectoris. Lancet I:697–702
25. Parkinson J, Bedford DE (1931) Electrocardiographic changes during brief attacks of angina pectoris. Lancet I:15–19
26. Peretz DI (1961) Variant angina pectoris of prinzmetal. Canad Med Ass J 85:1101–1102
27. Prinzmetal M, Kennamer R, Merliss R, Wada T, Bor N (1959) Angina pectoris. A variant form of angina pectoris. Am J Med 27:375–388
28. Rafflenbeul W, Lichtlen PR (1983a) Release of residual vascular tone in coronary artery stenoses with nifedipine and glyceril trinitrate. In: Kaltenbach M, Neufeld HN (eds) 5th International Adalat symposium. New therapy of ischemic heart disease and hypertension. Experta Medica Amsterdam/Oxford/Princeton, pp 300–308
29. Rafflenbeul W, Lichtlen PR (1983b) Quantitative coronary angiography: evidence of a sustained increase in vascular smooth muscle tone in coronary artery stenoses. Z Kardiol 72 (Suppl 3):87–91
30. Reiber JHC, Serruys PW, Kooijman CJ, Wijns W, Slager CJ, Gerbrands JJ, Schuurbiers JCH, den Boer A, Hugenholtz PG (1985) Assessment of short-, medium- and long-term variations in arterial dimensions from computer-assisted quantitation of coronary cineangiograms. Circulation 71:280–288
31. Schulz W, Kober G, Bamberg E, Kaltenbach M (1978) Kardiale und periphere Effekte von Nifedipin. Z Kardiol 67:196
32. Schulz W, Wendt T, Scherer D, Kober G (1983a) Weitenänderungen epikardialer Koronararterien und Koronarstenosen nach intrakoronarer Gabe von Sin-1, einem Molsidomin-Metaboliten. Z Kardiol 72:404–409
33. Schulz W, Anderten WV, Reiber JHC, Bernauer R, Kaltenbach M, Kober G (1983b) Active and passive coronary vasodilation after intracoronary and sublingual nitroglycerin. Z Kardiol 72 (Suppl 3):82–86
34. Schulz W, Wendt T, Kaltenbach M, Kober G (1983c) Active and passive changes in coronary artery diameters after vasodilation. In: Kaltenbach M, Neufeld HN (eds) 5th International Adalat symposium. New therapy of ischemic heart disease and hypertension. Experta Medica Amsterdam/Oxford/Princeton, pp 309–317
35. Schulz W, Kaltenbach M, Kober G (1983d) Chronotropic response after injection of nifedipine into the sinus node artery in man. In: Kaltenbach M, Neufeld HN (eds) 5th International Adalat symposium. New therapy of ischemic heart disease and hypertension. Experta Medica Amsterdam/Oxford/Princeton, pp 322–326
36. Schulz W, Kober G, Bernauer R, Kaltenbach M (1985) Active and passive changes in coronary diameter after vasodilation with SIN-1, the active metabolite of molsidomine. Am Heart J 109:694–699
37. Schulz W, Kaufhold A, Kaltenbach M, Kober G (1990) Der „vasospastische" Ruheherzschmerz. Herz + Gefäße 10:416–421
38. Sebening H, Sauer E (1983) Beeinflussung der Koronararterien und Hämodynamik durch Gallopamil. In: Kaltenbach M, Hopf R (Hrsg) Springer-Verlag Berlin, S. 117–119
39. Serruys PW, Steward R, Booman F, Michels R, Reiber JHC, Hugenholtz PG (1980) Can unstable angina pectoris be due to increased coronary vasomotor tone? Eur Heart J 1 (Suppl B): 71–85
40. Serruys PW, Deckers JW, Luijten HE, Reiber JHC, Tijssen JGP, Chadha D, Hugenholtz PG (1987) Long-acting coronary vasodilatory action of the molsidomine metabolite SIN-1: a quantitative angiographic study. Eur Heart J 8:263–270

41. Siegel M, Feil H (1931) Electrocardiographic studies during attacks of angina pectoris and of other paroxysmal pain. J Clin Invest 10:795–806
42. Sobolski J, Vandermoten P, Stoupel E, Berkenboom G, Degre S (1985) The new long-acting coronary dilator molsidomine and its metabolite SIN-1. Am Heart J 109:700–703
43. Wilson FN, Johnston FD (1941) The occurrence in angina pectoris of electrocardiographic changes similar in magnitude and in kind to those produced by myocardial infarction. Am Heart J 22:64–74

Author's address:

W. Schulz
Klinische Forschung CASSELLA A6,
Hanauer Landstraße 526,
W-6000 Frankfurt/M. 61
G. Kober
Klinik Nordrhein,
Ernst Ludwig Ring 2,
W-6350 Bad Nauheim

Subject Index